Integrating Nanorobotics with Biophysics for Cancer Treatment

Online at: https://doi.org/10.1088/978-0-7503-6019-7

About the Series

The Biophysical Society and IOP Publishing have forged a new publishing partnership in biophysics, bringing the world-leading expertise and domain knowledge of the Biophysical Society into the rapidly developing IOP ebooks program.

The program publishes textbooks, monographs, reviews, and handbooks covering all areas of biophysics research, applications, education, methods, computational tools, and techniques. Subjects of the collection will include: bioenergetics; bioengineering; biological fluorescence; biopolymers *in vivo*; cryo-electron microscopy; exocytosis and endocytosis; intrinsically disordered proteins; mechanobiology; membrane biophysics; membrane structure and assembly; molecular biophysics; motility and cytoskeleton; nanoscale biophysics; and permeation and transport.

Integrating Nanorobotics with Biophysics for Cancer Treatment

Rishabha Malviya
Department of Pharmacy, Galgotias University, Greater Noida, India

Deepika Yadav
Department of Pharmacy, Galgotias University, Greater Noida, India

Sonali Sundram
Department of Pharmacy, Galgotias University, Greater Noida, India

Seifedine Kadry
Department of Mathematics and Computer Science, Beirut Arab University, Beirut, Lebanon

Gurvinder Singh Virk
Endoenergy System Ltd, Cambridge, United Kingdom

IOP Publishing, Bristol, UK

ISBN 978-0-7503-6019-7 (ebook)
ISBN 978-0-7503-6017-3 (print)
ISBN 978-0-7503-6020-3 (myPrint)
ISBN 978-0-7503-6018-0 (mobi)

DOI 10.1088/978-0-7503-6019-7

Version: 20240501

IOP ebooks

British Library Cataloguing-in-Publication Data: A catalogue record for this book is available from the British Library.

Published by IOP Publishing, wholly owned by The Institute of Physics, London

IOP Publishing, No.2 The Distillery, Glassfields, Avon Street, Bristol, BS2 0GR, UK

US Office: IOP Publishing, Inc., 190 North Independence Mall West, Suite 601, Philadelphia, PA 19106, USA

Dear Healthcare Professionals,

We are dedicating this book to you. Our love for the profession shall live forever.

Contents

Preface

The detailed book 'Integrating Nanorobotics with Biophysics for Cancer Treatment' covers the domain where nanorobotics and biophysics converge and provides a comprehensive perspective. The bioelectrical profiling of malignant cells, molecule-targeting medical devices for tumor treatment, biosecurity in relation to biorobotics for healthcare, nanorobotics, robotics, nanobiology, nanotechnology, robotics and biophysics, nanorobots, nanomedicine, and nanotherapeutic approaches are just a few of the topics covered in this book.

The book opens with an introduction to nanorobotics, including its components, designs, and technological foundations. It then describes difficulties in creating and developing nanorobots, their adaptability in biomedical applications, and their particular applications in the fields of gene therapy, hematology, neurosurgery, dentistry, microbiology, and bioinspired design. In addition, it covers the function of robotics in biophysics, including the value of robots in biophysical study and its applications.

The book subsequently explores the fundamentals of the detection of telomerase and nuclear acids in malignant cells, therapeutic applications, and the clinical implications of using magnetomechanical systems on the micro- or nanoscale for cancer therapy. It also examines the application of active nanorobots in personalized medicine, encompassing neurology, cancer treatment, and diagnosis.

Foreword

'Integrating Nanorobotics with Biophysics for Cancer Treatment' is a book that explores the intersection of nanorobotics and biophysics in cancer treatment. Authored by Dr Rishabha Malviya, the book provides a holistic perspective on the innovative convergence of these technologies. It covers the design, material considerations, and technological intricacies of nanorobots, their versatility in various applications, and the convergence of robotics and biophysics, including soft robotics, biomimetic design, exoskeletons, prosthetics, and autonomous robots. The book also discusses ethical and regulatory considerations guiding their deployment.

Nanorobots, powered by magnets, ultrasound, biological mechanisms, or hybrid power sources, have the potential to revolutionize cancer therapy. However, challenges include scalability, cost, quality control, and regulatory hurdles. This book explores bioelectrochemical profiling, wireless medical microbots, and motile targeting devices, as well as the concept of cyborgs and cyberorgans in healthcare.

Dr Rishabha Malviya and contributing experts provide a symphony of knowledge, research, and foresight, illuminating a path towards innovative solutions and transformative progress. This book is an invaluable resource for researchers, scientists, clinicians, and those passionate about the future of healthcare.

With best wishes

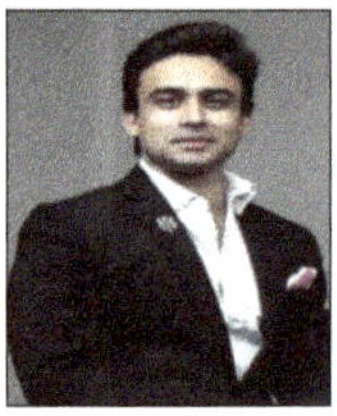

Dr Dhruv Galgotia
CEO, Galgotias University, Greater Noida, India

Author biographies

Rishabha Malviya

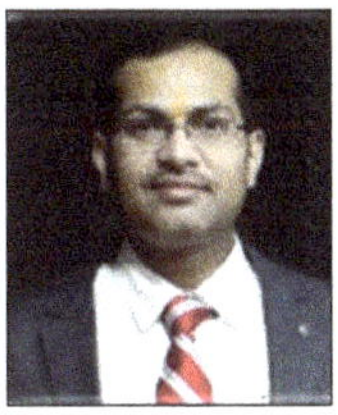

Rishabha Malviya completed his B. Pharmacy at Uttar Pradesh Technical University and his M. Pharmacy (Pharmaceutics) at Gautam Buddha Technical University, Lucknow, Uttar Pradesh. The topic of his PhD (Pharmacy) was novel formulation development techniques. He has 13 years of research experience and has worked as an associate professor in the Department of Pharmacy, School of Medical and Allied Sciences, Galgotias University for the last ten years. His areas of interest include formulation optimization, nanoformulation, targeted drug delivery, localized drug delivery and the characterization of natural polymers as pharmaceutical excipients. He has authored more than 150 research/review papers for national and international journals of repute. He has 51 patents (20 grants, 31 published), and publications in reputed national and international journals with a cumulative impact factor of more than 250. He has also received an Outstanding Reviewer award from Elsevier. He has authored, edited, or is editing 38 books (Wiley, CRC Press/Taylor and Francis, IOP Publishing, River Publisher, Springer Nature, Apple Academic Press, and OMICS Publishing Group) and authored 52 book chapters. His name was included in the world's top 2% scientist lists for 2020, 2021, and 2022 by Elsevier BV and Stanford University. He is a reviewer, editor, or editorial board member of more than 50 national and international journals of repute. He has been invited to write for Atlas of Science and a pharmacology magazine aimed at industry (B2B), Ingredient South Asia Magazines.

Deepika Yadav

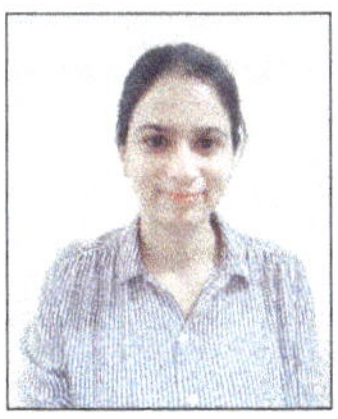

Deepika Yadav completed her B. Pharmacy at K R Mangalam University, Sohna Road, Gurugram, Haryana and her M. Pharmacy at Galgotias University, Greater Noida. She is currently working as an assistant professor in the Department of Pharmacy, Sushant University, Gurugram. She has authored two books with Apple Academic Press (Taylor and Francis Group) and John Wiley & Sons. She has authored many Science Citation Index manuscripts for reputed international publishers.

Sonali Sundram

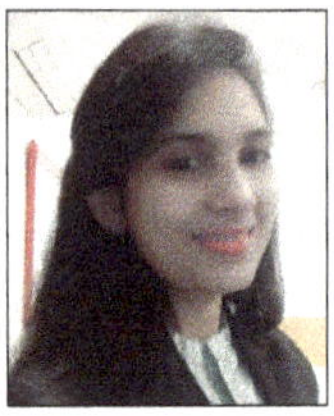

Sonali Sundram completed her B. Pharm and M. Pharm (Pharmacology) degrees at AKTU, Lucknow. She worked as a research scientist for the ICMR project at King George's Medical University, Lucknow; subsequently, she joined Babu Banarasi Das Northern India Institute of Technology (BBDNIIT); and she is currently working at Galgotias University, Greater Noida. Her PhD work was in the areas of neurodegeneration and nanoformulation. Her areas of interest are neurodegeneration, clinical research, and artificial intelligence. She has authored, edited, or is editing 18 books (Wiley, CRC Press/Taylor and Francis, River Publishers, Apple Academic Press/Taylor and Francis group). She has attended or organized more than 15 national and international seminars, conferences, and workshops. She has more than eight national and international patents to her credit.

Seifedine Kadry

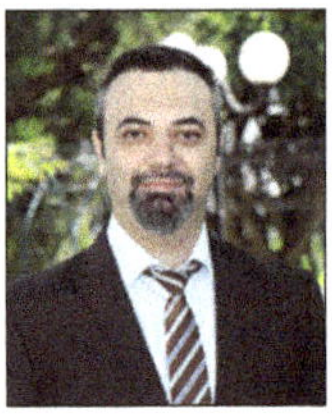

Seifedine Kadry is a professor of data science at the Faculty of Applied Computing and Technology at Noroff University College, Kristiansand, Norway. He is the author of 12 books published by prestigious publishers such as IGI Global, Elsevier, Springer, and Bentham. Some of these books are related to mathematical sciences, system simulation, system prognostics, and reliability engineering. He has also published more than 200 articles and organized numerous conference tracks and workshops. Professor Kadry is the editor-in-chief of the ARPN Journal of Systems and Software and the Maxwell Journal of Mathematics and Statistics. He is an IEEE senior member. His specialized areas of research include computing, software engineering, and systems reliability and safety.

Gurvinder Singh Virk

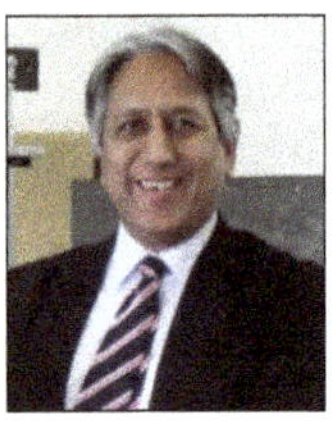

Professor Gurvinder Singh Virk is currently a managing director at Endoenergy Systems Limited, which aims to develop wearable assistive exoskeletons to help address the societal challenges of global ageing. Endoenergy has bases in Cambridge, United Kingdom and Mohali, India. He has carried out pioneering work in the field of robotics science and engineering and its application in addressing real-world challenges. He has published around 375 publications in robotics and control engineering, secured over £30M of research funding and led over 50 national and international projects. He has held 13 professorial positions in seven countries (the UK, France, New Zealand, China, Sweden, Germany, and India) and has been a leading actor in ISO/IEC robot standardization for the medical and nonmedical robot sectors since 2005. Professor Virk is a fellow of the IET (FIET), a chartered engineer (CEng), a fellow of the Institute of Mathematics (FIMA), a chartered mathematician (CMath), and a senior member of the IEEE (SMIEEE). He has been awarded the Freedom of the City of London and is a liveryman of the Worshipful Company of Information Technology.

About the book

The search for better methods to comprehend and treat cancer is more urgent than ever, since it is a tough opponent. We explore the novel combination of nanorobotics and biophysics in 'Integrating Nanorobotics with Biophysics for Cancer Treatment,' providing an overview of the transformational potential and intriguing possibilities that this convergence provides.

The discipline of nanorobotics, which combines the creative possibilities of robotics with the accuracy of nanotechnology, has the potential to completely transform how clinicians diagnose and treat cancer. This book takes the reader on an exciting tour through the complex world of nanorobots, including their materials, design, and technological advancements. It explains the complex issues involved in creating nanorobots and their extraordinary adaptability in a range of biological settings, including neurosurgery and microbiology.

The systematic book 'Integrating Nanorobotics with Biophysics for Cancer Treatment' discusses the relationship between nanotechnology and cancer treatment. The book opens with an introduction to nanorobotics, with an emphasis on its ability to understand cancer biology. After that, it addresses how robotics fits into biophysics, looking at both technological developments and ethical challenges. The book then highlights precision cancer diagnosis and treatment while exploring the engineered systems of nanorobots for the delivery of anticancer medications. In addition, it covers the application of magnetomechanical particles in cancer treatment.

It then examines the application of micro- and nanorobotics in individualized healthcare, encompassing imaging, diagnosis, and surgery. It also covers the potential uses of nanorobots in diabetes treatment and dentistry. The book also discusses the development of bioelectrochemical and biophysical profiling as a diagnostic tool for cancer, the potential uses of wireless medical microbots in biomedical applications, and the function of micro/nanorobots in precise drug delivery, surgery, and sensing in medicine. A case study on cyborgs and cyberorgans, as well as a summary of related patents, conclude the book.

Experts from a multitude of domains joined together to create this book, sharing their knowledge and ideas to encourage, inform, and push the envelope in healthcare innovation. It brings the reader up to date on the most recent developments, obstacles, and promising prospects that the combination of biophysics and nanorobotics represents in the battle against cancer.

For scientists, doctors, researchers, and everyone interested in the future of cancer diagnosis and treatment, 'Integrating Nanorobotics with Biophysics for Cancer Treatment' is an essential read. Join us on this amazing journey of innovation where compassion, science, and technology come together to impact the fight against cancer.

IOP Publishing

Rishabha Malviya, Deepika Yadav, Sonali Sundram, Seifedine Kadry and Gurvinder Singh Virk

Chapter 1

Nanorobotics: materials, design, and technology

Nanorobotics is a captivating domain within the field of medicine that has emerged as a result of advancements in nanotechnology and the utilization of sophisticated electrical materials. Nanorobots, which operate at the nanoscale, possess considerable potential for revolutionizing the healthcare domain. The potential applications of these technologies encompass a diverse range of domains, such as diagnostics, therapy, and surgical operations, that were previously deemed unattainable in terms of scale. Nanorobots are built with precision using specialized materials and design processes, ensuring their adherence to specific requirements connected with their wide array of functions. One notable benefit of nanorobots is their remarkable biocompatibility, which mitigates any potential toxicity concerns. This attribute facilitates the successful cellular penetration of nanoscale agents and the precise delivery of drugs to targeted areas, hence reducing potential damage to unaffected tissues. The significance of achieving such a high level of precision lies in its potential to greatly enhance the efficacy and reduce the invasiveness of medical therapies. Nanorobots effectively navigate the intricate network of the human bloodstream by harnessing Brownian motion, hence exhibiting unparalleled mobility. This ability to move allows them to accurately arrive at their intended locations. The nascent field of nanorobotics signifies a paradigm-shifting breakthrough in the realm of healthcare. The incorporation of cutting-edge materials, innovative design, and modern technology makes it possible to improve the safety and effectiveness of medical interventions while functioning at a level that is imperceptible to unaided human vision. Nanorobots possess the capacity to significantly transform the healthcare domain, offering considerable potential for improved precision in diagnostics, minimally invasive therapeutic approaches, and groundbreaking surgical methodologies.

1.1 Introduction

Nanorobotics is an emerging field within the realm of nanotechnology, which is dedicated to the construction and manipulation of machinery at the molecular, cellular, and

doi:10.1088/978-0-7503-6019-7ch1

subatomic scales. The hypothetical nanorobots in question possess dimensions so minuscule that they could traverse the human body's circulatory system inconspicuously. The potential use of nanorobots is based on their ability to detect specific molecules, leading to the diagnosis and treatment of several severe medical conditions [1]. At the nanoscale, specifically measuring 9–10 nm, nanorobots can be defined as intelligent structures that possess the capacity to perform various functions such as acting, sensing, signaling, processing information, exhibiting intelligence, manipulating objects, and operating collectively in swarms. Nanomedicine holds significant potential for the development of innovative approaches for the diagnosis and treatment of human diseases as well as the improvement of physiological processes in the human body. Nanomedicine encompasses the application of biochemical techniques in conjunction with a comprehensive comprehension of the human body, thereby assuming a pivotal function in the realms of medical diagnostics, treatment, and prevention, as well as the management of severe injuries. Furthermore, these technologies facilitate the management of pain and contribute to the maintenance and improvement of individuals' well-being [2].

To achieve precise manipulation at the nanoscale, technologists have developed nanorobots. Nanorobots are commonly designated as monoids in academic discourse. Nanorobots derive their design inspiration from bacterial models. It is likely that nanorobots would predominantly consist of carbon-based materials, specifically nanocomposites comprising diamond or diamondoid structures. These nanocomposites contain many forms of carbon allotropes, including pure diamond and crystalline carbon, alongside materials based on fullerene. It is possible to fabricate nanorobots utilizing ordinary mechanical components. Diamondoids are anticipated to be utilized in the construction of the outer casing of nanorobots due to their inert properties, elevated thermal conductivity, and durability. The presence of ultrasmooth surfaces may potentially reduce the probability of an adverse immune system response. Elements such as hydrogen, sulfur, oxygen, nitrogen, and silicon have been identified as potential candidates for use in the fabrication of nanoscale gears and other bespoke components [3].

Advancements in various domains such as manufacturing, computation, transducers, and manipulation have shown promise in enabling the future creation of nanorobots. The utilization of deep UV lithography in complementary metal–oxide–semiconductor (CMOS) **very-large-scale integration (VLSI)** design enabled the precise and large-scale manufacture of the early nanodevices and nanoelectronic systems [4]. The Verification Hardware Description Language (VHDL) has been widely adopted by the integrated circuit (IC) manufacturing industry as the standard approach for design verification and efficient implementation [5]. Figure 1.1 illustrates the components of nanorobots. Nanorobots can utilize sound sensors to engage in collective communication over extended distances by employing low-power CMOS technology and submicron system-on-chip (SoC) architecture [6].

1.2 Nanorobot design and development

Nanorobotics have diverse applications in healthcare. Advancements in biomolecular studies and manufacturing techniques have played a crucial role in enabling the

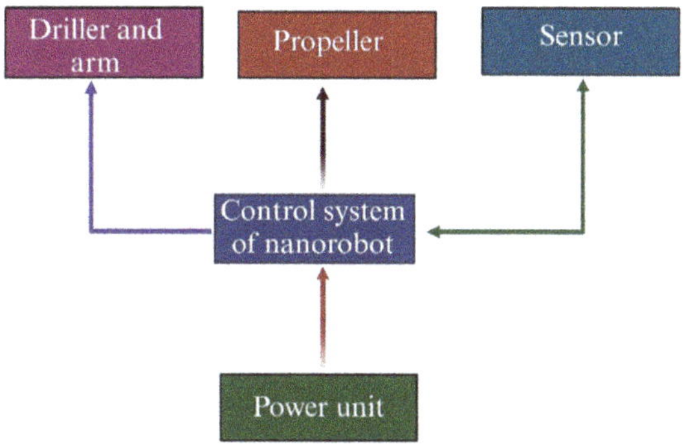

Figure 1.1. The components of a nanorobot.

transition from microelectronics to nanotechnologies. Microdevices have recently been employed to augment several medicinal and surgical procedures [7–9]. This section will elucidate the different challenges that scientists have encountered during their endeavors in the field of nanorobotics.

The successful execution of crucial functions, including targeting, energy provision, locomotion, operational capability, and compatibility with biological systems, is of the utmost importance for nanorobots. However, the operating conditions and potential applications of nanorobots present a notable barrier [10]. The prevailing approach used to integrate monitoring techniques in the IC manufacturing industry entails the utilization of VHDL to develop and produce nanorobots. The monitoring of patients necessitates the careful assessment of fluctuations in temperature and chemical concentrations within the bloodstream, as these factors play a critical role in determining the suitability of the monitoring approach for a certain application [11]. The fields of nanoelectronics and nanobiotechnology have witnessed significant progress in recent times. These advancements offer the potential to develop molecular machines that possess the capability to detect, perform actions, be remotely controlled, and transmit and receive data. These functionalities are crucial for the effective functioning of medical nanorobots [12]. Nanorobots, like conventional robots, are fabricated utilizing a structural framework and many components endowed with the capability to sense and manipulate their surroundings. Nanomotors can be readily manufactured utilizing a wide array of materials, encompassing inorganic substances, flagellar motors, DNA motors, viral protein linear (VPL) motors, and adenosine triphosphate (ATP). The fundamental structure of a nanorobot consists of its frame and the interconnections among its various components [13]. Both inorganic resources, such as metals, and biological materials, such as DNA and proteins, can be utilized to construct these components. The connecting components of the robot function to unite its various elements; in a similar manner, the driving component of the robot generates the necessary force to successfully execute a designated objective [14].

It is widely acknowledged that due to spatial constraints at the nanoscale, there is a need to reconsider the conventional robotics framework that relies on sensors, actuators, and control mechanisms. This implies that the diverse components (such as sensors, actuators, etc.) of nanorobots will collaborate and integrate into more extensive architectures. To minimize discrepancies between the intended and actual parameter values, the standard method of sensor analysis, data evaluation, and control strategy development used to transmit commands to actuators may not be applicable [15]. Nevertheless, it is imperative to investigate the novel approaches proposed for the regulation of a nanorobot's response or behaviors. Various imaging technologies can be employed to detect the interior location of the nanorobot. Subsequently, the control system can utilize this data to deliver instructions to the actuators or direct the nanorobot by manipulating magnetic fields of different strengths. This chapter will discuss the challenges encountered during the design and construction of nanoscale robotic components, such as sensors and actuators. Nevertheless, it is crucial to consider that the distinctive architecture of a nanorobot might require a completely novel methodology in the field of robotics. The development of nanorobots necessitates the creation of nanoscale components, which is of the utmost importance. However, advancements in the field have been impeded by many technical limitations [2]. Two primary challenges impede the production and application of nanorobots in the field of nanomedicine. The first hurdle pertains to the current level of technological advancement, while the second issue relates to the inherent limitations of nanorobots when operating within microfluidic environments [16]. The advancement of nanomechatronics has facilitated the removal of the initial obstacle, whereas the rapid expansion of nanobiotechnology and the emergence of molecular manufacturing have enabled the fabrication of minuscule devices. Nanorobots comprise crucial components such as drives, sensors, motors, data senders, power sources, and controllers [17, 18]. Significant progress has been made in the field of nanoelectronics through the utilization of CMOS technology, which has facilitated the fabrication of circuits with dimensions on the order of tens of nanometers [19]. Nanoprocessors have been deemed feasible for biological computers; their development has been made possible by recent advancements in molecular-level processing, genetic engineering, and nanotechnology [20]. In the realm of the medical applications of nanorobotics, the second limitation arises from the challenge associated with integrating a nanorobot into the fluidic milieu. A significant number of researchers are currently focusing their efforts on the advancement of microbots, often known as microrobots or 'swimmers,' that can perform efficient aquatic navigation. Like their biological counterparts, microbots exhibit optimal functionality when provided with a suitable food or energy source [21].

1.3 Nanorobots designed for a broad spectrum of healthcare uses

During the latter half of the 1950s, Richard introduced the concept of 'ingesting a surgeon' as a way of performing microsurgery on an individual [22]. The domains of biomaterials, engineering, and medicine have experienced significant advancements, leading to notable discoveries in micro/nanotechnology and the development of numerous miniature robots. Various propulsion methods have been developed to improve the effectiveness of locomotion, by taking account of the intricate nature of physiology and the influence of viscous forces rather than inertia on the movement of microscopic robots in the low-Reynolds-number domain. Various forms of external propulsion include ultrasonic, optical, thermal, electrical, and magnetic forces, either individually or in combination. Another alternative is the utilization of internal chemical propulsion [23]. Micro/nanorobots have advanced significantly; nonetheless, they have encountered several challenges in their journey toward clinical implementation for the treatment of a wide array of medical ailments. These challenges encompass, among others, the complexities associated with the integration of various medical treatments, the inefficiency of real-time visual surveillance, and insufficient biocompatibility [24].

The utilization of nanorobots with magnetic actuation has garnered considerable interest due to their ability to operate remotely, i.e. without the need for physical connections, and navigate without the need for motors or fuel. This has led to their recognition as superior to micro- or nanorobots powered by alternative actuation methods, owing to their numerous advantages. Moreover, these robotic systems demonstrate a lack of sensitivity towards organic substances and feature highly precise positioning capabilities. Consequently, they have garnered significant attention within the realm of scholarly investigation and advancement. Considerable attention and progress have been observed in recent years [25]. Moreover, magnetic micro/nanorobots have a wide range of potential applications due to the adaptability of synthetic materials, their diverse structural configurations, and unique magnetic manipulation mechanisms. The classification of contemporary magnetic micro/nanorobots can vary based on one's perspective. These robots can be categorized into three distinct classes, according to their design philosophy: natural/biological, artificial, and biohybrid [26, 27]. Magnetic robots exhibit a diverse range of forms and dimensions, encompassing wires, coils, U-shapes, rods, spheres, helixes, and piscine configurations; each configuration is specifically engineered to fulfill certain operational tasks [28]. Robots can also be categorized into three main types based on their physical characteristics: soft/flexible, stiff, or rigid with flexible joints/tails. These classifications are directly associated with the level of complexity in handling different textures, as indicated by previous research [29]. Magnetic micro/nanorobots have employed the locomotion patterns observed in nematodes, bacterial flagella, inchworms, and sperm [30]. Nevertheless, the paramount and pressing characteristic in the development of micro/nanorobots is the ability to mobilize and perform designated functions.

The rapid expansion of magnetically controlled micro/nanorobots has been identified as a significant factor contributing to numerous recent advancements. Previous literature on magnetic micro/nanorobots has predominantly concentrated on singular applications, such as imaging technology [31], cargo transport robots [32], or cell measurement applications [33]. The focus has primarily been the realization of various functionalities and the practical applications that have been achieved thus far. Magnetic micro/nanorobots can be used in imaging techniques and applications in the fields of biomedicine and biosafety. Studies have examined the synthesis procedures used for micro/nanorobots from the perspective of micro/

nanomaterials, with a specific focus on their magnetic properties [33]. The areas of study also encompass magnetic actuation technologies, various forms of movement, and monitoring approaches. The advancement of magnetic micro/nanorobots has contributed to various biomedical applications, including targeted delivery, minimally invasive surgery, cellular and intracellular monitoring, intelligent sensing, detoxification, and antibacterial treatment.

1.4 The applications of nanorobots in the field of biomedicine

The potential impact of nanorobots in the field of biomedicine is significant since they can bring about a transformative shift in healthcare via their ability to perform precise and minimally intrusive operations at the nanoscale. The following sections discuss various prominent domains in which nanorobots are now being investigated for their potential biomedical applications (figure 1.2).

1.4.1 Microbiology

The initial robotic capabilities of nanobiotechnology were advanced by collaborating with the field of microbiology. Although the construction and functionality of microrobots and nanorobots are feasible, challenges related to transportation and propulsion hinder their extensive utilization within the vascular system. The enhancement of microrobot and nanorobot propulsion could potentially be achieved through the integration of magnetotactic bacteria such as *Magnetococcus* spp and *Magnetospirillum magneticum* [34]. The fundamental constituent of these nanorobots would mostly comprise magnetotactic bacteria, encompassing the cellular structure of the bacterial organism. The marine magnetotactic spirillum is acknowledged as the smallest known species of magnetotactic bacteria that has been documented thus far. The dimensions of each bacterium are approximately 0.5 μm, which is comparable to 500 nm. This length falls slightly above the upper limit set by the National Nanotechnology Initiative for classifying objects as falling

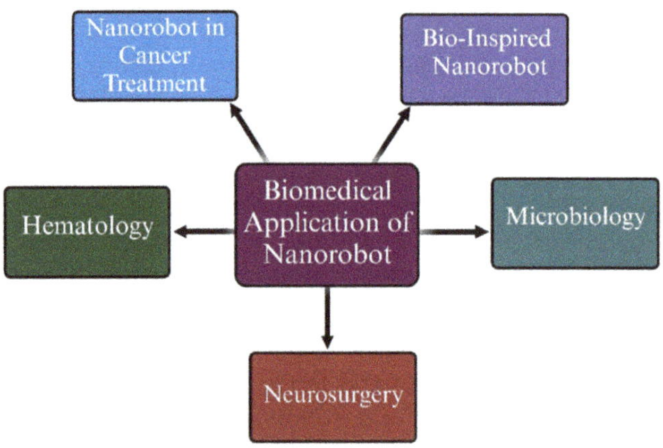

Figure 1.2. The biomedical applications of nanorobots.

within the nanoscale range. According to [35], marine magnetotactic spirillum is of limited use due to its speed, which is more suitable for intravascular functions.

The utilization of magnetic fields has the potential to manipulate the movement of magnetotactic microorganisms in a specific direction. Magnetosomes are specialized organelles found in magnetotactic bacteria that possess the ability to perceive and react to magnetic fields. The formation of magnetosomes, prokaryotic pseudo-organelles, involves the encapsulation of around 15–20 magnetite crystals within an invagination of the bacterial cell membrane. These magnetite crystals have an estimated diameter of 50 nm. Magnetite crystals are composed of the iron oxide Fe_3O_4. The phenomenon of magnetotactic cocci migration has been observed to align with recognized geomagnetic lines [36].

Numerous prospective uses have been posited for the innovations in nanorobotics. Therapeutic substances, such as pharmaceuticals and synthetic antibodies, can be encapsulated within a flexible framework that can be affixed to bacteria, enabling targeted delivery to the intended site of action. These devices can also function as sensors [37], enabling the collection of data. Larger robotic systems exhibit enhanced capabilities in navigating and functioning inside broader pathways, in contrast to smaller robotic systems which are limited to performing constrained tasks within capillary and minuscule vascular structures [38]. The utilization of nanorobots has proven to be highly advantageous for capillary settings and microvasculature, whereas their effectiveness is limited in larger vessels due to their restricted speed range. To enhance practical advancements in the field, a dual-component robotic system has been suggested in which the smaller components would be released from bigger containers following the deployment of the larger system for control and transportation.

1.4.2 Cancer therapy using nanorobots

The efficacy of cancer treatment is contingent upon the advancement of novel medical technologies. The prognosis of a cancer patient is conventionally considered to be contingent upon the promptness of disease detection. The timely identification of cancer before the onset of metastasis is of paramount importance to optimize the efficacy of cancer treatment. The integration of chemical biosensors within nanorobots has the potential to facilitate the early detection of tumors. E-cadherin, a constituent of the transmembrane protein family, functions as a tumor suppressor. Cadherin-1, a cell adhesion molecule alternatively referred to as CAM 120/80, is reliant on calcium ions for its proper physiological functioning. Nanorobots have the potential to monitor the intensity of e-cadherin, a protein involved in cell adhesion, and this capability could be utilized for the early detection of cancer [39]. The use of nanorobots has the potential to enhance tumor excision techniques. Radioisotope-guided lymph node dissection is employed as a more efficient approach for identifying metastases in comparison to open lymph dissection. Before the resection procedure, a radioactive intraprostatic colloid injection is administered to the patient. The utilization of nanorobots, which possess the capability to operate without requiring hospitalization, has the potential to enhance the efficiency of this procedure [40].

Tailored drug administration has the potential to enhance the tolerability of chemotherapy, a widely employed therapeutic approach for cancer. As previously mentioned, nanorobots possess the capability to traverse constricted blood vessels to accurately deliver pharmaceutical substances to targeted locations. The utilization of nanorobots in cancer treatment shows considerable potential. Due to its nonselective cytotoxicity, conventional chemotherapy exhibits a limited threshold for safe administration, as it adversely affects both healthy and malignant cells. The selectivity of treatment locations exhibited by nanotechnology will enable it to surmount this obstacle. Nanorobots possess the ability to autonomously locate cancer cells and deliver therapeutic agents to the specific places impacted by the disease. Nanorobots can be designed with a specific and directed reaction to particular cell surface receptors, hence enabling highly accurate and controlled contact. Furthermore, the amount of payload that is supplied can be precisely calibrated. The nanorobots proposed for this use would be constructed using a genetically modified DNA strand that possesses a distinct tertiary structure. Upon attachment to the tumor cells, the nanorobot deploys an opening mechanism to liberate the therapeutic payload. A 'pharmacy' refers to an artificially designed nanorobot that possesses the ability to traverse the bloodstream and deliver medication precisely to the desired location. The nanorobot can transport a therapeutic payload across cell membranes and tissues by utilizing its energy production and locomotion skills [41].

1.4.3 Biologically inspired nanorobots

Nanorobots have the potential to autonomously combine and form a functional entity, or they can be externally validated for their interconnection [42]. Recent research has focused on the development of nanorobots that draw inspiration from biological systems. Bionanorobots are constructed using a diverse array of biological components and can execute cellular activities following predetermined instructions. The structural connections, power sources, and biosensors of a nanorobotic system necessitate the presence of DNA, carbon nanotubes, and proteins. The conversion of chemical energy into kinetic energy enables a bionanobot to move molecules [43]. The popularity of biomolecular motors has increased due to their rapidity, versatility, and extensive capabilities in molecular identification and reproduction [43]. The primary obstacle encountered in the advancement of these micromachines is the establishment of a reliable interface between their organic and inorganic constituents.

The coupling of DNA strands to a VPL engine can be achieved through the utilization of sodium thiosulfate and amino carbamate or by employing a carbon nanotube with modified hydroxyl terminals [44]. One study employed hydrophilic DNA strands to establish a connection to single-walled carbon nanotubes (SWNTs) that exhibited hydrophobic properties. This was accomplished by enclosing a peptide nucleic acid (PNA) molecule within each SWNT [45]. The difficulty of interconnecting components and the assessed system resilience are considered significant in the manufacture of components. Despite these challenges, the use of organic nanorobots is gaining traction due to their notable advantages compared to their inorganic counterparts [46]. These attributes have led to the emergence of techniques for fabricating organic nanorobots, including the integration of genetic sequences with nanomaterials and the adaptation of machine surfaces to meet the needs of biological entities [47].

Biohybrids, also known as organism-based motors, are an intriguing concept that involves the combination of naturally existing organisms, such as bacteria, with artificial components. Such integration fulfills the requirements for propulsion and responsiveness to environmental stimuli [48]. The development of nanorobotic systems has been facilitated through the utilization of propulsion principles observed in microorganisms. In the context of mobility and the monitoring of temperature and concentration, it may be argued that the utilization of spinning flagella offers the highest degree of propulsion efficiency. Flagella exhibit various characteristics in terms of their structure, protein content, and propulsion mechanism. According to the research literature, cells can be categorized into two main types: eukaryotic and prokaryotic [49]. The latter term pertains to slender protein filaments that carry out the propulsive process, while the former indicates cells that undergo flexion to create microtubules and cause directional movement through clockwise or counterclockwise rotation. As a result, groups of objects come together and move collectively for a finite period before breaking apart and transitioning into the next iteration [50]. The emergence of these technologies has prompted numerous researchers to expand their scope, resulting in enhanced medication administration through improved control and navigation mechanisms.

Biohybrid micromotors demonstrate a notable level of velocity and can be made to adopt different speeds. The movement of these systems is governed by the influence of a magnetic field and accelerated by the force exerted by motile cells. The development of biohybrid nanorobots which utilize magnetotactic bacteria and flagellum nanomotors has mainly been achieved in human capillaries [51]. However, ensuring the viability and stability of the biohybrid machine's living component while maintaining its physiological properties poses a challenge. The integration of varied components at the micro and nanoscale levels has grown progressively challenging, leading to increased complexity in the fabrication of intricate micro and nanoscale devices [52]. Therefore, it is imperative to simplify these devices while conserving the essential functions of nature [53]. Despite these challenges, many bioinspired nanorobots have been successfully engineered to fulfill various objectives. These nanorobots exhibit characteristics such as flexible filaments, malleable magnetic alloys, and catalytic capabilities.

1.4.4 The prospects of nanorobots for use in hematology

The field of hematology presents a plethora of prospects for the advancement of nanomedicine and nanorobotics. The field of hematology offers a wide array of possible applications for nanorobotics, encompassing many areas such as the emergency delivery of non-blood oxygen-carrying molecules and the restoration of primary hemostasis. The respirocyte, a nanorobot, is an example of a technology currently being developed. This robot has three distinct objectives as it navigates the circulatory system. Initially, the respiratory system is responsible for the acquisition of oxygen, which is subsequently transported to the various tissues and organs of the body via the circulatory system. In addition, it facilitates the transportation of carbon dioxide from the tissues to the lungs, where it is subsequently exhaled. The final stage involves the utilization of glucose obtained from the circulatory system as a primary source of energy. The dimensions of the robot are approximately one micron or 1000 nm. The encased components, on the other hand, are constructed at the nanoscale level. The onboard system incorporates a microprocessor with a diameter of 58 nm, with loading rotors for oxygen/CO2 with a diameter of 14 nm. Respirocytes exhibit a significantly enhanced oxygen transport capacity, surpassing that of red blood cells by a factor of 236 in terms of oxygen volume transportation. In the future, this methodology could perhaps replace perilous blood transfusions [54].

Nanorobotics could potentially be applied in the context of hemostasis. The complex phenomenon of hemostasis encompasses a diverse array of factors that both facilitate and impede the delicate equilibrium between thrombosis and fibrinolysis. The efficacy of hemostasis in halting hemorrhage and promoting vascular repair is significantly augmented when it operates optimally. Nevertheless, nanorobotics has the potential to address several intrinsic limitations of physiological hemostasis, such as the time it takes for an average individual to achieve hemostasis, which is approximately 5 min. Moreover, there are risks linked to the current methodologies employed by researchers to reinstate proper hemostasis following an interruption of physiological hemostatic mechanisms, such as thrombocytopenia. Patients who receive platelet transfusions are susceptible to pathogenic infections and may experience immune responses. Discussion is taking place about the potential utilization of a nanorobot known as a 'choanocyte,' a term derived from 'artificial mechanical platelet,' to perform the functions of a platelet. A proposed design parameter for this nanorobot is a two-micron size with a mesh scale of 0.8 nm, equipped with proteins that facilitate blood coagulation. Hemostasis could be achieved by directing these nanorobots toward sites of vascular injury [55].

In addition, nanorobots have the potential to serve as phagocytic agents. The term 'microbivores' has been assigned to diminutive robotic entities that consume microorganisms. The robots would possess a diverse array of binding sites on their exteriors, which could be programmed to selectively attach to specific antigens or illnesses, such as those present in HIV or *Escherichia coli*. In theory, the introduction of microbivores might potentially remove septicemia within a short time, as they are believed to be around 80 times more effective than natural phagocytes. Considering the escalation in antibiotic resistance, it is plausible that novel avenues for addressing infection could emerge through the use of nanorobotic capabilities [56].

1.4.5 The neurosurgical prospects of nanorobots

Nanotechnology has seen significant development, progressing from the realm of theoretical speculation to a fertile field that fosters the generation of novel ideas and drives active research. The field of neurosurgery, characterized by its focus on intricate procedures, is perfectly positioned to use numerous advancements in the realm of nanotechnology. Several advantages can be identified, including the capability to detect diseases at an earlier stage, the capacity to monitor the intracranial region with minimal disruption, and the potential to administer medicines. Advancements in the manufacture of microelectromechanical systems (MEMS) have significantly enhanced their ability to function at progressively smaller dimensions. These advancements have the potential to facilitate manipulation at the cellular and molecular levels in the near future [57].

The field of neurosurgery places significant emphasis on spinal cord injuries and nerve damage due to its substantial implications for patients' quality of life. The restoration of function to severed nerves has been a practice that has spanned more than a century, witnessing advancements in both technique and technology with each successive decade. Two contemporary approaches being investigated to optimize and augment nerve reconnection outcomes involve the utilization of growth factors and enriched scaffolds to facilitate axon regeneration. The process of reestablishing connections between damaged axons is a critical component in the restoration of functionality following an injury. The ability to perform large-scale surgery is subject to technical limits [58]. The development of nanoscale devices has facilitated the manipulation of individual axons, due to significant technological progress. Successful axon surgery has been accomplished by the utilization of a nanoknife possessing a diameter of 40 nm. The efficacy of dielectrophoresis in achieving accurate control over axonal mobility within a surgical setting has been demonstrated. This methodology utilizes electric fields to alter the polarization of objects within a specific spatial framework. Studies have examined several fusion techniques, namely electrofusion, polyethylene-glycol-mediated fusion, and laser-induced cell fusion, as potential ways for facilitating fusion following the controlled transection of axons. These techniques have been considered in conjunction with the positioning of the two severed ends using dielectrophoresis. The reconnection of nerves facilitated by nanodevices introduces an enhanced degree of accuracy and manipulation [59].

The management of cerebral aneurysms before rupture is considered a highly effective approach in the field of neurosurgery for the prevention of morbidity and mortality. Ruptured cerebral aneurysms are significantly related to a notable probability of death [60]. The mortality rate associated with the rupture of an aneurysm is considerable, as evidenced by the fact that 10% of patients expire before hospital arrival, 25% expire within the initial 24 h period, and more than 50% expire within a month. There is currently a lack of recognized efficient recommendations for the screening of cerebral aneurysms. Nanorobotics has the potential to offer a unique approach for the detection of aneurysms and the continuous monitoring of preexisting ones. The potential of an intravascular nanorobot lies in its ability to detect the progression of aneurysms by monitoring higher levels of nitric oxide synthase protein within the compromised blood vessel. To mitigate the substantial costs associated with screening protocols such as imaging and multiple subsequent appointments, it is conceivable that these nanorobots may be endowed with the capability to convey pertinent vascular alterations wirelessly to healthcare practitioners. Significantly, the establishment of the fundamental infrastructure for such a device would provide the potential for horizontal expansion into various additional applications, including detecting tumors and monitoring changes in ischemia [61].

1.5 The prospects of nanorobots for use in dentistry

The utilization of nanorobots in the field of dentistry is becoming more prevalent, leading to the flourishing development of nanodentistry. Nanorobots possess numerous prospective applications within the field of dentistry, encompassing a range of operations such as cleaning, cosmetic dental interventions such as tooth whitening, therapy for root canals, hypersensitivity treatment, tooth alignment, reinforcement of tooth durability, and alleviation of oral pain. The restoration of a compromised tooth necessitates the utilization of a diverse range of tissue engineering methodologies. The induction of oral analgesia may be achieved by ingesting a solution containing a vast number of nanorobots that can traverse the mucosa and access the gingival sulcus and pulp. Nanorobots can be employed to administer the medication in a controlled fashion to the specific areas of interest. The encapsulation of nanorobots within a capsule, enabling their interaction and detection, holds significant potential for the advancement of root canal treatments and the treatment of dental infections. The utilization of nanorobots that are equipped with miniature cameras to visualize damaged roots during root canal therapy has been demonstrated to result in a notable enhancement in the success rate of the procedure. Based on data from the National Health Service, it was observed that the efficacy of root canal therapy showed a notable rise to 70% in the year 2011. The utilization of nanostructured composite materials in autologous, full-tooth replacement has significantly transformed the approach to dentition replacement treatment from a biological standpoint. Sapphire, which is covalently bonded, has been utilized as a replacement for the enamel in an artificial tooth. This material exhibits a hardness that is 200 times that of ceramic and standard whitening sealant. The fundamental constituents of a nanocomposite are resin-dispersed nanoparticles. The refractive index of the nanofiller is 1.503, and it comprises a mixture of aluminum and silicon powder. In contrast to conventional composites, its ability to blend more seamlessly with natural teeth is a distinguishing characteristic. There has been an increase in scholarly attention to the utilization of nanorobots as a potential solution for addressing dentine hypersensitivity. Teeth that are hypersensitive exhibit a heightened concentration of dentinal tubules. Nanorobots, when introduced into the dentinal tubules, perform targeted ablation, effectively inhibiting the transmission of pain signals to the central nervous system. The application of nanorobots in dental hygiene contributes to the realignment of teeth through the direct manipulation of the periodontal tissues [62]. The potential integration of nanorobots into mouthwash and toothpaste has been proposed to enhance dental hygiene.

1.6 The use of nanorobots in gene therapy

Nanorobots play a crucial role in the treatment of genetics-based disorders. Through a comprehensive examination of the molecular composition of DNA and protein sequences, it is plausible that medical nanorobots could identify the underlying factors responsible for genetic ailments and subsequently administer appropriate therapeutic interventions. Aberrations or irregularities could potentially be addressed through nanoscale alterations to the genetic composition. Empirical evidence demonstrates that the application of chromosomal replacement treatment holds promise in effectively replacing cell repair mechanisms.

The nucleus of the human cell functions as the conduit for the maintenance of genetic material. A study compared the molecular structure of DNA and protein sequences and analyzed the data stored in a nanocomputer's database. In the event of an identified defect, the DNA strand underwent a repair process wherein suitable proteins were reattached to the chain, therefore restoring its original orientation.

1.7 The biocompatibility and toxicity of nanorobots

Micro/nanomotors are commonly employed *in vivo* for many applications such as drug delivery and cargo movement. However, these motors must overcome immune system clearance. Therefore, it is imperative to optimize the management of pharmaceuticals and their therapeutic efficacy while concurrently developing approaches to circumvent the host's immune response. Moreover, nanorobots must deliver medication with utmost accuracy at the precise location of contact. The successful implementation of the task necessitates the integration of a motorized mechanism that possesses the ability to traverse the cellular and tissue barriers within the host organism, hence facilitating the exploration of remote organs and systems. The strategic advancement of micro/nano vehicles is of the utmost importance in attaining the desired goals in diverse biological scenarios [64]. Therefore, it is crucial to carefully consider the design, composition, and power supply of nanorobots if they are to be seen as effective sensors or delivery systems for theragnostic applications [65, 66]. Traditional methods of drug administration face substantial limitations in efficiently distributing therapeutic substances, especially to specific cells that are affected, even when the amounts involved are quite minimal. The capacity of autonomous micro/nanomotors to demonstrate directed motion, tissue adherence, and penetrating capabilities facilitates the active deployment of these motors to the intended site. Consequently, the approach frequently involves the encapsulation of pharmaceuticals, genes, or proteins within micro/nanorobots which are subsequently deployed to the intended site; the payload is subsequently released in response to physiological or environmental stimuli [67, 68].

1.8 Conclusions

The significance of nanorobots in the prevention and treatment of common diseases, as well as their potential to enhance diverse human capacities, holds substantial academic value. However, ongoing research into, and testing of the dynamic properties of nanorobots continue due to the inherent difficulties involved in programming these robots to interact efficiently with their biological environment at the nanoscale. To enhance the mobility and guidance of nanorobots operating at the nanoscale, it is essential to incorporate minute motors and other propulsion technologies within these minuscule entities. The creation of a diverse range of nanoscale sensors is important. Despite the seeming difficulty of the endeavor, numerous research teams are currently engaged in the active pursuit of the biomimetic approach. Despite the current perception of its impossibility, it is plausible that future advancements resulting from the collaborative efforts of diverse research teams could render it achievable. To realize medical nanorobotics, it is imperative to overcome the obstacles that currently hinder nanomanufacture. The field of nanorobotics exhibits promising prospects for use as a groundbreaking medical technique. The scientific community expresses a high level of confidence in the emergence of several novel improvements in the form of both academic reports and commercial products. This optimism stems from the rapid progress observed in the field of nanorobotics in recent years. Significant advancements have been achieved by scientists and engineers in the field of nanoscale mechanisms and devices. In recent times, there have been notable advancements in the development of robots that possess dimensions smaller than the average width of a human hair. These robots possess the capability to rotate and move in both the forward and reverse directions by utilizing a magnetic field. They can be programmed to perform a range of functions, including the administration of medication, the destruction of malignant tumors, or the removal of plaque. Ongoing development is underway to design a nanorobot for ocular placement and extended residence to deliver therapeutic interventions to mitigate or eliminate the pathological neovascularization responsible for a specific disease. In the near future, individuals will be able to see their bodies host a multitude of miniature robots that are equipped to deliver diagnostic and therapeutic functionalities.

References and further reading

[1] Nistor M T and Rusu A G 2019 Nanorobots with applications in medicine *Polymeric Nanomaterials in Nanotherapeutics* (Amsterdam: Elsevier) 123–49

[2] Varadan V K, Chen L and Xie J 2008 *Nanomedicine: Design and Applications of Magnetic Nanomaterials, Nanosensors and Nanosystems* (New York: Wiley)

[3] Ma Y, Zhang F and Lively R P 2020 Manufacturing nanoporous materials for energy-efficient separations: application and challenges *Sustainable Nanoscale Engineering* (Amsterdam: Elsevier) 33–81

[4] Radamson H H *et al* 2020 State of the art and future perspectives in advanced CMOS technology *Nanomaterials* **1555** 1555

[5] Liu J and Deng Z S 2009 Nano-cryosurgery: advances and challenges *J. Nanosci. Nanotechnol.* **9** 4521–42

[6] Gannon C J, Patra C R, Bhattacharya R, Mukherjee P and Curley S A 2008 Intracellular gold nanoparticles enhance non-invasive radiofrequency thermal destruction of human gastrointestinal cancer cells *J. Nanobiotechnol.* **6** 1–9

[7] Torney F, Trewyn B G, Lin V S Y and Wang K 2007 Mesoporous silica nanoparticles deliver DNA and chemicals into plants *Nat. Nanotechnol.* **2** 295–300
[8] Polla D L, Erdman A G, Robbins W P, Markus D T, Diaz-Diaz J, Rizq R, Nam Y, Brickner H T, Wang A and Krulevitch P 2000 Microdevices in medicine *Annu. Rev. Biomed. Eng.* **2** 551–76
[9] Schurr M O, Schostek S, Ho C N, Rieber F and Menciassi A 2007 Microtechnologies in medicine: an overview *Minim. Invasive Ther. Allied Technol.* **1** 76–86
[10] Feynman R P 1961 There's plenty of room at the bottom *Miniaturization* ed H D Gilbert (New York: Reinhold) 282–96
[11] Giri G, Maddahi Y and Zareinia K 2021 A brief review on challenges in design and development of nanorobots for medical applications *Appl. Sci.* **5** 10385
[12] Martel S 2008 Nanorobots for microfactories to operations in the human body and robots propelled by bacteria *Facta Univ. Ser. Mech. Autom. Control Robot.* **7** 1–8
[13] Blakemore R 1975 Magnetotactic bacteria *Science* **190** 377–9
[14] Lefèvre C T, Schmidt M L, Viloria N, Trubitsyn D, Schüler D and Bazylinski D A 2012 Insight into the evolution of magnetotaxis in *Magnetospirillum* spp., based on mam gene phylogeny *Appl. Environ. Microbiol.* **78** 7238–48
[15] Xia F, Tian Y C, Li Y and Sun Y 2007 Wireless sensor/actuator network design for mobile control applications *Sensors 9* 2157–73
[16] Farsad N, Yilmaz H B, Eckford A, Chae C B and Guo W 2016 A comprehensive survey of recent advancements in molecular communication *IEEE Commun. Surv. Tutor.* **11** 1887–919
[17] Hu Y and Wang Z L 2015 Recent progress in piezoelectric nanogenerators as a sustainable power source in self-powered systems and active sensors *Nano Energy* **1** 3–14
[18] Freitas R A Jr 2009 Computational tasks in medical nanorobotics *Nanoscale and Bio-Inspired Computing* ed M M Eshaghian-Wilner (New York, NY: Wiley) 29 15 391–428
[19] Ceyhan B, Alhorn P, Lang C, Schuler D and Niemeyer C M 2006 Semisynthetic biogenic magnetosome nanoparticles for the detection of proteins and nucleic acids *Small* **2** 11
[20] Rosen J, Hannaford B and Satava R M 2011 *Surgical Robotics: Systems Applications and Visions* (Berlin: Springer)
[21] Bogunia-Kubik K and Sugisaka M 2002 From molecular biology to nanotechnology and nanomedicine *Biosystems* **65** 123–38
[22] Shah J, Vyas A and Vyas D 2014 The history of robotics in surgical specialties *AJRS* **1** 12–20
[23] Freitas R A 1998 Exploratory design in medical nanotechnology: a mechanical artificial red cell *Artif. Cells, Blood Substit., Biotechnol.* **26** 411–30
[24] Hassouna H I 2000 Blood stasis, thrombosis, and fibrinolysis *Hematol. Oncol. Clin. North Am.* **14** xvii–xxii
[25] Peterson P, Hayes T E, Arkin C F, Bovill E G, Fairweather R B, Rock W A Jr, Triplett D A and Brandt J T 1998 The preoperative bleeding time test lacks clinical benefit: College of American Pathologists and American Society of Clinical Pathologistsapos; position article *Arch Surg.* **133** 134–9
[26] Ricotti L, Trimmer B, Feinberg A W, Raman R, Parker K K, Bashir R, Sitti M, Martel S, Dario P and Menciassi A 2017 Biohybrid actuators for robotics: a review of devices actuated by living cells *Sci. Robot.* **29** eaaq0495
[27] Fernández-Colino A, Kiessling F, Slabu I, De Laporte L, Akhyari P, Nagel S K, Stingl J, Reese S and Jockenhoevel S 2023 Lifelike transformative materials for biohybrid implants inspired by nature, driven by technology *Adv. Healthcare Mater.* **8** 2300991

[28] Sandhiya S, Dkhar S A and Surendiran A 2009 Emerging trends of nanomedicine–an overview *Fundam. Clin. Pharmacol.* **23** 3
[29] Freitas R A Jr 2005 Microbivores: artificial mechanical phagocytes using digest and discharge protocol *J. Evol. Technol.* **14** 55–106
[30] Freitas R A Jr 2005 What is nanomedicine? *Nanomedicine* **1** 2–9
[31] Sahoo S, Parveen S and Panda J 2007 The present and future of nanotechnology in human health care *Nanomed. Nanotechnol. Biol. Med.* **3** 1
[32] Berg H C 2003 The rotary motor of bacterial flagella *Annu. Rev. Biochem.* **72** 19–54
[33] Wang L, Meng Z, Chen Y and Zheng Y 2021 Engineering magnetic micro/nanorobots for versatile biomedical applications *Adv. Intell. Syst.* **3** 2000267
[34] Saadeh Y and Vyas D 2014 Nanorobotic applications in medicine: current proposals and designs *Am. J. Robot. Surg.* **1** 4–11
[35] Jeutter D C 1994 Spinal Cord Society. Position Sensitive Power Transfer Antenna *U.S. Patent* **5**,314,453
[36] Giri G, Maddahi Y and Zareinia K 2021 A brief review on challenges in design and development of nanorobots for medical applications *Appl. Sci.* **11** 10385
[37] Al-Arif S M R 2012 Control system for autonomous medical nanorobots *In Proc. of the Int. Conf. on Biomedical Engineering (ICoBE)* vol 27 *(Penang, Malaysia)* 161–4
[38] Xiong P, Molnar S V, Moerland T S, Hong S and Chase P B 2006 Biomolecular-based actuator *US Patent Specification* 7014823
[39] Tripathi R, Kumar A and Kumar A 2020 Architecture and application of nanorobots in medicine *Control Systems Design of Bio-Robotics and Bio-mechatronics with Advanced Applications* (New York: Academic) 1 445–64
[40] Yan X, Wang F, Zheng B and Huang F 2012 Stimuli-responsive supramolecular polymeric materials *Chem. Soc. Rev.* **41** 6042–65
[41] Agrahari V, Agrahari V, Chou M L, Chew C H, Noll J and Burnouf T 2020 Intelligent micro-/nanorobots as drug and cell carrier devices for biomedical therapeutic advancement: promising development opportunities and translational challenges *Biomaterials* **1** 120163
[42] Ohm C, Brehmer M and Zentel R 2010 Liquid crystalline elastomers as actuators and sensors *Adv. Mater.* **22** 3366–87
[43] Wang Y, Tu Y and Peng F 2021 The energy conversion behind micro-and nanomotors *Micromachines* **22** 222
[44] Huang H W, Sakar M S, Petruska A J, Pané S and Nelson B J 2016 Soft micromachines with programmable motility and morphology *Nat. Commun.* **7** 12263
[45] Wang W, Yao C, Zhang M J, Ju X J, Xie R and Chu L Y 2013 Thermo-driven microcrawlers fabricated via a microfluidic approach *J. Phys. D: Appl. Phys.* **46** 114007
[46] Filippi M, Garello F, Yasa O, Kasamkattil J, Scherberich A and Katzschmann R K 2022 Engineered magnetic nanocomposites to modulate cellular function *Small* **18** 2104079
[47] Tregubov A A, Nikitin P I and Nikitin M P 2018 Advanced smart nanomaterials with integrated logic-gating and biocomputing: dawn of theranostic nanorobots *Chem. Rev.* **20** 10294–348
[48] Camacho-Lopez M, Finkelmann H, Palffy-Muhoray P and Shelley M 2004 Fast liquid-crystal elastomer swims into the dark *Nat. Mater.* **3** 307–10
[49] Zeng H, Wasylczyk P, Parmeggiani C, Martella D, Burresi M and Wiersma D S 2015 Light-fueled microscopic walkers *Adv. Mater.* **27** 3883–7
[50] Palima D and Glückstad J 2013 Gearing up for optical micro-robotics: micromanipulation and actuation of synthetic microstructures by optical forces *Laser Photonics Rev.* **7** 478–94

[51] Shivalkar S, Chowdhary P, Afshan T, Chaudhary S, Roy A, Samanta S K and Sahoo A K 2022 Nanoengineering of biohybrid micro/nanobots for programmed biomedical applications *Colloids Surf.* B **24** 113054

[52] Tabatabaei S N, Lapointe J and Martel S 2011 Shrinkable hydrogel-based magnetic microrobots for interventions in the vascular network *Adv. Robot.* **25** 1049–67

[53] Yang C S, Wu H C, Sun J S, Hsiao H M and Wang T W 2013 Thermo-induced shape-memory PEG-PCL copolymer as a dual-drug-eluting biodegradable stent *ACS Appl. Mater. Interfaces* **5** 10985–94

[54] Suhail M, Khan A, Rahim M A, Naeem A, Fahad M, Badshah S F, Jabar A and Janakiraman A K 2022 Micro and nanorobot-based drug delivery: an overview *J. Drug Target.* **21** 349–58

[55] Piovanelli M, Fujie T, Mazzolai B and Beccai L A 2012 *4th IEEE RAS & EMBS Int. Conf. on Biomedical Robotics and Biomechatronics (BioRob) Bio-inspired approach towards the development of soft amoeboid microrobots* **24** *(Rome, Italy)* 612–6

[56] Lämmermann T and Sixt M 2009 Mechanical modes of 'amoeboid'cell migration *Curr. Opin. Cell Biol.* **21** 636–44

[57] Terentjev E M and Weitz D A 2015 *The Oxford Handbook of Soft Condensed Matter* (Oxford: Oxford Handbooks)

[58] Rubinstein L 2000 *8th Foresight Conf. on Molecular Nanotechnology A practical nanorobot for treatment of various medical problems (Bethesda, MD)* (draft)

[59] Van den Heuvel M G and Dekker C 2007 Motor proteins at work for nanotechnology *Science* **317** 333–6

[60] Toth G and Cerejo R 2018 Intracranial aneurysms: review of current science and management *Vasc. Med.* **23** 276–88

[61] Suntornsuk W and Suntornsuk L 2020 Recent applications of paper-based point-of-care devices for biomarker detection *Electrophoresis* **41** 287–305

[62] Viswa Chandra R 2023 Nanorobotics in dentistry *Nanomaterials in Dental Medicine* (Singapore: Springer Nature Singapore) vol 4 121–39

[63] Hede S and Huilgol N 2006 Nano': the new nemesis of cancer *J. Cancer Res. Therap.* **2** 186–95

[64] Wickline S A, Neubauer A M, Winter P, Caruthers S and Lanza G 2006 Applications of nanotechnology to atherosclerosis, thrombosis, and vascular biology *Arter. Thromb. Vasc. Biol.* **26** 435–41

[65] Katz E, Riklin A, Heleg-Shabtai V, Willner I and Bückmann A F 1999 Glucose oxidase electrodes via reconstitution of the apo-enzyme: tailoring of novel glucose biosensors *Anal. Chim. Acta* **385** 45–58

[66] Ricotti L, Cafarelli A, Iacovacci V, Vannozzi L and Menciassi A 2015 Advanced micro-nano-bio systems for future targeted therapies *Curr. Nanosci.* **1** 144–60

[67] Cavalcanti A, Rosen L, Shirinzadeh B and Rosenfeld M 2006 Nanorobot for treatment of patients with artery occlusion *In Proc. of Virtual Concept* 1–10

[68] Cavalcanti A, Shirinzadeh B, Fukuda T and Ikeda S 2007 Hardware architecture for nanorobot application in cerebral aneurysm *7th IEEE Conf. on Nanotechnology* (IEEE: Piscataway, NJ)

[69] Iacovacci V, Lucarini G, Ricotti L, Dario P, Dupont P E and Menciassi A 2015 Untethered magnetic millirobot for targeted drug delivery *Biomed. Microdevices* **17** 1–2

IOP Publishing

Integrating Nanorobotics with Biophysics for Cancer Treatment

Rishabha Malviya, Deepika Yadav, Sonali Sundram, Seifedine Kadry and Gurvinder Singh Virk

Chapter 2

Robotics and biophysics: technology advances and challenges in organic and inorganic domains

The integration of biophysics and robotics is a rapidly developing and promising domain that is positioned to revolutionize several realms within the fields of scientific inquiry and technological advancement. The field of biophysics, which involves the application of physical ideas to biological structures, is experiencing a productive collaboration with automation. This partnership has facilitated the development of novel robotic devices and structures that possess the ability to comprehend and engage with human beings in significant manners. The adoption of a multidisciplinary strategy is fundamentally transforming various domains, including medical care, ecological surveillance, the space program, and other related professions. The utilization of biophysics-based robotics has the capacity to enhance healthcare diagnostics, therapy, and recuperation, concurrently fostering the progression of our comprehension of environmental systems and diversification. Nevertheless, this captivating expedition is not devoid of obstacles, encompassing ethical deliberations, regulatory structures, and the imperative for proficient interdisciplinary cooperation. As we contemplate the forthcoming years, the indisputable possibilities for biophysics-based robots emerge, offering vast opportunities to tackle complex difficulties, enhance the well-being of humans, and expand the frontiers of understanding within science. In the forthcoming era, the symbiotic relationship between biophysics and automation will persistently propel advancements and cultivate a more profound integration of technological advances with the environment.

2.1 Introduction

Within the current context of interdisciplinary exploration and innovations in technology, the convergence of robots and biological physics presents itself as a domain of exceptional potential and intricacy. The integration of several fields of study presents a wide range of possibilities for leveraging the capabilities of

doi:10.1088/978-0-7503-6019-7ch2

mechanical components in comprehending, reproducing, and cooperating with biological entities, while simultaneously acknowledging the complexities associated with communicating with nonliving entities [1]. The objective of the study we are conducting, titled 'Robotics and Biophysics: Technological Advancements and Constraints in Organic and Inorganic Materials Aspects,' is to present a thorough and all-encompassing analysis of this rapidly changing and developing discipline.

Within the organic domain, one may observe the captivating amalgamation of automation and biological processes, wherein robots are purposefully engineered to imitate, aid, or potentially enhance the functioning of biological systems. The potential of this interaction to revolutionize healthcare, aid those with impairments, and expand our comprehension of the human condition is significant [2]. The field of robotics research has yielded a wide range of remarkable achievements, such as robotic surgical assistants that improve the accuracy of complicated surgical procedures and bioinspired robots that imitate animals' movement patterns to aid in search-and-rescue efforts [3].

Conversely, the inclusion of the inanimate component acquaints us with the complex domain of materials science and biophysics. The primary foci of this research are the development of innovative materials capable of interacting with biological structures and the investigation of the underlying fundamental physical concepts that control these interactions. The integration of inorganic and organic domains has led to the emergence of several advancements, including bioelectronic gadgets, intelligent prosthetic devices, and medication administration systems [4]. Nevertheless, the difficulties related to the development of biocompatible components, the guarantee of long-term stability, and the establishment of seamless interactions with live creatures are substantial and necessitate meticulous deliberation.

In this chapter, we shall explore the innovative developments that are driving progress in this domain, encompassing the utilization of intelligent machines for the management of robots, the evolution of soft robotics, and the downsizing of sensing. Concurrently, we shall address the ethical, safeguarding, and regulatory problems, alongside the imperative of multidisciplinary cooperation, to effectively tackle the complex issues inherent in this convergence.

The article titled 'Robotics and Biophysics: Technological Advancement and Constraints in Organic and Inorganic Dimensions' invites readers to enter an extraordinary domain where the distinctions between the biological and mechanical realms become indistinct [5]. The subject in question is characterized by a harmonious relationship between creativity and comprehension, giving rise to significant inquiries and presenting exceptional resolutions. Our expedition through this complex realm of exploration holds the potential to be informative and captivating.

2.2 An introduction to the use of robots in the field of biophysics

The integration of robotics within the domain of biophysics has assumed a pivotal position in the progression of our comprehension of biological structures and their inherent physical attributes. This multidisciplinary scientific discipline integrates ideas from the biological and physical disciplines, alongside other related subjects, to investigate the physical, electrical, and structural characteristics of living creatures. The field of robotics plays a crucial role in the study of biomechanical assessment, enabling thorough investigation into the functioning of biological organisms. This capability proves to be of immense value in various domains, including prosthetics and rehabilitation [6]. Furthermore, this technology facilitates the accurate manipulation of cells and the examination of individual molecules, thereby offering valuable insights into essential biological mechanisms and contributing to the advancement of drug administration and techniques for sorting cell types. Robotics plays a pivotal role in augmenting laboratories' automated processes, high-throughput capabilities for drug assessment, and biological image processing, thereby significantly enhancing the effectiveness and accuracy of experimental processes. Surgical robots play a crucial role in healthcare by facilitating less invasive operations, hence enhancing the precision of surgery and expediting patient recuperation. In addition, the burgeoning discipline of automation investigates the development of robotics that draw inspiration from biological systems, thereby enhancing our comprehension of biomechanics and biomimicry. Robots play a crucial role in the field of biological physics, contributing to advancements and improvements in various areas such as data processing, the administration of medications, recuperation, and biophysical approach modeling. This varied range of applications has a significant impact on both scientific endeavors and medical outcomes [7].

2.2.1 The importance of robots in the field of biophysical research

The scientific discipline of biophysics relies heavily on integration with automation, as it serves a crucial and central role in the study of the fundamental physical principles that regulate the functioning of biological systems. This multidisciplinary field of study integrates principles and concepts from the domains of both biology and physics to explore and analyze the mechanical, electronic, and structural properties exhibited by biological organisms [8]. The integration of robotics has significantly enhanced the field of biophysical study through several means. The utilization of this technology enables the examination of biomechanical processes, thus enabling investigators to accurately recreate and thoroughly examine the mechanical maneuvers and functionalities of biological structures. This has significant implications for the advancement of prosthetics, rehabilitative equipment, and the field of locomotion study. The field of robotics also facilitates accurate manipulation of cells and the study of individual molecules, including deoxyribonucleic acid (DNA) as well as proteins, thereby improving our understanding of cellular mechanics, medication administration, and molecular relationships [9]. Moreover, the implementation of autonomous robotic systems in laboratory settings has been found to optimize several aspects of operations in laboratories, encompassing specimen transportation and data processing. This integration has demonstrated a notable enhancement in the overall effectiveness and precision of experimental procedures. Within the field of medicine, the utilization of robotic surgical instruments has led to significant advancements in the field of less invasive operations, hence enhancing both surgical accuracy and patient recuperation. Moreover, within the field of automation, there is a category of robotics that draws inspiration from biological systems, hence facilitating the investigation of biomechanical and biological mimicry. Robotics plays a crucial role in advancing biological physics by facilitating high-throughput capabilities for medication assessment, enabling precise biological imaging, and promoting proficient biological information technology. This integration of automation into biophysics leads to inventiveness, enhancing both the academic as well as medical care sectors. Furthermore, it contributes to a more comprehensive comprehension of the complex physical mechanisms inherent in biological organisms [10].

2.2.2 The possible application of robots in areas of biophysical investigation

The field of automation presents a wide range of possible applications in the realm of physicochemical investigation, thereby greatly augmenting our comprehension of the underlying physical laws that regulate biological processes. The field of biomechanics derives significant advantages from the integration of automation, as it facilitates the precise examination of the mechanical features within organisms. This integration consequently opens avenues for progress in the development of prostheses and orthopedics and provides important insights into the mechanics of movement [11]. At both the molecular and cellular scales, the field of automation enables accurate manipulations and study, hence facilitating the investigation of cell behavior, mechanobiology, and interactions between molecules. The domain of drug development is significantly enhanced by the implementation of advanced screening, a method that effectively evaluates the impacts of several substances on biological processes, therefore accelerating the process of identifying prospective medications. Moreover, the implementation of automation in laboratories serves to streamline a multitude of investigative tasks, whilst the integration of healthcare robots contributes to the enhancement of surgical excellence and the facilitation of fewer invasive treatments, ultimately leading to improved outcomes for patients. The utilization of robots in imaging and microscopy provides a high level of accuracy and surveillance, which in turn facilitates the visualization of complex biological components. Automation plays a crucial role in biophysical modeling by enabling the simulation of intricate biological processes. In addition, it offers valuable insights into the fields of biomechanics and biomimicry [12]. Moreover, robots assume a crucial role in the advancement of rehabilitative and assistive equipment, as well as in the fields of statistical analysis and biological information technology, facilitating the management of the vast amount of data produced in biophysical research [13]. In general, the implementation of robots in several fields enables scientists to enhance the accuracy, effectiveness, and ingenuity of their investigations, thus contributing to the expansion of knowledge about biological structures and supporting progress in medical care and innovation.

2.2.3 Biophysical applications of robot-based systems

A variety of robotics devices and technologies are utilized in the field of biophysics to enhance the processes of investigation, experimentation, and information acquisition. Presented below are several illustrations of automated devices employed in several biophysical applications:

Optical tweezers: the utilization of optical tweezers involves the employment of concentrated laser light to control and confine minute objects, such as particular cells or macromolecules. Scientists utilize these tools to investigate the mechanical features and interplay of molecules in biological systems [14]. **Atomic force microscopes (AFMs)** are automated devices that employ a finely pointed probe to meticulously examine the topography of biological specimens at the nanometer level. These instruments are employed for the quantification of intermolecular forces, the investigation of cellular mechanics, and the visualization of the topographical characteristics of biological samples [15]. **Liquid handling robots** are specifically engineered to provide accurate automated dispensing of liquids in applications such as advanced screening and laboratory automated processes. These entities play a vital role in various activities, including drug testing, DNA sequencing, and sample preparation [16].

Robotic surgical systems: robotic surgical systems, such as the da Vinci Surgical System, have been developed to facilitate less invasive surgical procedures by offering improved precision. Robotic arms are utilized by physicians to execute surgeries with diminished incisions, hence mitigating patient recuperation durations and minimizing damage [17]. **Lab-on-a-chip (LOC) systems:** LOC systems encompass microfluidic instruments that effectively consolidate diverse laboratory functionalities into a condensed chip format. Robotic equipment can exert oversight over them, hence enabling the automation of sample processing. This attribute renders them highly advantageous in the realms of biomolecular investigation and diagnosis [18]. **Automated microscopy:** Automatic microscopes, specifically robotic microscopes, provide accurate positioning and focusing capabilities that allow images of biological specimens to be captured at high resolution. These devices have a vital role in the fields of cellular biology, neurology, and genetics studies [19]. Microarrayers are automated systems employed in the production of microarrays, which are utilized to assess gene expression, genome sequencing, and protein analyses. These technologies facilitate the simultaneous investigation of hundreds of genomes or proteins, resulting in improved efficiency.

Testing methodologies based on biomechanics: robotic systems, such as materials evaluation machines, are commonly employed in scientific research to investigate and analyze the mechanical characteristics of various biological entities, including cell membranes, tissues, and biological materials. Our comprehension of the behavior of biological components under conditions of strain and stress is due to their availability. Autonomous pipetting technologies are robotic devices designed to automate the highly precise and repetitive process of pipetting fluids [20]. By doing so, these systems effectively minimize human error and enhance the effectiveness of investigations that include the manipulation of materials [20]. **Exoskeletons**

and rehabilitation robots: robotic exoskeletons are employed within the realm of rehabilitative and physical therapy to facilitate the restoration of motion and muscular endurance for individuals following injury or surgical procedures. According to studies, these gadgets are beneficial for improving walking technique and muscular development [21]. **Bioinformatics pipelines** involve the development and implementation of computational workflows for the analysis and interpretation of biological data. Bioinformatics pipelines frequently employ automated scripts and algorithms to handle and examine extensive biological data sets, thereby facilitating the comprehension of proteomics, genomics, and other 'omics' data. Although these systems are not embodied as tangible automated machines, they effectively contribute to the processing and analysis of such information. These examples demonstrate the multifunctionality of automated devices in the field of biological physics, facilitating the execution of accurate investigations, streamlining repetitive operations, and acquiring crucial data that is pivotal in furthering our comprehension of biological structures and their physical characteristics [19].

2.3 Technology advances of soft robotics in the organic domain

Soft automation has emerged as a prominent discipline within the realm of biological physics, focusing on the creation and advancement of robotics constructed from pliable and adaptable substances. This area has gained considerable recognition because of its distinctive attributes, which closely replicate the properties that characterize biological cellular tissue and organisms. The utilization of soft robotics has found numerous uses in various significant areas of biological physics, such as biomechanics. In this field, scientists employ soft robotics to investigate the biomechanics of human and animal movement, as well as the complicated architecture of soft tissues such as muscles and ligaments [21]. Soft robotics plays a crucial role in the field of medicine by facilitating the development of surgical equipment and customizable exoskeletons that improve surgical precision and assist persons with restricted movement in recovering their physical strength and mobility. These robots possess a high level of compliance, making them particularly suitable for performing intricate activities such as biomedical sampling, organ transplantation, and biopsies. Scholars are currently exploring biohybrid technologies that integrate biological tissues and cells with soft robotics frameworks, thereby advancing the frontiers of biological engineering and regenerative healthcare [19, 20]. These robots are utilized to replicate biological components such as arteries and blood vessels, to conduct biological *in vivo* studies, and to monitor aquatic environments. In addition, they serve as a more convenient and flexible option in the fields of prosthetics and rehabilitation [22]. The inherent compliance of soft robotics enables a nuanced and flexible engagement with biological systems, hence facilitating a deeper comprehension of biophysical fundamentals and the development of groundbreaking medical solutions.

2.3.1 The applications of soft robots in medical and biological settings

The utilization of soft robotics in healthcare and biological environments has been extensive, mostly due to their inherent characteristics of versatility, adaptability, and capacity to engage with biological components delicately and responsively. Several significant uses include soft **robotic devices**, which are frequently employed in less invasive surgical procedures and have numerous benefits within medical environments [23]. The compliance of these devices enables them to adapt to and gently engage with fragile tissues, hence mitigating the potential for injury to tissues and minimizing patient trauma [23]. Soft robotic devices can be manipulated by physicians with an elevated level of accuracy, rendering them well suited for surgical procedures such as laparoscopic surgeries. This is particularly advantageous when access is restricted or the manipulation of delicate organs necessitates careful handling. Soft robots have been utilized in medical operations, including prostatectomies and gynecological surgery, to improve the results of surgical procedures [18]. The utilization of soft robotics in endoscopic treatments has demonstrated significant advantages. The inherent attributes of flexibility and controllability possessed by these entities facilitate the navigation of intricate and convoluted biological structures, such as the gastrointestinal tract. **Endoscopes** possess the ability to conform to the inherent curvatures of the body's interior pathways, hence enhancing visualization and facilitating access to anatomical regions that present difficulties for conventional rigid endoscopes. The utilization of this technology has substantial consequences for the timely identification and management of gastrointestinal ailments, hence mitigating patient suffering and minimizing the requirement for sedation [24]. **Rehabilitation exoskeletons** are wearable devices that are specifically designed to offer support and aid to those who experience mobility limitations. These devices are characterized by their soft exoskeleton structure. The pliable and malleable constituents of these devices provide a more organic and adaptable range of motion, hence assisting in the recuperation of individuals undergoing rehabilitation following injury or surgical procedures [25]. The customization of exoskeletons allows for the targeting of specific muscle areas, rendering them highly advantageous for individuals with neurological disorders or those undergoing orthopedic rehabilitation. **Assistive gadgets**: the utilization of soft robotics is observed in assistive gadgets designed to aid those with disabilities. This encompasses soft grippers and prosthetic devices that provide a heightened level of user engagement by offering a more authentic and ergonomic interface [23]. The purpose of these devices is to replicate the dexterity and versatility of human hands and limbs, hence enhancing the overall well-being of individuals who have experienced limb loss or who have restricted mobility [26]. **Biohybrids:** the coupling of biological tissues and cells with soft robotic components, leading to the development of biohybrid networks, is currently being investigated by scientists. Such structures integrate the benefits of both natural and synthetic materials to create novel approaches in the fields of tissue restoration, regenerative healthcare, and disease modeling. Soft robots have the potential to contribute to the development of computer-generated organs and tissues for transplantation and drug evaluation, as evidenced by previous research [27]. **Telemedicine:** the utilization of soft robotic systems is highly advantageous in the field of telemedicine due to their ability to be manipulated and controlled from a remote location. They can aid in many duties such as monitoring vital signs, administering rehabilitation therapy, participating in telemedicine consultations, and facilitating the delivery of medical services to individuals residing in rural or underdeveloped areas [28]. Soft robots have distinct attributes such as conformity mobility, and flexibility, which render them highly versatile in various medical and biological contexts. Consequently, they hold great potential for enhancing patient treatment, rehabilitative practices, and surgery, thereby offering substantial advancements in these domains. Ongoing progress in the discipline of soft robotics is expected to make significant contributions to the advancement of new approaches that prioritize the needs of patients

2.3.2 Biomimetic design

2.3.2.1 Biomimetic design in robotics

The utilization of mimetic principles for design in the field of automation is an intriguing methodology that involves deriving inspiration from the structures within the body and the behavioral patterns and functional mechanisms observed in biological networks. This technique aims to develop robotics that precisely emulates the characteristics found naturally [29]. This methodology encompasses the replication of diverse attributes exhibited by biological beings, including their anatomical structure, modes of movement, sensing mechanisms, and regulatory tactics.

2.3.2.2 Morphology and structure

Biomimetic design frequently involves the construction of robots that mimic the physical qualities and frameworks observed in the natural world. As an illustration, certain robotics are engineered to possess adaptable and responsive structures that emulate the inherent flexibility observed in living organisms. The utilization of compliant constructions facilitates the safe interaction of robotics with their surroundings and allows them to successfully execute activities that would cause difficulties for stiff robotics [30].

2.3.2.3 Locomotion

Biomimetic robots aim to replicate the locomotive techniques observed in mammals. For example, robots with four legs imitate the walking patterns of mammals, while robots designed to resemble snakes employ serpentine motion [31]. By imitating the locomotive patterns exhibited by organisms, these robotic systems acquire the ability to adjust to diverse landscapes and efficiently traverse complex surroundings.

2.3.2.4 Sensors

Biomimetic robots frequently integrate sensors that draw inspiration from organic sensory systems. For example, robots can employ sensors and image-processing algorithms that simulate the functionality of the human visual system to perform tasks such as recognizing objects and navigating [32]. In addition, the integration of tactile detectors that mimic the structure and function of whiskers or other biological sensory organs allows robots to gain perception of their environment via the sense of touch.

2.3.2.5 Behavior and its regulation

Biomimetic robots can imitate and reproduce behaviors as well as regulate strategies that are observed in the natural environment. Swarm robotics draws inspiration from the collective behaviors exhibited by social organisms such as termites and honeybees [33]. Decentralized control strategies are commonly used in various robotic tasks, including but not limited to collaborative scavenging exploration and monitoring the environment.

2.3.3 The benefits of biomimetic design in biophysics

Enhanced adaptability: biomimetic robots demonstrate exceptional proficiency in maneuvering intricate and ever-changing surroundings, rendering them highly suitable for biophysical investigations, particularly in the context of monitoring wildlife. The capacity to adjust to unforeseen circumstances is of great significance in the realm of ecological and behavioral research [34]. **Bioinspired sensing:** the sensing performed by biomimetic sensors closely resembles the sensing abilities observed in living organisms. This facilitates the acquisition of knowledge by scientists in a manner that closely emulates the sensory experiences of animals. This confers notable benefits in the context of research about the behavior of animals, ecological surveillance, and ecosystem assessment. **Energy efficiency:** biomimetic robots frequently emulate the cost-effective modes of mobility and navigation observed in natural organisms. This reduces the power consumed by these devices during their operation, thus giving them the capability to endure prolonged missions, rendering them suitable for extensive field investigations and data acquisition in remote or arduous settings [35]. **Bioinspired control:** the biomimetic algorithms used for control purposes offer valuable insights into the mechanisms by which biological entities effectively execute intricate tasks. Through the replication of control techniques observed in natural phenomena, investigators can acquire a more profound comprehension of the fundamental principles that drive these behaviors. This, in turn, facilitates the comprehension of biological systems.

2.3.4 The challenges of applying biomimetic design principles in the field of biophysics

Complexities: the endeavor of emulating the complex nature of biological phenomena in robotic entities might be a formidable challenge. An interdisciplinary approach is frequently required, encompassing skills in mechanics, electronic devices, materials science, and biological processes, hence demanding significant resources. **Biological variability:** biological networks can demonstrate substantial variety in both their anatomical frameworks and physiological behaviors. The task of developing mimetic robots capable of properly functioning in diverse conditions and scenarios presents a significant challenge. **Ethical and regulatory issues:** the utilization of biomimetics or robotics in the field of biological physics investigation has the potential to give rise to ethical and regulatory considerations, especially in cases involving studies of or interactions with living beings [36]. Ethical considerations encompass the prospect of adverse effects on mammals or ecological systems, giving rise to inquiries regarding the ethical dimensions of the investigation and the well-being of animals. **The resource-intensive process** of biomimetic design can impose significant demands on resources, including time, finances, and specialized knowledge and skills. The faithful replication of biological processes in the development of robots may impose limitations on their extensive use in some research settings [37]. **Constraints imposed by technology:** despite recent advancements, it is arguable that modern technologies may not possess the ability to completely reproduce the multifaceted abilities exhibited by biological systems. Our ability to mimic some qualities, such as the sensory acuity of specific animals or the complexity of brain networks, is constrained by both physical and technological restrictions. In brief, the use of biomimetic design principles in the field of automation presents numerous advantages in the biophysical realm. These advantages encompass improved versatility, bioinspired sensing capabilities, more efficient use of energy, and valuable perspectives on biological control systems [38]. Nevertheless, this phenomenon also presents a set of obstacles, such as intricacy, the unpredictability of biological systems, ethical considerations, resource constraints, and the intrinsic limitations of existing technology. When making decisions regarding the use of biomimetic designs in their research projects, scientists in the field of biophysics are required to thoroughly evaluate these variables.

2.4 Developments in inorganic measurement technology

Significant progress in the study of inorganic substances has fueled innovations in several fields in recent decades. Carbon-based materials and transition-metal dichalcogenides (TMDs) are two examples of the growing interest in two-dimensional materials [39] due to their unique mechanical as well as electrical properties, which show potential for use in semiconductors and photonics. Displays, solar power plants, and healthcare imaging are just some of the fields in which nanometer-sized semiconductors, known as quantum dots, have benefited from advances in production methods. In addition to their widespread use in gas storage, segregation, and catalysis, metal–organic frameworks (MOFs) are also being studied for potential new roles in pharmaceutical delivery and sensors [40]. Progress in the effectiveness and reliability of polycrystalline solar cells may alter the alternative energy landscape [41]. Drug delivery and cancer therapy have benefited from developments in inorganic nanoparticles, including customized nanoparticles for personalized treatments. Improvements are also being made in the areas such as functional porcelain, superhard substances, and inorganic polymers, which will have uses in areas such as energy harvesting, cutting instruments, and flame-resistant materials. New avenues for optical communication, wearable devices, and commercial uses are also being opened by the development of photonic crystals, composite substances, and improved coatings. These inorganic dimensional advances are a promising new area of research in materials that may have far-reaching effects across a range of businesses and enterprises.

2.4.1 The integration of advanced prosthetic limbs and biophysics

In recent decades, significant progress has been made in the areas of exoskeletal and limb prostheses, resulting in notable breakthroughs in recuperation, locomotion support, and the effective merging of advanced prosthetic limbs and biophysics [42]. Exoskeletons made of robotic components have become indispensable instruments in the realm of physical rehabilitation, assisting persons who experience limitations in their movement. Prosthetic devices emulate the inherent motions of human joints and possess the ability to be customized to accommodate the unique walking patterns of individuals. This adaptability promotes the reconditioning of muscles and aids in the restoration of both physical endurance and flexibility. In addition to their rehabilitative purposes, exoskeletons have demonstrated their usefulness in medical facilities by alleviating the mental and physical strain on medical personnel. Furthermore, they have experienced significant progress in their use within the defense and manufacturing industries [43].

Simultaneously, there has been notable advancement in the field of limb prostheses, as they have become increasingly integrated with the principles of biophysics to achieve improved usefulness and convenience. Sophisticated prosthetic arms and legs are engineered to closely mimic the biomechanical characteristics of organic limbs, hence facilitating a more seamless and instinctive integration with the user's physique. The utilization of myoelectric control mechanisms has become increasingly widespread, allowing individuals to manipulate their prosthetic devices using muscular impulses. Feedback-sensing methods facilitate the provision of tactile sensations for individuals, hence enhancing their ability to communicate with the environment. The process of bone formation, which involves the direct anchoring of a prosthetic leg to the user's bone, has been found to significantly improve both the durability and the performance of the prosthetic [44]. The utilization of biocompatible substances serves to mitigate inconvenience and allergic responses. Furthermore, the advancement of periprosthetics exhibits the potential to reinstate senses as well as promote organic motor function, hence enhancing the level of integration between the individual and the prosthetic limb. Powered exoskeleton prosthetics can blur the distinction between exoskeletons and prostheses, as they provide individuals with enhanced mobility and physical ability, particularly in demanding environments. This progress highlights the integration of biophysics and technology, which aims to establish a more seamless and empowering interface between humans and their prosthetic limbs, thereby enhancing their standard of life and movement.

2.4.2 Robotics in diagnostic imaging and laboratory tasks

The utilization of clinical robotics has become increasingly prevalent within the medical field, serving as an influential instrument that can significantly impact operations and diagnostic activities. The advent of surgical robots has significantly transformed the field of minimally invasive surgery (MIS), prioritizing accuracy and minimizing patient trauma [45]. The da Vinci surgical framework, a type of automation, provides doctors with exceptional degrees of precision, equilibrium, and manual skill [46]. Consequently, there has been a notable boom in the utilization of robotic aids in a wide range of surgical specialties, including gynecology, urological surgery, neurological surgery, and cardiology. Patients benefit from smaller surgical incisions, as they experience a decrease in postoperative pain and an expedited recovery process. Surgical robots serve to augment the proficiency of surgeons while also enabling the practice of telecommunications—allowing qualified surgeons to conduct operations from a distance, thereby extending their abilities to underserved or geographically isolated regions.

The incorporation of healthcare robotics also offers significant advantages in the field of diagnostic imaging. Robotic assistance is employed in medical procedures such as magnetic resonance imaging (MRI) and computed tomography (CT) scans to ensure accurate positioning of patients [47]. This phenomenon enhances the quality of images and diminishes the necessity for multiple scans as well as guaranteeing an accurate diagnosis. In addition, the implementation of automated equipment has been found to improve patient comfort and mitigate the risk of individual errors, especially in the context of extended scanning operations. Medical robots are utilized in laboratories to carry out various duties, such as specimen management, high-throughput screening, and sample processing. These methodologies offer a reliable and replicable strategy for carrying out these procedures, thereby enhancing the dependability and effectiveness of the laboratory's operations. The incorporation of robots into the healthcare industry has a broader scope than their use in surgical settings and diagnostic laboratories alone. It has a profound influence on the entirety of patient healthcare, spanning from the initial evaluation stage to the subsequent medical care and recovery processes. The near future holds the potential for more breakthroughs in robotics, which will result in a wider range of sophisticated uses. These developments are expected to have a positive impact on healthcare and eventually improve outcomes for patients.

2.5 Challenges in integration

Autonomous robots have become essential in several domains, since they are utilized for robotic investigations as well as information acquisition in demanding settings. Within the domain of robot exploration, these devices have assumed important functions in the field of aerospace research. Notably, spacecraft such as Carrasco and Perseverance have demonstrated the ability to independently traverse the Martian landscape, execute scientific investigations, and relay invaluable data back to Earth. In a similar vein, autonomous underwater vehicles (AUVs) and remotely operated vehicles (ROVs) have been deployed to the profound depths of the sea to research marine organisms, examine geographical characteristics, and investigate shipwrecks [48]. In the terrestrial setting, these machines valiantly navigate harsh environments such as arid regions, Arctic regions, and erupting volcanoes to gather data and conduct research in areas that might have restricted or hazardous accessibility for humans.

Artificial intelligence (AI) plays an important part in the operation of autonomous machines within the realm of biophysics and its associated disciplines. It also plays a crucial role in enhancing the evaluation and comprehension of data gathered by robotic systems [48]. This integration allows for the effective handling of extensive data sets, permitting the identification of trends, deviations, and noteworthy discoveries. This capability plays a crucial role in ecological research, as it facilitates the examination of animal behavior, the surveillance of migration patterns, and the evaluation of ecosystem health. Furthermore, AI enables autonomous robots to make instantaneous judgments in changing and uncertain settings, enabling them to adjust their techniques for gathering data and successfully monitor biological species [48]. Within the field of the science of genomics, AI has assumed a pivotal function in the analysis and interpretation of DNA information acquired through robotic means. This involvement includes the recognition of organisms, the analysis of genetic variation, and the inference of evolutionary links [49]. AI-driven autonomous robots have proven to be advantageous in the fields of healthcare and medical robotics. These machines can perform a variety of assignments, including monitoring patients, medication exploration, and genetic evaluation. Their contributions in these areas are crucial in advancing disease diagnosis and the advancement of treatments. The integration of AI and robot autonomy has been essential in driving progress in the field of the science of biophysics and has led to significant breakthroughs in our comprehension of the natural environment, ecological dynamics, and clinical studies [49].

2.5.1 Ethical and regulatory issues

The incorporation of robots into the field of biophysical investigation raises a variety of concerns regarding ethics that necessitate thorough scrutiny and contemplation. The implementation of robots in studies involving individuals necessitates adherence to the basic ethical tenet of well-informed consent. Those participating must be provided with comprehensive information regarding the study's characteristics, the application of automation, any hazards, and their entitlement to discontinue their participation in the research. It is crucial to ensure that participants possess a full understanding of the utilization of robots. The preservation of confidentiality and the safeguarding of sensitive data are crucial considerations in the realm of robots, given the frequent acquisition and examination of delicate information about individuals, such as healthcare records, genealogical information, and biometric information. The ethical obligation entails the implementation of comprehensive data protection measures, compliance with relevant data protection rules, and the protection of personal data.

Ensuring impartiality and promoting equity is of utmost importance, especially in the context of utilizing computational intelligence and algorithmic learning algorithms in biophysics research [50]. These algorithms have the potential to unintentionally sustain biases that are present within the training data. The fulfillment of ethical responsibilities involves the routine examination and revision of algorithms to mitigate bias, particularly in the context of healthcare decision-making. Furthermore, it is of utmost importance to prioritize integrity in research practices and ensure responsible application of robotic technologies. Moral dilemmas emerge when investigators neglect to divulge conflicts of interest, engage in results manipulation, or abuse information. It is of the utmost importance to maintain moral standards in biophysics research that incorporates robots. This is crucial not only to preserve the integrity of the research but also to safeguard the physical and mental health and liberties of those participating, as well as to adhere to the overarching moral principles that govern scientific investigation [51].

2.5.2 Regulatory challenges in the development of biophysics-based robotic systems

The emergence of biophysics-based robotic systems poses a variety of regulatory hurdles due to the distinctive and transdisciplinary characteristics associated with these technologies. The degree of complexity present in these systems and the need for cross-disciplinary collaboration pose a considerable challenge, as they frequently incorporate elements from the disciplines of biology, physics, and technology. This degree of complexity makes it difficult for regulatory bodies to stay abreast of the rapid advances in technology and develop appropriate standards. Safeguarding patients is of the utmost importance, especially in the healthcare industry where these automated instruments are utilized. The assurance of safeguarding, dependability, and precision of these systems necessitates the implementation of thorough testing, confirmation, and continuous evaluation. Data security and privacy concerns are significant problems, particularly in healthcare and research contexts, where the collection and analysis of personally identifiable patient information occurs [52]. Ensuring adherence to data privacy legislation and the preservation of patient information is of the utmost importance. The absence of standards for the creation, evaluation, and functioning of different applications, coupled with the wide range of uses and the rapid rate of invention, gives rise to regulatory complications. It is imperative to tackle concerns regarding ethics, specifically those about well-informed permission and the fair treatment of study topics, particularly in cases involving human participation.

The presence of international legislation presents significant obstacles in the context of cooperative investigation and the advancement in international technology. The job of achieving the harmonization of rules and regulations across international boundaries is a multifaceted endeavor. The consideration of environmental impacts and compliance with environmental standards is of the utmost importance in the context of biophysics-based robotic systems, which may have significant ecological implications. The prolonged procedures involved in obtaining regulatory permission can hinder the prompt progress of research and the development of medical remedies. Moreover, the identification of possible hazards and the development of complete risk management systems are complex endeavors that require meticulous evaluation of the risks to individuals, administrators, and the surrounding environment [49]. Furthermore, the absence of precise regulatory frameworks customized for biophysics-based robotic systems can give rise to uncertainty and difficulties for researchers and innovators endeavoring to efficiently navigate the regulatory environment. To effectively tackle these regulatory obstacles, it is imperative to foster strong cooperation among diverse stakeholders, such as researchers, developers, regulatory agencies, ethicists, and policymakers. This aim of such collaboration is to establish flexible frameworks that effectively reconcile safety, ethical concerns, and technological advancements within the field of biophysics-based robotics.

2.5.3 Interdisciplinary collaboration

2.5.3.1 Bridging the gap between biophysicists and robotics engineers

The significance of collaborative efforts across multiple disciplines in the realm of biophysics and robotics is of the utmost relevance and should not be underestimated. These disciplines possess unique and complementary knowledge and skills, and it is imperative to foster cooperation between biophysicists and robotics engineers to effectively tackle the complex obstacles that emerge within this multidisciplinary domain. Multidisciplinary groups provide an integrative approach to devising solutions, as they leverage the expertise of biophysicists who possess a deep comprehension of biological systems, alongside robotics technologists who provide creative technical solutions [53]. This collaborative effort facilitates the cultivation of innovative thinking and creativity, enabling the amalgamation of varied perspectives in ways that result in pioneering methodologies and original resolutions that may not be achievable inside the confines of a solitary field. Through collaboration, interdisciplinary teams can address difficulties with greater effectiveness and acquire a thorough comprehension of the complexities they encounter. This, in turn, facilitates informed decision-making and the creation of more streamlined and customized solutions. Effective interpersonal interaction plays a crucial role in facilitating team cohesion, as it establishes a common vocabulary among team members, fosters mutual understanding of diverse perspectives, and enables seamless collaboration [54]. In the realm of biophysics-based robotics, the integration of multiple disciplines within a team is crucial to optimize research findings, foster creativity, and facilitate the effective application of theoretical understanding in practical contexts. This collaborative approach serves as a fundamental pillar of advancement in this field.

To facilitate communication and collaboration between biophysicists and robotic engineers, it is imperative to build a common lexicon, foster mutual respect through cross-training programs, and cultivate collaborative environments [55]. Centers of interdisciplinary study play a pivotal role in facilitating collaborative endeavors by serving as central hubs that offer valuable assets and comprehensive assistance for joint initiatives. Such centers serve as platforms for the sharing of expertise and the collaboration of professionals from many sectors to work through complex difficulties. Collaborative research endeavors that encompass participants from multiple disciplines foster active cooperation and the utilization of collective expertise. Furthermore, it is imperative to offer promotions, acknowledgment, and funding opportunities as a means of acknowledging the significance of collaborating across disciplines. These measures will serve to motivate academics to take an active role in bridging the separation between the fields of biophysics and robotics. The resulting projects will aim to effectively utilize the collaborative efforts of biophysicists and robotic engineers to propel progress at the dynamic intersection of these disciplines, resulting in the development of novel solutions that have tangible effects in practical settings [56].

2.6 Future prospects

The future potential of biophysics-based robotics appears highly encouraging, presenting a wide range of captivating possibilities. Sophisticated medical robotics is an essential domain of development. Robotic surgical instruments are anticipated to exhibit heightened precision and less invasiveness, hence transforming medical processes and augmenting patient results [57]. In a similar vein, the field of robotics for rehabilitation is poised to experience significant advancements, as exoskeletal and robotic prosthetics become increasingly accessible and proficient. This development holds immense potential for enhancing the mobility and overall well-being of those who have suffered limb loss or disability [58]. The domain of biomechanically inspired robots is anticipated to undergo significant growth, leading to the development of machines proficient at traversing complex surroundings and engaging in seamless interactions with human beings. Consequently, these robots are expected to become indispensable in several domains, such as search-and-rescue operations and space exploration. The incorporation of microscopic and tiny robots into the field of healthcare holds great potential for revolutionizing the management of illnesses through customized drug administration and minimally invasive therapies [59]. The ongoing development of AI is expected to maintain its pivotal position in the advancement of biophysics-based robotics as it further enhances their capacity for adaptation and decision-making capabilities. Consequently, these robotic devices are anticipated to become increasingly adaptable and proficient in acquiring knowledge from their interactions. Furthermore, these robotic systems will have the capacity to expand their impact in the realm of ecosystem surveillance and environmental study, thereby offering important data for the advancement of conservation initiatives, climate investigations, and catastrophe management. Furthermore, they will continue to play a crucial role in the field of space exploration, aiding in the examination of remote planets and celestial entities.

The establishment of collaboration between disciplines among biophysicists, robotics technologists, computational scientists, and medical professionals is of the utmost importance to facilitate the development of innovative solutions and tackle complex difficulties [59]. The proper safeguarded utilization of such technologies will necessitate a growing emphasis on ethical issues and regulatory measures. The progression of biophysics-based robotics necessitates the implementation of educational recruitment and retention programs to adequately prepare the upcoming cohort of specialists in this interdisciplinary domain. In general, the potential of biophysics-based robotics for healthcare, research, and exploration is poised to bring about significant advancements that can greatly benefit society and enhance our understanding of the natural world.

2.7 Conclusions

The integration of biophysics and robotics signifies an emerging and promising future within the realm of technological and scientific advancement. The utilization of physical principles in the study and manipulation of biological creatures is a multidisciplinary strategy with broad applications in multiple domains. The potential for transformative impacts in various fields, such as medical services, surveillance of the environment, and the exploration of space, is evident in the inventive and cooperative characteristics of biophysics-based robotics. With the advancement of robotic systems, there is a growing potential to tackle complex problems, enhance human well-being, and broaden our understanding of the natural world. Nevertheless, this exhilarating expedition is not devoid of its obstacles. To guarantee the dependable, safe, and useful research and deployment of biophysics-based robotics, it is imperative to address concerns related to ethics and regulatory frameworks and to foster collaboration between disciplines. The subject of biophysics-based robotics holds immense promise for the near future, and as we delve further into this domain, it is imperative to uphold ethical principles, foster collaboration, and sustain the innovative drive that propels advancements in this discipline. By adopting this approach, it is possible to anticipate a future in which the fields of biophysical and robotics collaborate synergistically to surmount complex obstacles, enhance human welfare, and push the boundaries of scientific understanding.

References

[1] Rollié S, Mangold M and Sundmacher K 2012 Designing biological systems: systems engineering meets synthetic biology *Chem. Eng. Sci.* **69** 1–29

[2] Adlakha R, Price J and Heidari S 2017 Disability and sexuality: claiming sexual and reproductive rights *Reprod. Health Matters* **25** 4–9

[3] Goldfield E C 2018 *Bioinspired Devices: Emulating Nature's Assembly and Repair Process* (Cambridge, MA: Harvard University Press) https://www.hup.harvard.edu/books/9780674967946

[4] Vijayan V M, Mathai S and Thomas V 2022 Polymeric biomaterials and current trends for advanced applications *Progress in Polymer Research for Biomedical, Energy and Specialty Applications* (Boca Raton, FL: CRC Press) 15–34

[5] Sharon T 2013 *Human Nature in an Age of Biotechnology: The Case for Mediated Posthumanism* (Berlin: Springer Science & Business Media) p 14

[6] Orban M, Guo K, Yang H, Hu X, Hassaan M and Elsamanty M 2023 Soft pneumatic muscles for post-stroke lower limb ankle rehabilitation: leveraging the potential of soft robotics to optimize functional outcomes *Front. Bioeng. Biotechnol.* **11** 1251879

[7] Puranik A, Dandekar P and Jain R 2022 Exploring the potential of machine learning for more efficient development and production of biopharmaceuticals *Biotechnol. Progr.* **6** e3291

[8] Gouvea, Svoboda J, Sawtelle V, Geller B D and Turpen C 2013 A framework for analyzing interdisciplinary tasks: implications for student learning and curricular design *CBE—Life Sci. Educ.* **12** 187–205

[9] Mestre R, Patiño T and Sánchez S 2021 Biohybrid robotics: from the nanoscale to the macroscale *Wiley Interdiscip. Rev. Nanomed. Nanobiotechnol.* **13** e1703

[10] Soheilmoghaddam F, Rumble M and Cooper-White J 2021 High-throughput routes to biomaterials discovery *Chem. Rev.* **121** 10792–864

[11] Xu K and Qin S 2023 An interdisciplinary approach and advanced techniques for enhanced 3D-printed upper limb prosthetic socket design: a literature review *Actuators* **12** 223

[12] Banerjee D, Pratap Singh Y, Datta P, Ozbolat V, O'Donnell A, Yeo M and Ozbolat I T 2022 Strategies for 3D bioprinting of spheroids: a comprehensive review *Biomaterials* **291** 121881

[13] Wiśniowski Z 2021 International conference cybernetic modelling of biological systems MCSB *Bio-Algorithms Med-Syst.* **17** eA1–eA45

[14] Sapci, Hasan A and Aylin Sapci H 2019 Innovative assisted living tools, remote monitoring technologies, artificial intelligence-driven solutions, and robotic systems for aging societies: systematic review *JMIR Aging* **2** e15429
[15] Arbore C, Perego L, Sergides M and Capitano M 2016 Probing force in living cells with optical tweezers: from single-molecule mechanics to cell mechanotransduction *Biophys. Rev.* **11** 765–82
[16] Liang W, Shi H, Yang X, Wang J, Yang W, Zhang H and Liu L 2021 Recent advances in AFM-based biological characterization and applications at multiple levels *Soft Matter* **16** 8962–84
[17] Vitiello V, Lee S-L, Cundy T P and Yang G-Z 2012 Emerging robotic platforms for minimally invasive surgery *IEEE Rev. Biomed. Eng.* **6** 111–26
[18] Yeo Leslie Y, Chang H-C, Chan P P Y and Friend J R 2011 Microfluidic devices for bioapplications *Small* **7** 12–48
[19] Arrasate M and Finkbeiner S 2005 Automated microscope system for determining factors that predict neuronal fate *Proc. Natl Acad. Sci.* **102** 3840–5
[20] Whitehead E 2017 *A software system for automating lab experiments with liquid-handling robots* ETH Zurich https://doi.org/10.3929/ethz-b-000244796
[21] Rodríguez-Fernández A, Lobo-Prat J and Font-Llagunes J M 2021 Systematic review on wearable lower-limb exoskeletons for gait training in neuromuscular impairments *J. Neuroeng. Rehab* **18** 1–21
[22] Yeo J C and Teck Lim C 2016 Emerging flexible and wearable physical sensing platforms for healthcare and biomedical applications *Microsyst. Nanoeng.* **2** 1–19
[23] Runciman M, Darzi A and Mylonas G P 2019 Soft robotics in minimally invasive surgery *Soft Robot.* **6** 423–43
[24] Abad S-A, Arezzo A, Homer-Vanniasinkam S and Wurdemann H A 2022 Soft robotic systems for endoscopic interventions *Endorobotics* (New York: Academic) 61–93
[25] Pan M, Yuan C, Liang X, Dong T, Liu T, Zhang J, Zou J, Yang H and Bowen C 2022 Soft actuators and robotic devices for rehabilitation and assistance *Adv. Intell. Syst.* **4** 2100140
[26] Arslan-Yildiz A, El Assal R, Chen P, Guven S, Inci F and Demirci U 2016 Towards artificial tissue models: past, present, and future of 3D bioprinting *Biofabrication* **8** 014103
[27] Avgousti S, Christoforou E G, Panayides A S, Voskarides S, Novales C, Nouaille L, Pattichis C S and Vieyres P 2016 Medical telerobotic systems: current status and future trends *Biomed. Eng. Online* **15** 1–44
[28] Habib Maki K 2011 Biomimetics: innovations and robotics *Int. J. Mechatron. Manuf. Syst.* **4** 113–34
[29] Heng W, Solomon S and Gao W 2022 Flexible electronics and devices as human–machine interfaces for medical robotics *Adv. Mater.* **34** 2107902
[30] Cho K-J and Wood R 2016 Biomimetic robots *Springer Handbook of Robotics* (Cham: Springer) 543–74
[31] Wang J, Chen W, Xiao X, Xu Y, Li C, Jia X and Meng M Q-H 2021 A survey of the development of biomimetic intelligence and robotics *Biomim. Intell. Robot.* **1** 100001
[32] Majid M H A, Arshad M R and Mokhtar R M 2022 Swarm robotics behaviors and tasks: a technical review *Control Engineering in Robotics and Industrial Automation* (Cham: Springer) 99–167
[33] Stevens R, Taylor V, Nichols J, Maccabe A B, Yelick K and Brown D 2020 *AI for Science: Report on the Department of Energy (DOE) Town Halls on Artificial Intelligence (AI) for*

Science. No. ANL-20/17 (Argonne, IL: Argonne National Lab. (ANL)) https://publications.anl.gov/anlpubs/2020/03/158802.pdf

[34] Kashiri N, Abate A, Abram S J, Albu-Schaffer A, Clary P J, Daley M and Faraji, th S 2018 An overview on principles for energy-efficient robot locomotion *Front. Robot. AI* **5** 129

[35] 2018 A roadmap for living machines research *Living Machines: A Handbook of Research in Biomimetics and Biohybrid Systems* ed T J Prescott, N Lepora and P F M J Verschure (Oxford: Oxford University Press) 3 26–48

[36] Marcos-Pablos S and García-Peñalvo F J 2022 More than surgical tools: a systematic review of robots as didactic tools for the education of professionals in health sciences *Adv. Health Sci. Educ.* **27** 1139–76

[37] Kondoyanni Maria D L, Chrysanthos Maraveas C D and Konstantinos G 2022 Bio-inspired robots and structures toward fostering the modernization of agriculture *Biomimetics* **7** 69

[38] Bhimanapati Ganesh R, Lin Z, Meunier V, Jung Y, Cha J, Das S and Xiao D *et al* 2015 Recent advances in two-dimensional materials beyond graphene *ACS Nano* **9** 11509–39

[39] Karmakar A, Samanta P, Desai A V and Ghosh S K 2017 Guest-responsive metal–organic frameworks as scaffolds for separation and sensing applications *ACC. Chem. Res.* **50** 2457–69

[40] Rajagopal A, Yao K and Jen A K Y 2018 Toward perovskite solar cell commercialization: a perspective and research roadmap based on interfacial engineering *Adv. Mater.* **30** 1800455

[41] Nizamis K, Athanasiou A, Almpani S, Dimitrousis C and Astaras A 2021 Converging robotic technologies in targeted neural rehabilitation: a review of emerging solutions and challenges *Sensors* **21** 2084

[42] Stone P, Brooks R, Brynjolfsson E, Calo R, Etzioni O, Hager G, Julia and Hirschberg *et al* 2022 Artificial intelligence and life in 2030: the one-hundred-year study on artificial intelligence arXiv preprint arXiv:2211 06318

[43] Hagberg K, Häggström E, Jönsson S, Rydevik B and Brånemark R 2008 Osseoperception and osseointegrated prosthetic limbs *Psych Prosthetics* (London: Springer) 131–40

[44] Li L, Li X, Ouyang B, Mo H, Ren H and Yang S 2023 Three-dimensional collision avoidance method for robot-assisted minimally invasive surgery *Cyborg Bionic Syst.* **4** 0042

[45] Bloom Matthew B, Salzberg A D and Krummel T M 2002 Advanced technology in surgery *Curr. Prob. Surg.* **39** 745–830

[46] Habuza T, Navaz A N, Hashim F, Alnajjar F, Zaki N, Adel Serhani M and Statsenko Y 2021 AI applications in robotics, diagnostic image analysis and precision medicine: current limitations, future trends, guidelines on CAD systems for medicine *Inform. Med. Unlocked* **24** 100596

[47] Mohsan Syed A H, Mazinani A, Othman N Q H and Amjad H 2022 Towards the internet of underwater things: a comprehensive survey *Earth Sci. Inf.* **15** 735–64

[48] Lam Tommy T Y, Yi Guan H Z and Holmes E C 2016 Genomic analysis of the emergence, evolution, and spread of human respiratory RNA viruses *Annu. Rev. Genom. Hum. Genet.* **17** 193–218

[49] Tripathi S and Musiolik T H 2023 Fairness and ethics in artificial intelligence-based medical imaging *Research Anthology on Improving Medical Imaging Techniques for Analysis and Intervention* (Hershey, PA: IGI Global) 79–90

[50] Amadio J, Bi G-Q, Boshears P F, Carter A, Devor A, Doya K and Garden H 2018 Neuroethics questions to guide ethical research in the international brain initiatives *Neuron* **100** 19–36

[51] Abouelmehdi K, Beni-Hessane A and Khaloufi H 2018 Big healthcare data: preserving security and privacy *J. Big Data* **5** 1–18
[52] Roy M and Roy A 2021 The rise of interdisciplinarity in engineering education in the era of industry 4.0: implications for management practice *IEEE Eng. Manage. Rev.* **49** 56–70
[53] Hurlock-Chorostecki C, van Soeren M, MacMillan K, Sidani S, Donald F and Reeves S 2016 A qualitative study of nurse practitioner promotion of interprofessional care across institutional settings: perspectives from different healthcare professionals *Int. J. Nurs. Sci.* **3** 3–10
[54] 2010 *Research at the Intersection of the Physical and Life Sciences.* (Washington, DC: National Academies Press (US))
[55] Dunaway N and Berger K M 2021 The changing face of biological research and the growing role of biosecurity *Applied Biosecurity: Global Health, Biodefense, and Developing Technologies* (Cham: Springer International Publishing) 88–119
[56] Camarillo David B, Thomas M K and Kenneth Salisbury J 2004 Robotic technology in surgery: past, present, and future *Am. J. Surg.* **188** 2–15
[57] Cooper Rory A and Cooper R 2019 Rehabilitation engineering: a perspective on the past 40 years and thoughts for the future *Med. Eng. Phys.* **72** 3–12
[58] Li J, Esteban-Fernández de Ávila B, Gao W, Zhang L and Wang J 2017 Micro/nanorobots for biomedicine: delivery, surgery, sensing, and detoxification *Sci. Robot.* **2** eaam6431
[59] Murday J, Bell L, Heath J, Kong C H, Chang R, Fonash S and Baba M 2013 Implications: people and physical infrastructure *Convergence of Knowledge, Technology and Society. Science Policy Reports.* (Cham: Springer) 287–370

Chapter 3

Nanorobots: a primer for deciphering the biophysics of cancer

Over the last decade, there has been a significant increase in investigations into the impact of alterations in the biophysical characteristics of cells and subcellular structures on the development and advancement of many human illnesses, as well as the reciprocal effect of these diseases on the same characteristics. In the domain of cancer biophysics, significant effort has been committed to examining the differences in mechanical properties between normal and cancerous cells. Cancer is a complicated and progressive disease that exhibits biochemical and physical abnormalities. There is an increasing recognition that the presence of physical irregularities in cancerous cells and their surrounding microenvironment, which exist across several scales of measurement, have a significant role in promoting the development and spread of cancer. Nanorobots have the potential to transport and administer significant amounts of anticancer medications to malignant cells, while simultaneously minimizing injury to healthy cells, thus decreasing the adverse effects of traditional chemotherapy. The objective of this chapter is to provide a comprehensive assessment of the current state of nanorobotics in the field of cancer treatment. Nanorobotics is seen as a promising prospect for the future of medicine. Nanorobots are sophisticated submicron devices mainly composed of bionanocomponents. Nanorobots combine nanotechnology and robotics and show great potential for cancer investigations and therapy. This chapter explains the principles of nanorobots, describing their construction, propulsion, and remote-control capabilities. It then describes their vital significance in cancer research, including early diagnosis, targeted medication administration, precision surgery, and real-time monitoring. Investigations of the biophysical aspects of cancer, such as the microenvironment of tumors, the mechanical characteristics of cancer cells, hemodynamics, and tissue stiffness, can be enhanced by utilizing the accuracy and flexibility of nanorobots.

doi:10.1088/978-0-7503-6019-7ch3

3.1 Introduction

Nanorobotics, like the broader field of nanoelectromechanical systems (NEMS) study, encompass several aspects, including design, which often draws inspiration from biological systems, prototyping, manufacturing, programming, and potential uses in biomedical nanotechnology. Sensing, controlling, acting, propelling, powering, communicating, interfacing, programming, and coordinating are all essential to robotics at any scale. The focus is activity, which is an important capability of robots. One significant challenge currently encountered by this kind of innovation is the absence of efficient methodologies for constructing the nanoscale structures necessary for the intended applications. Nanorobots are very small, with dimensions similar to those of organelles and cells in living organisms. The potential uses of this technology in monitoring the environment and medical diagnosis are considerable. A fundamental change from treatment to prevention may be required if this amounts to a programmed system with broad implications in medicine. The emerging concept of a physically connected improved information infrastructure also calls for miniaturized sensors and actuators. Molecularly focused medical care has evolved as a collaborative method to overcome the lack of specificity of traditional cancer therapeutic drugs [1]. Using both passive and active targeting methodologies, nanoparticles may boost the intracellular concentration of medication in cancer cells while sparing normal cells from harm [2].

Cancer is a multifaceted illness that results from a complicated progression of events that promotes the degeneration of healthy cells into tumors. It is known that malignancies are not solely comprised of rapidly dividing cells, but rather can be characterized as heterogeneous tissues consisting of various cell types that are accepted during the development of the malignancy and contribute to its progression. These cell types include endothelial cells, pericytes, immune-inflammatory cells, and fibroblasts associated with cancer [3]. During the process of cancer advancement, cells seem to have distinct characteristics that may be identified as their defining features, which significantly impact their condition and activities. These cells can independently respond to signals that promote development, exhibit insensitivity to signals that inhibit growth, challenge programmed cell death, possess unlimited capacity for replication, cause new blood vessels to be produced, permeate surrounding tissues, and generate metastases [4]. In recent times, there has been a growing recognition of the significance of the extracellular matrix (ECM) in governing various cellular responses [5–7]. Hence, it is evident that the investigation of tumorigenic mechanisms and treatment strategies should not just focus on cancer as a disorder of individual cells, but rather should embrace the involvement of the microenvironment. This entails evaluating the biochemical and biophysical characteristics of the ECM [8].

Cancer has traditionally been attributed to function-altering genetic mutations that affect cell proliferation, survival, metabolism, migration, metastasis, and responsiveness to treatment [9–12]. However, there is an increasing acknowledgment among researchers in the field of malignancy that there exists an incontrovertible physiological foundation for the factors that contribute to the genesis, development, and therapeutic response of cancer [13]. In most solid tumors, there is a coexistence of malignant cells and non-cancerous host tissue, which is often referred to as either the tumor's stroma or tumor microenvironment [14]. Solid tumor formation and progression are linked to physical abnormalities in cancerous cells and the tumor microenvironment. These abnormalities have been shown to modify the prometastatic functions of cancerous cells [15–17]. According to Abhilash [18], a multidisciplinary strategy has been suggested to ensure the realization of the promising potential of nanotechnology at many levels, as supported by subsequent studies. Cell mechanics is a crucial biophysical characteristic of a cell and has received significant attention as a valuable quantitative instrument for comprehending cellular mechanisms in various domains, including regenerative medicine, tissue engineering [19], and the diagnosis of numerous pathological states, such as cancer [20, 21]. Cell mechanics can distinguish between healthy and cancerous states in cancer biology since malignant cells exhibit significant stiffness changes relative to their normal state. Several methodologies may be used to investigate cell mechanics. For instance, micropipette aspiration (MPA) and optical stretchers have been utilized to measure the mechanical properties of whole cells in suspension [22, 23]. In addition, atomic force microscopy (AFM) has been employed to analyze the mechanical characteristics of individual adherent cells [24–26].

3.2 Multiscale cancer biophysics

Chronic alterations and irregularities in cancer, including mechanical forces and structural characteristics, are seen across several length scales, including the tissue; multi-, single-, and subcellular; and molecular scales (figure 3.1). At the cellular

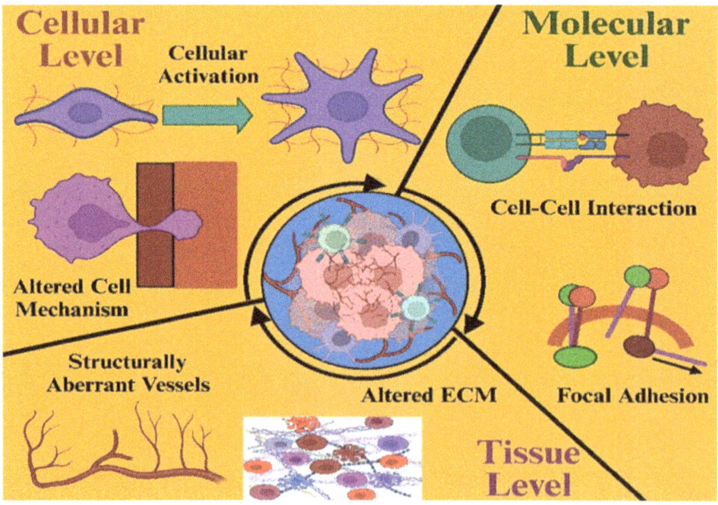

Figure 3.1. The multiscale biophysics of malignancy. At the tissue level, the tumor microenvironment exhibits an altered ECM and abnormal vasculature. Cancer cells have been seen to possess a lower degree of cellular rigidity compared to normal cells, but activated fibroblasts exhibit an overproduction of ECM proteins. Adapted from [31] John Wiley & Sons. [© 2021 The Authors. Advanced NanoBiomed Research published by Wiley-VCH GmbH.]

level, medical professionals can identify the enhanced morphological flexibility or rigidity of malignancies using palpation and elastography. This characteristic may potentially function as a prognostic biomarker for metastasis [27]. The elevated rigidity of tissues in many cancer types may be attributed to an atypical presence of structural ECM components, including fibrillar collagen and nonfibrillar hyaluronan [27]. It has been shown that making the ECM stiffer can help cancer cells grow and metastasize, activate fibroblasts, and make new blood vessels [28, 29]. Alterations in the microstructures of the ECM such as modifications in collagen filament diameter and alignment, as well as changes in pore size, have the potential to facilitate the process of localized tumor cell propagation and migration into adjacent healthy tissue [30]. Besides impacting the way in which cells move, the ECM's pores and microstructures also control the mass transport characteristics (such as diffusion and convection) of drugs and molecules that carry signals.

Dysfunctional blood and lymph vasculatures are also seen in solid malignant tumors [32, 33]. Tumors are often characterized by the presence of blood vessels that exhibit a high degree of tortuosity and increased permeability, resulting in bleeding [34]. The field of multiscale cancer biophysics encompasses a multidisciplinary framework that aims to explain the complicated and ever-changing characteristics of cancer across several dimensions, ranging from the molecular and cellular level to the broader levels of tissues and organisms. Investigators attempt to elucidate the complex mechanisms behind the origin, development, and therapeutic resistance of cancer by synthesizing insights from several disciplines including physics, biology, and medicine. This methodology facilitates the investigation of the influence of physical factors, such as cellular mechanical characteristics and the microenvironment, on the progression of cancer, metastatic disease, and the efficacy of therapeutic interventions. The multiscale biophysics of cancer can provide significant knowledge about innovative approaches to diagnosis and treatment, therefore enhancing our capacity to effectively address the serious consequences of this ailment. These malignant blood artery features contribute to inefficient nutrition and medication delivery as well as abnormal levels of plasma fluid that extravasate and collect in the tumor tissue, resulting in increased interstitial fluid pressure (IFP). High IFP in tumors may promote interstitial fluid outflow into surrounding tissue, but new contrast-enhanced magnetic resonance imaging research shows that the direction of flow at the tumor boundary is not necessarily outward [35, 36]. Previous studies have shown that interstitial flow has a significant role in the stimulation of cancer growth via the activation of fibroblasts, induction of angiogenesis, and promotion of cancer cell migration [37–40].

The presence of intratumoral solid pressures, resulting from uncontrolled growth inside a confined tumor, exacerbates vascular dysfunction in tumors [41]. The application of significant forces to permeable and delicate blood and lymphatic vessels results in their collapse. The collapse of blood vessels worsens the elevated IFP, impairs perfusion and medication transportation, and leads to hypoxia. Interestingly, it has been found that the amplitude of solid stress is correlated with tumor size, although no such relationship is seen for rigidity and interstitial flow [36, 42].

The tissue-level abnormalities that are indicative of cancer may also impact the cellular and molecular responses that regulate the development of tumors. An example of this phenomenon is the coactivation of fibroblasts that forms cancer-associated fibroblasts (CAFs) via the interaction between the regulating cytokine transforming growth factor beta (TGF-β) and matrix stiffness. Fibroblast activation results in increased ECM deposition, leading to the development of fibrosis and subsequent tissue stiffness [43]. Moreover, heightened ECM stiffness facilitates the process of epithelial–mesenchymal transition (EMT) in cells [44]. In addition, analyses have demonstrated that cancerous cells are more malleable than healthy cells [45], which improves their capacity to move in the constrained ECM and between constricting endothelial junctions. At the molecular level, endothelial junctions, such as adhesion and tight junctions, are crucial in the processes of angiogenesis, the regulation of vascular permeability, and the intravasation of cancer cells in metastasis [46, 47]. Moreover, the focal adhesion (FA) proteins present on cellular membranes serve as mechanotransducers, enabling them to perceive flow forces as well as the stiffness and alignment of the adjacent matrix. Consequently, these proteins can trigger cell cycle arrest or control migration [48, 49]. FA proteins are known to have a significant impact on EMT processes as well as on cellular movement within three-dimensional matrices [50]. These examples show how cancer growth and metastasis depend on a web of interactions between biophysical systems operating at various scales. Table 3.1 presents an overview of the essential features of several micro- and nanoscale experimental instruments that have been used to investigate the biophysical properties of cancer. These techniques have been used to research cancer biophysics and give valuable insights into cancer biology. Their engineering concepts and their implementation are also explained in table 3.1.

3.3 The biology of cancer cells

Cancer is a pathological condition that originates from abnormal biological cells. The abnormal cells undergo uncontrolled proliferation, leading to the disruption of tissue organization. Biopolymeric proteins are the basic components of the cellular cytoskeleton. The following section provides a detailed description of the internal scaffolding, which plays an essential role in determining the cellular form and mechanical stiffness. Proteins that are released into the intercellular spaces make up the ECM, a structural framework that facilitates cell clustering and adhesion, ultimately leading to tissue formation. Integrins are transmembrane receptors located on the cell surface that facilitate the formation of focal adhesions, which function as sites of interaction between the cell interface and the ECM [51].

Cancer induces alterations in the architectural organization of both the cytoskeleton and the ECM. Modified protein structures may also impact the mechanical properties of cancer cells and thus alter their capacity to contract or stretch during deformation. Consequently, the movement of cancer cells may exhibit significant disparities compared to that of healthy cells, leading to their ability to traverse tissue and propagate to various locations throughout the human body, ultimately

Table 3.1. The advantages and drawbacks of strategies used to analyze the biophysics of cancer [31].

S. No.	Concepts	Method	Benefit(s)	Limitation(s)
1.	IFP and movement	Microfluid dynamics	Controls the movement of mass and changes in pressure. Maximum throughput. Relevant to physiological length scales.	Needs modern fabrication resources and specific training.
2.	Solid stress	Transwell system	Adjustable pressure. Commercially accessible. Co-culture studies are possible.	2D conditions for culture. Minimal throughput.
		Flexible microsystem	Applies pressure with precision. Three-dimensional tissue culture environments.	Needs modern manufacturing tools and specific training. The pressure distribution is not uniform.
3.	Biomechanics of cells	MPA	Appropriate for analyzing the mechanics of cells and adherence. Facilitates the implementation of regulated elevated levels of suction pressure.	Needs special training. Advanced microfluidic systems are required in manufacturing facilities.
		AFM	Appropriate for research into ECM, cell mechanics, and adhesion. Provides subnanometer precision. Compatible with a wide variety of microscopy methods.	Difficult 3D measurements. Substrate plating is necessary.
		Traction force microscopy (TFM)	Does not need complicated instruments. Modular design for use with a variety of microscopy and fabrication methods. Enables greater spatial sensitivity.	Measuring and analyzing in three dimensions can be difficult.

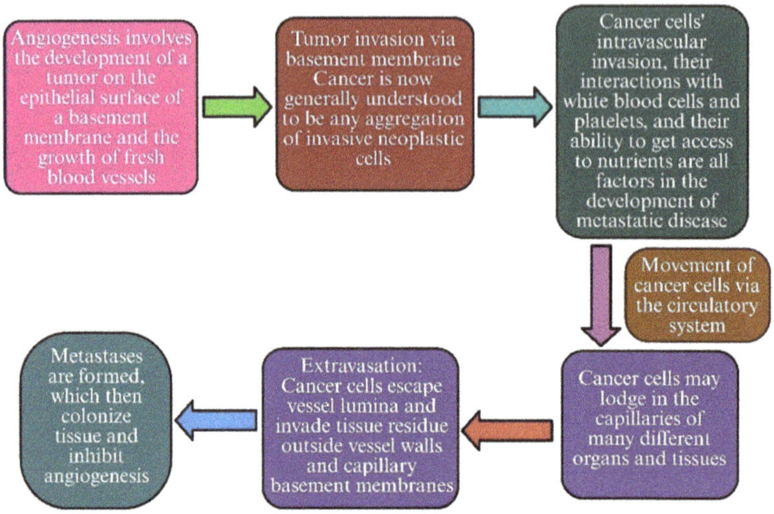

Figure 3.2. The several stages of the process of cancer cell invasion and metastasis [51] Taylor & Francis Ltd (http://tandfonline.com).

activating the process of tumor metastasis. Cancer cells possess the ability to generate internal signals that facilitate continuous proliferation and replication. These signals are transmitted between proteins via a biological mechanism known as signal transduction.

The development and division of cells are regulated by a control circuit composed of proteins, which they can reprogram. The signals within this circuit are exchanged bidirectionally via a communication pathway that connects the ECM with the intracellular environment, including the cytoplasm and nucleus. This communication is facilitated by integrins and focal adhesions, which establish a binding connection between the cell and the ECM. Varmus and Bishop [51] attributed the beginnings of cancer to the proto-oncogene in their seminal finding, which described the involvement of chemicals and genes in the development of human cancer.

The identification of proto-oncogenes prompted the recognition that the genomes of normal vertebrate cells include a gene that has the capacity, in some cases, to promote the conversion of a healthy cell into a cancerous cell [52]. A schematic representation of the invasive–metastatic pathway is shown in figure 3.2, which illustrates the several sequential stages involved in this process.

3.4 The reason for a biophysical strategy for cancer

Even though advances in cancer research and treatment continue, there is still much that needs to be done to enhance clinical outcomes. The use of a biophysical framework in the study of cancer is important to understand the complex and dynamic characteristics of the illness, since it involves both physical and mechanical elements. Biophysics, as opposed to conventional biological techniques that largely concentrate on genetics and molecular biology, investigates the physical qualities and forces that influence cancer's start, development, and response to therapy. Through an examination of the mechanical properties of cancer cells and their interactions within the tumor microenvironment, this methodology offers significant insights into the mechanisms behind disease dissemination and treatment resistance. Developing a comprehension of the biomechanical stimuli that impact cellular activities, including migration, adhesion, and signaling, is vital to advance novel treatment approaches and diagnostic instruments. In addition, adopting a biophysical approach allows investigators to explore the inherent physical characteristics of tumors, which may be used to enhance imaging techniques, facilitate early identification, and develop more effective treatment methods. The biophysical method provides an integrated comprehension of cancer that supplements conventional biological investigations, hence facilitating the development of more efficacious therapies as well as personalized medical strategies in combating this intricate and destructive ailment. Two main types of challenges can be summarized, as follows:

(1) A precise and practical diagnosis. Currently, the ability to accurately detect cancer in its early stages and accurately forecast its future progression remains limited. Prostate cancer is a clear example in which differentiating between tumors that will advance to malignancy and those that will exhibit delayed growth has proven to be very challenging. Pancreatic cancer poses a significant challenge in terms of early detection, since it is characterized by a lack of discernible symptoms in its early stages. Ovarian cancer is often denoted as the 'silent killer' for the same reason.

(2) Long-term, successful treatment. Although some types of cancer may be efficiently treated with hormonal and/or cytotoxic medications, these treatments often result in substantial and severe adverse effects. Importantly, cancer cells frequently develop resistance to such drugs over time, likely due to cancer's inherent 'stemness.' As an example, the efficacy of hormone-based therapy, namely androgen downregulation, in managing prostate cancer is limited to a finite duration of a few years. Subsequently, the cancer reemerges in a very aggressive manner and is resistant to hormone-based treatments; this may lead to mortality due to the spread of the illness to other parts of the body within a few months.

Our comprehension of the molecular pathways underlying cancer is of the greatest significance in each of these aspects. However, a multitude of genes undergo alterations throughout cancer development. These alterations can appear as either the activation or reduction of gene expression. However, deciphering whether these changes are directly responsible for the malignant transformation or serve as incidental outcomes is a challenge in some cases. Therefore, prioritizing the early examination of genes may not result in the most valuable data [53]. The rationale for this phenomenon is readily apparent due to the existence of several dynamic processes that occur between gene expression (or its disruption) and the development of disease.

$$\text{Gene} \rightarrow \text{Protein} \rightarrow \text{Signal} \rightarrow \text{Process/Illness}$$

Moreover, the process of gene expression, which includes the pathway from gene to protein, is subject to the effect of several stimuli within the microenvironment. It is important to understand that not all transcription events result in protein synthesis. For instance, messenger RNA (mRNA) can undergo a process known as docking inside cellular structures, where it is selectively translated into protein only under circumstances that need it, sometimes occurring at a precise subcellular position [54, 55]. Even when mRNA is translated into protein, it may not always reach its ultimate destination, such as the plasma membrane, and become functional. Therefore, it is common for mature proteins to undergo internalization inside cells and thereafter be transported out when required. The trafficking of proteins, which includes ion channels, is a dynamic process that is partially regulated by the activity of the protein itself [56–59].

3.5 Nanorobots

Nanorobots are little robots that can perform the same functions as larger machines; more specifically, the advancement of this new technology has positive implications for the fields of medicine, manufacture, and other fields [60]. Nanorobotics is growing as a difficult discipline that deals with small molecules at the molecular level. Nanorobots are tiny mechanical devices that are very carefully engineered to carry out precise tasks at the nanoscale level. The primary benefit of this alternative approach in comparison to traditional therapy is its compactness. Particle size has an impact on both the duration of serum presence in the body and the way in which particles are deposited. This phenomenon enables the use of nanoscale medicines at reduced concentrations, resulting in a prompter initiation of therapeutic effects. In addition, it facilitates the production of materials for controlled medication administration by the precise guidance of carriers to a designated target [61]. The anticipated medical nanodevices are expected to be robots of micron-scale dimensions, constructed by assembling nanoscale components.

Nanorobots possess the ability to collectively respond to environmental inputs and execute programmed principles, hence yielding outcomes at the macro scale. Nanorobots with dimensions similar to those of bacteria have the potential to provide a multitude of innovative functionalities through their capacity to see and manipulate inside minuscule surroundings. Of particular importance are their applications in biomedical engineering, as shown by scholarly sources [62, 63]. These applications include the use of nanorobots and nanoscale-structured materials inside the human body, leading to notable advancements in illness detection and treatment [64, 65]. Rapid advancements in the field of nanoscale device engineering are expected to provide a diverse array of functionalities. For instance, continuous advancement [66, 67] in the field of molecular-scale electronics, sensors, and motors has yielded essential components that may be used in the construction of nanorobots [68]. Programmable microorganisms have been shown to possess the capacity to provide computational capabilities for nanodevices [69].

Using catalytic nanomotors, nanodevices may be used to solve energy conversion issues; contemporary research is looking for ways to boost the speed, force, and longevity of synthetic nanomotors; and some nanomotors can even move on their own, surpassing 100 body lengths per second. To generate electricity in chip microsystems driven by autonomous transportation, it is crucial to enhance the speed, motion control, and lifespan of catalytic nanomotors. Additionally, this innovation may be used to develop a 'lab on a chip' [70] gadgets. Infertility treatment is yet another field of use. German engineers have developed a nanorobot that can be attached to the male reproductive tract and used as a power source, with the goal of making affordable and successful fertility treatments widely available [71]. Nanorobots have the potential to be used in a variety of ways to combat environmental issues, including pollution [72]. For example, engineers at the University of California are using nanorobots to remove excess carbon dioxide from water sources such as lakes, rivers, and seas.

The advancement of nanosystems designed to regulate nanorobots in the execution of precise medical activities might potentially lead to enhancements in the automation of nanotechnology [73]. It is quite probable that carbon will serve as the primary constituent of a medical nanorobot, mostly in the form of diamond or diamondoid/fullerene nanocomposites. Various light elements, including hydrogen, sulfur, oxygen, nitrogen, fluorine, silicon, and others, are anticipated to be used for specific applications in nanoscale gears and other components. Nanorobot construction may include a range of components, such as internal sensors, motors, manipulative devices, power supplies, and molecular processors. The ribosome stands out as a significant biological demonstration of molecular machinery, being the only nanoscale assembler now in existence that has the capability of unrestricted programmability. The process by which a protein interacts with a particular receptor site might potentially serve as a model for the development of a molecular robotic arm. The manipulator arm may be operated by a precise sequence of control signals, which is similar to the reliance of the ribosome on mRNA for guidance in its functioning. The control signals for the robotic arm are detected by an onboard sensor, which utilizes a 'broadcast architectural' approach [74, 75]. These signals are externally generated and may be auditory, electrical, or chemical in nature. In addition, this technology can be used to facilitate power transfer. The biological cell may be seen as an instance of a broadcast architecture, whereby the cell nucleus transmits messages to ribosomes in the form of mRNA to synthesize proteins inside the cell.

3.6 Nanorobots for the detection and treatment of cancer

Cancer is a collection of disorders that are characterized by the unregulated proliferation and dissemination of atypical cells inside the body. The incidence of cancer has been steadily increasing, with a reported rise in the number of afflicted persons each year [76]. Cancer is the subject of most studies because it harms people and costs a lot of money. According to the Global Oncology Trend Report published by the IMS Institute for Healthcare Informatics, expenditure on cancer drugs worldwide reached $100 billion in 2014 [77]. The advancement of nanorobotics has mainly been driven by its potential use in the treatment of cancer.

Nanorobotics has shown promise in effectively treating cancer using existing medical technology and therapeutic instruments. To ascertain the prognosis of a patient diagnosed with cancer, many factors should be taken into consideration: the timing of illness progression is a crucial factor to consider, particularly the timing of diagnosis. Early detection of a disease often leads to a more favorable prognosis. In addition, an essential feature of successful patient therapy is the advancement of targeted drug delivery methods, which may effectively reduce the negative effects of chemotherapy [78]. The use of nanorobots as bloodborne sensors has significant potential in facilitating crucial treatment procedures for complicated illnesses via early detection and intelligent medication administration [79].

Nanorobots have the potential to provide an effective means of early cancer detection and facilitate targeted medication administration for intelligent chemotherapy. The use of nanorobots as carriers for drugs to provide timely dosages enables the retention of chemical compounds within the bloodstream for an extended duration, as required. This facilitates the attainment of the required pharmacokinetic characteristics in chemotherapy or other anticancer therapies [80–82]. It prevents the currently observed resultant extravasations toward tumors that are not localized in the reticuloendothelial system, which are associated with significant levels of degenerative side effects during the chemotherapy procedure [83]. Nanorobots equipped with chemical nanobiosensors can be programmed to detect varying amounts of E-cadherin and beta catenin, which are considered important medical targets throughout both the primary and metastatic stages [77, 84].

This technological advancement aids in the identification of targets and facilitates the administration of drugs. The administration of nanorobots for diagnostic, therapeutic, and surgical applications in clinical settings is often achieved by intravenous injection. Consequently, nanorobots can be directly introduced into the circulatory system of an individual. The primary cancer treatment regimen for chemotherapy pharmacokinetics includes the processes of absorption and metabolism, followed by a period of rest to allow the body to recover before the subsequent chemotherapy session. Patients are often treated at regular intervals of two weeks for small tumors [85]. For medical purposes, nanorobots must have the capability to conduct an analysis of the body and provide a diagnosis within a week. This may be achieved using proteomic-based sensors. The distribution of protein medicines to solid tumors may be predicted by analyzing the uptake kinetics of a low-molecular-weight magnetic resonance contrast agent [86]. Therefore, the use of a comparable methodology is advantageous to validate the activation of a nanorobot's biosensor *in vivo* by specific antigen detection [87].

Examination and diagnostic procedures play a crucial role in the investigation of nanorobotics. This technology facilitates expeditious testing and diagnosis at the first consultation, obviating the need for further follow-up visits after laboratory testing. In addition, it allows for the identification of illnesses at earlier stages. Nanorobots cannot be used in living things because they need energy to move. Increased amounts of energy are necessary due to the combination of low inertia and high viscous forces, which are associated with poor efficiency and limited convective motion [88]. Nanomotors based on chemical propulsion use hazardous fuels.

The proliferation of renewable energy sources, such as vibrations and light, has prompted a surge in research into the *in vivo* use of nanorobots, resulting in a corresponding rise in patent filings.

The creation of ultrasonic-wave-powered materials that are safe for living systems led to research into nanomotors, such as that described in 'Acoustic Acceleration of Nanorod Motors Inside Living Cells' [89]. Gao *et al* [90] presented an *in vivo* model of live artificial micromotors. After the micromotors had been orally administered to mice, the model analyzed their distribution, retention, cargo delivery, and acute toxicity. Subsequently, the medical nanorobots selectively eliminated specific cells, only targeting them. The following control strategies may be considered:

Random: nanorobots traveling passively with the fluid only reach their destination if they happen to collide with it due to Brownian motion.

Maintain gradient: the concentration strength of E-cadherin signals is monitored by the nanorobots. Upon detection, the nanorobots proceed to measure and track the gradient until they reach their specified destination. If, after signal detection, the gradient estimation process does not detect any further signal within a period of 50 milliseconds, the nanorobot concludes that the detected signal is a false positive and proceeds to move along with the fluid.

Following gradient using an attractant: as previously stated, when nanorobots reach the target, they emit a new chemical signal that other nanorobots can utilize to increase their ability to discover the target. Therefore, the use of a greater gradient of signaling intensity of E-cadherin serves as a chemical parameter that directs nanorobots in the identification of malignant tissues. Integrated nanosensors may be employed to determine the strength of E-cadherin signals. Therefore, they may be efficiently used for the treatment of cancer [91].

3.7 Conclusions

This chapter presented the conceptual structure of the causes and effects of physical characteristics in cancer. These physical characteristics of cancer complement its biological characteristics and have become important areas of study for physical investigators, engineers, scientists, and oncologists involved in the field of cancer research. Micro- and nanoscale technologies, methodologies, and sensors with physiological integration have been emphasized here for their roles in advancing our knowledge of the observable characteristics of cancer. The exploration of the physics underlying cancer via the use of micro- and nanoscale methodologies is a very promising topic within the field of cancer study. With continued financing from sponsors, the physical aspects of cancer are set to achieve greater acceptance in the cancer research community. While hurdles persist for cancer biophysics research expansion, we see them as possibilities rather than limitations. Although significant progress has been made, the tools used to investigate cancer physics at the nanoscale are limited compared to the many biological instruments and assays used in prevalent cancer research. This chapter provided a comprehensive analysis of the current state of nanorobotics in the field of cancer therapy. Given the significant impact of cancer on human life and the economic burden it creates, extensive research has been conducted into various strategies that utilize nanorobots for cancer treatment. The advancement of nanorobotics has enabled the effective treatment of several medical conditions using existing medical technology and therapeutic techniques.

References and further reading

[1] Ross J S *et al* 2004 Targeted therapies for cancer 2004 *Am. J. Clin. Pathol.* **122** 598–609

[2] Maeda H 2001 The enhanced permeability and retention (EPR) effect in tumor vasculature: the key role of tumor-selective macromolecular drug targeting *Adv. Enzyme Regul.* **41** 1898–207

[3] Egeblad M, Nakasone E S and Werb Z 2010 Tumors as organs: complex tissues that interface with the entire organism *Dev. Cell* **18** 884–901

[4] Hanahan D and Weinberg R A 2000 The hallmarks of cancer *Cell* **100** 57–70

[5] Hanahan D and Weinberg R A 2011 Hallmarks of cancer: the next generation *Cell* **144** 646–74

[6] Weigelt B, Ghajar C M and Bissell M J 2014 The need for complex 3D culture models to unravel novel pathways and identify accurate biomarkers in breast cancer *Adv. Drug Deliv. Rev.* **69** 42–51

[7] Pickup M W, Mouw J K and Weaver V M 2014 The extracellular matrix modulates the hallmarks of cancer *EMBO Rep.* **15** 1243–53

[8] Lu P, Weaver V M and Werb Z 2012 The extracellular matrix: a dynamic niche in cancer progression *J. Cell Biol.* **196** 395–406

[9] Vogelstein B, Papadopoulos N, Velculescu V E, Zhou S, Diaz Jr L A and Kinzler K W 2013 Cancer genome landscapes *Science* **339** 1546–58

[10] Wendel H G, Stanchina E D, Fridman J S, Malina A, Ray S, Kogan S, Cordon-Cardo C, Pelletier J and Lowe S W 2004 Survival signalling by Akt and eIF4E in oncogenesis and cancer therapy *Nature* **428** 332–7

[11] Vander Heiden M G, Chandel N S, Williamson E K, Schumacker P T and Thompson C B 1997 Bcl-xL regulates the membrane potential and volume homeostasis of mitochondria *Cell* **91** 627–37

[12] Hidalgo-Carcedo C, Hooper S, Chaudhry S I, Williamson P, Harrington K, Leitinger B and Sahai E 2011 Collective cell migration requires suppression of actomyosin at cell–cell contacts mediated by DDR1 and the cell polarity regulators Par3 and Par6 *Nat. Cell Biol.* **13** 49–59

[13] Rahbari N N *et al* 2016 Anti-VEGF therapy induces ECM remodeling and mechanical barriers to therapy in colorectal cancer liver metastases *Sci. Transl. Med.* **8** pp. 360ra135–365

[14] McAllister S S and Weinberg R A 2010 Tumor-host interactions: a far-reaching relationship *J. Clin. Oncol.* **28** 4022–8

[15] Cao X, Moeendarbary E, Isermann P, Davidson P M, Wang X, Chen M B, Burkart A K, Lammerding J, Kamm R D and Shenoy V B 2016 A chemomechanical model for nuclear morphology and stresses during cell transendothelial migration *Biophys. J.* **111** 1541–52

[16] Trimboli A J *et al* 2009 Pten in stromal fibroblasts suppresses mammary epithelial tumors *Nature* **461** 1084–91

[17] Friedl P and Alexander S 2011 Cancer invasion and the microenvironment: plasticity and reciprocity *Cell* **147** 992–1009

[18] Abhilash M 2010 Nanorobots *Int. J. Pharm. Bio Sci.* **1** 1–10

[19] Shieh A C and Athanasiou K A 2003 Principles of cell mechanics for cartilage tissue engineering *Ann. Biomed. Eng.* **31** 1–11

[20] Suresh S, Spatz J, Mills J P, Micoulet A, Dao M, Lim C T, Beil M and Seufferlein T 2005 Connections between single-cell biomechanics and human disease states: gastrointestinal cancer and malaria *Acta Biomater.* **1** 15–30

[21] Suresh S 2007 Biomechanics and biophysics of cancer cells *Acta Biomater.* **3** 413–38

[22] Lee L M and Liu A P 2014 The application of micropipette aspiration in molecular mechanics of single cells *J. Nanotechnol. Eng. Med.* **5** 040902

[23] Pachenari M, Seyedpour S M, Janmaleki M, Shayan S B, Taranejoo S and Hosseinkhani H 2014 Mechanical properties of cancer cytoskeleton depend on actin filaments to microtubule content: investigating different grades of colon cancer cell lines *J. Biomech.* **47** 373–9

[24] Guck J *et al* 2005 Optical deformability as an inherent cell marker for testing malignant transformation and metastatic competence *Biophys. J.* **88** 3689–98

[25] Radmacher M, Tillmann R W, Fritz M and Gaub H E 1992 From molecules to cells: imaging soft samples with the atomic force microscope *Science* **257** 1900–5

[26] Lekka M, Pogoda K, Gostek J, Klymenko O, Prauzner-Bechcicki S, Wiltowska-Zuber J, Jaczewska J, Lekki J and Stachura Z 2012 Cancer cell recognition–mechanical phenotype *Micron* **43** 1259–66

[27] Fenner J, Stacer A C, Winterroth F, Johnson T D, Luker K E and Luker G D 2014 Macroscopic stiffness of breast tumors predicts metastasis *Sci. Rep.* **4** 5512

[28] Wirtz D, Konstantopoulos K and Searson P C 2011 The physics of cancer: the role of physical interactions and mechanical forces in metastasis *Nat. Rev. Cancer* **11** 512–22

[29] Bordeleau F *et al* 2017 Matrix stiffening promotes a tumor vasculature phenotype *Proc. Natl. Acad. Sci.* **114** 492–7

[30] Provenzano P P, Inman D R, Eliceiri K W, Trier S M and Keely P J 2008 Contact guidance mediated three-dimensional cell migration is regulated by Rho/ROCK-dependent matrix reorganization *Biophys. J.* **95** 5374–84

[31] Beshay P E, Cortes-Medina M G, Menyhert M M and Song J W 2022 The biophysics of cancer: emerging insights from micro- and nanoscale tools *Adv. NanoBiomed Res.* **2** 2100056

[32] Kerbel R S 2008 Tumor angiogenesis *New Engl. J. Med.* **358** 2039–49

[33] Swartz M A and Lund A W 2012 Lymphatic and interstitial flow in the tumor microenvironment: linking mechanobiology with immunity *Nat. Rev. Cancer* **12** 210–9

[34] Nagy J A, Chang S H, Dvorak A M and Dvorak H F 2009 Why are tumor blood vessels abnormal and why is it important to know? *Br. J. Cancer* **100** 865–9

[35] Heldin C H, Rubin K, Pietras K and Östman A 2004 High interstitial fluid pressure—an obstacle in cancer therapy *Nat. Rev. Cancer* **4** 806–13

[36] Kingsmore K M, Vaccari A, Abler D, Cui S X, Epstein F H, Rockne R C, Acton S T and Munson J M 2018 MRI analysis to map interstitial flow in the brain tumor microenvironment *APL Bioeng.* **2** 3

[37] Ng C P, Hinz B and Swartz M A 2005 Interstitial fluid flow induces myofibroblast differentiation and collagen alignment *in vitro J. Cell Sci.* **118** 4731–9

[38] Song J W and Munn L L 2011 Fluid forces control endothelial sprouting *Proc. Natl. Acad. Sci.* **108** 15342–7

[39] Shields J D, Fleury M E, Yong C, Tomei A A, Randolph G J and Swartz M A 2007 Autologous chemotaxis as a mechanism of tumor cell homing to lymphatics via interstitial flow and autocrine CCR7 signaling *Cancer Cell* **11** 526–38

[40] Polacheck W J, Charest J L and Kamm R D 2011 Interstitial flow influences the direction of tumor cell migration through competing mechanisms *Proc. Natl Acad. Sci.* **108** 11115–20

[41] Stylianopoulos T *et al* 2012 Causes, consequences, and remedies for growth-induced solid stress in murine and human tumors *Proc. Natl. Acad. Sci.* **109** 15101–8
[42] Nia H T *et al* 2016 Solid stress and elastic energy as measures of tumour mechanopathology *Nat. Biomed. Eng.* **1** 0004
[43] Nia H T, Munn L L and Jain R K 2020 Physical traits of cancer *Science* **370** eaaz0868
[44] Leight J L, Wozniak M A, Chen S, Lynch M L and Chen C S 2012 Matrix rigidity regulates a switch between TGF-β1–induced apoptosis and epithelial–mesenchymal transition *Mol. Biol. Cell* **23** 781–91
[45] Lekka M, Laidler P, Gil D, Lekki J, Stachura Z and Hrynkiewicz A Z 1999 Elasticity of normal and cancerous human bladder cells studied by scanning force microscopy *Eur. Biophys. J.* **28** 312–6
[46] Dejana E 1996 Endothelial adherens junctions: implications in the control of vascular permeability and angiogenesis *J. Clin. Invest.* **98** 1949–53
[47] Ahirwar D K *et al* 2018 Fibroblast-derived CXCL12 promotes breast cancer metastasis by facilitating tumor cell intravasation *Oncogene* **37** 4428–42
[48] Velez D O, Tsui B, Goshia T, Chute C L, Han A, Carter H and Fraley S I 2017 3D collagen architecture induces a conserved migratory and transcriptional response linked to vasculogenic mimicry *Nat. Commun.* **8** 1651
[49] Chang S F, Chang C A, Lee D Y, Lee P L, Yeh Y M, Yeh C R, Cheng C K, Chien S and Chiu J J 2008 Tumor cell cycle arrest induced by shear stress: roles of integrins and Smad *Proc. Natl. Acad. Sci.* **105** 3927–32
[50] Cicchini C, Laudadio I, Citarella F, Corazzari M, Steindler C, Conigliaro A, Fantoni A, Amicone L and Tripodi M 2008 TGFβ-induced EMT requires focal adhesion kinase (FAK) signaling *Exp. Cell. Res.* **314** 143–52
[51] Weinberg R A 2006 *The Biology of Cancer* (New York, NY: Garland Science) vol 850
[52] Stehelin D, Varmus H E, Bishop J M and Vogt P K 1976 DNA related to the transforming gene(s) of avian sarcoma viruses is present in normal avian DNA *Nature* **260** 170–3
[53] Hayden E C 2008 Cancer complexity slows quest for cure *Nature* **455** 148
[54] Wu C W K, Zeng F and Eberwine J 2007 mRNA transport to and translation in neuronal dendrites *Anal. Bioanal. Chem.* **387** 59–62
[55] Roberts Jr C T and Kurre P 2013 Vesicle trafficking and RNA transfer add complexity and connectivity to cell–cell communication *Cancer Res.* **73** 3200–5
[56] Dargent B and Couraud F 1990 Down-regulation of voltage-dependent sodium channels initiated by sodium influx in developing neurons *Proc. Natl Acad. Sci.* **87** 5907–11
[57] Paillart C, Boudier J L, Boudier J A, Rochat H, Couraud F and Dargent B 1996 Activity-induced internalization and rapid degradation of sodium channels in cultured fetal neurons *J. Cell Biol.* **134** 499–509
[58] Brackenbury W J and Djamgoz M B 2006 Activity-dependent regulation of voltage-gated Na+ channel expression in Mat-LyLu rat prostate cancer cell line *J. Physiol.* **573** 343–56
[59] Chioni A M, Shao D, Grose R and Djamgoz M B 2010 Protein kinase A and regulation of neonatal Nav1. 5 expression in human breast cancer cells: activity-dependent positive feedback and cellular migration *Int. J. Biochem. Cell Biol.* **42** 346–58
[60] Schwartz E E 1966 *The Biological Basis of Radiation Therapy* (Philadelphia, PA: J.B. Lippincott Company) 210–6
[61] Chan V S 2006 Nanomedicine: an unresolved regulatory issue *Regul. Toxicol. Pharm.* **46** 218–24

[62] Leary S P, Liu C Y and Apuzzo M L 2006 Toward the emergence of nanoneurosurgery: part III—nanomedicine: targeted nanotherapy, nanosurgery, and progress toward the realization of nanoneurosurgery *Neurosurgery* **58** 1009–26
[63] Couvreur P and Vauthier C 2006 Nanotechnology: intelligent design to treat complex disease *Pharm. Res.* **23** 1417–50
[64] Freitas R A 1999 *Nanomedicine, Volume I: Basic Capabilities* (Georgetown, TX: Landes Bioscience) vol 1 210–9
[65] Hood E 2004 Nanotechnology: looking as we leap *Environ. Health Perspect.* **112** A740–9
[66] Montemagno C, Bachand G, Stelick S and Bachand M 1999 Constructing biological motor powered nanomechanical devices *Nanotechnology* **10** 225–31
[67] Cavalcanti A, Wood W W, Kretly L C and Shirinzadeh B 2006 Computational nanomechatronics:a pathway for control and manufacturing nanorobots *2006 Int. Conf. on Computational Intelligence for Modelling Control and Automation and Int. Conf. on Intelligent Agents Web Technologies and Int. Commerce (CIMCA'06)* (Piscataway, NJ: IEEE) 185–5
[68] Cavalcanti A and Freitas R A 2005 Nanorobotics control design: a collective behavior approach for medicine *IEEE Trans. Nanobiosci.* **4** 133–40
[69] Weiss R and Knight Jr T F 2000 Engineered communications for microbial robotics *DNA Computing. DNA 2000.* Lecture Notes in Computer Science 2054 1–16
[70] Medina-Sánchez M, Schwarz L, Meyer A K, Hebenstreit F and Schmidt O G 2016 Cellular cargo delivery: toward-assisted fertilization by sperm-carrying micromotors *Nano Lett.* **16** 555–61
[71] Wang J 2009 Can man-made nanomachines compete with nature biomotors? *ACS Nano* **3** 4–9
[72] Uygun M, Singh V V, Kaufmann K, Uygun D A, de Oliveira S D S and Wang J 2015 Micromotor-based biomimetic carbon dioxide sequestration: towards mobile microscrubbers *Angew. Chem. (Int.)* **54** 12900–4
[73] Zhang M, Sabharwal C L, Tao W, Tarn T J, Xi N and Li G 2004 Interactive DNA sequence and structure design for DNA nanoapplications *IEEE Trans. Nanobiosci.* **3** 286–92
[74] Drexler K E 1992 *Nanosystems: Molecular Machinery, Manufacturing, and Computation* (New York: Wiley)
[75] Merkle R C 1995 Design-ahead for nanotechnology *Proceedings of the first general conference on Nanotechnology : development, applications, and opportunities: development, applications, and opportunities*; M Krummenacker and J Lewis (New York, NY: Wiley) 23–52
[76] World Health Organization 2007 *Cancer Control: Knowledge into Action: WHO Guide for Effective Programs* (Geneva: World Health Organization) vol 2
[77] da Silva Luz G V, Barros K V, de Araújo F V, da Silva G B, da Silva P A, Condori R C and Mattos L 2016 Nanorobotics in drug delivery systems for treatment of cancer: a review *J. Mater. Sci. Eng.* A*6 167–80*
[78] Kshirsagar N, Patil S, Kshirsagar R, Wagh A and Bade A 2014 Review on application of nanorobots in health care *World J. Pharm. Pharm. Sci.* **3** 472–80
[79] Freitas R A 2006 Pharmacytes: an ideal vehicle for targeted drug delivery *J. Nanosci. Nanotechnol.* **6** 2769–75
[80] Mutoh K, Tsukahara S, Mitsuhashi J, Katayama K and Sugimoto Y 2006 Estrogen-mediated post transcriptional down-regulation of P-glycoprotein in MDR1-transduced human breast cancer cells *Cancer Sci.* **97** 1198–204
[81] Lagzi I 2013 Chemical robotics—chemotactic drug carriers *Cent. Eur. J. Med.* **8** 377–82

[82] Xu X, Kim K and Fan D 2015 Tunable release of multiplex biochemicals by plasmonically active rotary nanomotors *Angew. Chem.* **127** 2555–9
[83] Couvreur P 2006 Nanotechnologies for drug delivery: application to cancer and autoimmune diseases *Prog. Solid State Chem.* **34** 231–5
[84] Janda E, Nevolo M, Lehmann K, Downward J, Beug H and Grieco M 2006 Raf plus TGFBeta-dependent EMT is initiated by endocytosis and lysosomal degradation of E-Cadherin *Oncogene* **25** 7117–30
[85] Osterlind K 2001 Chemotherapy in small cell lung cancer *Eur. Respir. J.* **18** 1026–43
[86] Artemov D, Solaiyappan M and Bhujwalla Z M 2001 Magnetic resonance pharmacoangiography to detect and predict chemotherapy delivery to solid tumors *Cancer Res.* **61** 3039–44
[87] Cavalcanti A, Shirinzadeh B, Freitas Jr R A and Hogg T 2007 Nanorobot architecture for medical target identification *Nanotechnology* **19** 015103
[88] Sharma N N and Mittal R K 2008 Nanorobot movement: challenges and biologically inspired solutions *Int. J. Smart Sens. Intell. Syst.* **1** 87–109
[89] Wang W, Li S, Mair L, Ahmed S, Huang T J and Mallouk T E 2014 Acoustic propulsion of nanorod motors inside living cells *Angew. Chem. Int. Ed.* **53** 3201–4
[90] Gao W, Dong R, Thamphiwatana S, Li J, Gao W, Zhang L and Wang J 2015 Artificial micromotors in the mouse's stomach: a step toward *in vivo* use of synthetic motors *ACS Nano* **9** 117–23
[91] Cavalcanti A, Hogg T, Shirinzadeh B and Liaw H C 2006 Nanorobot communication techniques: a comprehensive tutorial *2006 9th Int. Conf. on Control, Automation, Robotics and Vision* (Piscataway, NJ: IEEE) 1–6
[92] Abbott J J, Nagy Z, Beyeler F and Nelson B J 2007 Robotics in the small, part I: microbotics *IEEE Robot. Autom. Mag.* **14** 92–103

IOP Publishing

Rishabha Malviya, Deepika Yadav, Sonali Sundram, Seifedine Kadry and Gurvinder Singh Virk

Chapter 4

The biophysics of cancer: management at the nanoscale

The early recognition and evaluation of numerous kinds of malignancics pose significant challenges. The detection of cancer in its advanced stages consistently results in elevated fatalities. The development of innovative and highly sensitive diagnostic and therapeutic approaches for cancer therapy is thus of the utmost importance. The growth of medical research has discovered novel cancer remedies that are urgently required. Nanobots, which are regarded as one of the most promising implementations of nanomedicines, now occupy a prominent position in the realm of interdisciplinary research. Advancements at the nanoscale have facilitated the application of nanobots for the construction and implementation of functional molecular and nanoscale machines. These nanobots are currently being used in cancer diagnostics and therapeutic interventions. In the last decade, there has been significant development in this field, and these developments have changed from theoretical concepts to practical implementations that employ nanobots in cancer therapies. This transition encompasses the progression from conducting research solely in the laboratory setting to deploying these nanobots within living organisms. This chapter provides a deep investigation and analysis of recent developments in the field of nanobots for cancer treatment. It particularly focuses on the fundamental characteristics of these nanobots and their multiple uses in drug delivery, tumor recognition and assessment, personalized therapy, minimally invasive procedures, and other comprehensive therapeutic approaches. Simultaneously, we discuss the obstacles and prospective avenues for studying nanobots in their transformative role in cancer therapeutics. It is anticipated that in the future, medical nanobots will undergo advancements in sophistication and functionality, finally transforming into genuine nanosubmarines within the bloodstream.

doi:10.1088/978-0-7503-6019-7ch4

4.1 Introduction

Nanotechnology-based medicines have been developed by leveraging techniques at the nano or molecular scale and a biological understanding of the human body. These innovative treatments have been devised to address illnesses and promote the preservation and enhancement of human health [1, 2]. The rapid advancement of nanomedicines in recent decades can be attributed to their enormous potential for research and use in tumor therapy [3, 4]. Nanorobots are regarded as a very promising implementation of nanomedicines which can navigate and operate within distant and challenging anatomical parts of the human body, hence facilitating a diverse range of medicinal functions [5–7] (figure 4.1).

Healthcare nanorobots are nanoscale devices that are not attached to anything and possess an internal combustion engine or the ability to convert various forms of potential energy into mechanical energy to carry out a healthcare function [8–13]. Nanorobots can engage with cells and effectively infiltrate them, due to their diminutive dimensions. This enables them to directly interface with intricate cellular mechanisms [14, 15]. Nanorobotics, an interdisciplinary technology, is concerned with developing and utilizing functioning machinery at the nano to molecular scale. It has developed substantial applications in the realm of malignant tumor analysis and treatment. Nanorobots are miniature machines that possess the potential to transport various substances, such as medications and genetic material, and to recognize molecules. These micron-sized devices are designed to perform specific biomedical functions, including diagnosis and therapeutic actions. In addition, nanorobots possess the ability to target specific tumors or disease sites within the body. They are equipped with either an autonomous or passive power system, enabling them to receive externally supplied power, such as ultrasonic sound, near-infrared (NIR) illumination, or a magnetic driving force. On the other hand, these devices have the option to use existing media or a blood flow present in a biological system. Among the main distinctions between nanorobotic devices and nanocarriers is their respective active power systems. Nanotechnology-based medicines or nano-carriers that fall within the category under discussion are tiny robotic devices that

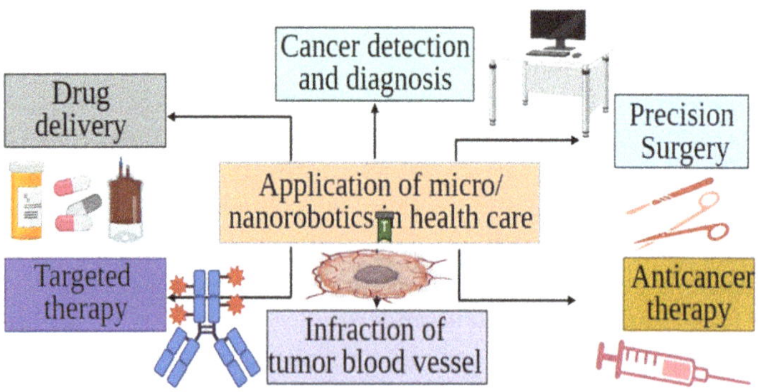

Figure 4.1. An analysis of the prospective applications of micro/nanorobots in the field of chemotherapy for cancer.

lack a functional source of energy. Scientists globally have dedicated their efforts to the investigation and advancement of malignancy-targeting nanorobotics to integrate them into healthcare environments and achieve breakthroughs in medicine. One of the main challenges that remains unresolved in the field of nanorobotic technology is the successful integration of these nanorobotic technologies into practical therapeutic applications.

In the last few years, there has been a notable advancement in the utilization of micro- and nanorobots in cancer therapy, transitioning from theoretical concepts to practical implementations. These advancements encompass a range of research conducted in both controlled laboratory settings (*in vitro*) and within living organisms (*in vivo*). The dimensions of individual biological molecules are often within the range of a nanometer and hence impose constraints on the functionality of microrobots. The manipulation and modification of biomolecules via robotics requires the use of nanorobots that possess comparable or analogous nanoscale characteristics [16–19]. Nanorobots have the potential to fulfill a range of health-related tasks in the field of cancer treatment as they transition from laboratory research to clinical applications. These tasks include drug administration, tumor detection and diagnostics, personalized therapy, minimally invasive surgical procedures, and other substantial responsibilities, as supported by scholarly sources [20–27]. The convergence of miniaturized robotic technology with modern medical technologies has facilitated the exploration of several applications in medicine, such as the administration of precise medicine. These programs are designed to address and overcome distinct challenges in the field of cancer therapy. While several previous investigations have discussed various aspects of micro- and nanorobots in the field of healthcare [10, 15, 20, 28, 29], the majority of these summaries have focused mainly on the biomedical uses of microrobots. However, there is a notable absence of reviews that specifically examine the recent advancements and endeavors related to the utilization of nanorobots in cancer treatments. This chapter begins with a concise investigation of biologically inspired nanotechnologies and the fundamental principles of nanorobotics. It subsequently offers a thorough analysis of the latest advancements in nanorobots, with a specific emphasis on their application in cancer treatments within the biomedical field. In addition, the assessment identifies and emphasizes the most auspicious research prospects that hold the potential to significantly influence cancer treatment in the upcoming decades. In future years, we can expect significant advancements in medical nanorobotics, leading to their enhanced sophistication and expanded capabilities in executing diverse medical tasks. Eventually, these nanorobots may evolve into fully functional nanosubmarines capable of navigating inside the bloodstream.

4.2 Important aspects of nanorobots for cancer therapy

Nanorobots, being diminutive in size, possess the ability to carry out predetermined duties. They exhibit distinct disparities when compared to their larger robotic counterparts. The creation and management of small-scale electromechanical or robotic elements pose significant hurdles to their advancement. These devices function inside a small-scale environment that exhibits physical features with different characteristics from those that typical robots encounter. The homogeneity of nanorobots' structural and chemical makeup is contingent upon their designated purpose, as well as the materials and methods employed during their fabrication. The discipline of nanorobotics is characterized by continuous progress and significant developments. In this context, we present a comprehensive overview of the fundamental elements and configurations frequently observed in nanorobots and offer an accessible compilation of representative examples of health-related nanorobots (table 4.1), as documented in the research conducted by Suhail *et al* [30].

Table 4.1. Several common examples of health-related nanorobots.

Forms of nanorobots	Essential features	References
Pharmacy	These healthcare nanorobots possess dimensions ranging from 1 to 2 μm. Molecular indicators, also known as chemical detection systems, are employed to assure the accuracy of the targeted mechanism. The elimination or recovery of these entities can be achieved by the application of centrifugal nanophoresis after the completion of the assigned activities.	[31]
Microchips	Nanorobots are equipped with microchips capable of transmitting electrical impulses upon the detection of disease-causing chemicals. The advantages of this system are its low cost of implementation and ease of operation.	[32]
Respirocyte	One example of a nanorobot is a synthetic hemoglobin cell that functions by transporting oxygen. Power is obtained from internalized blood sugar.	[33]
Microbivores	The nanorobot has a planar and spherical morphology, specifically designed for applications in the field of nanomedicine. The primary axis of the object has a length of 3.4 μm, while the minor axis has a length of 2.0 μm. The phagocytic capability of this entity is over 80 times more competent than that of other macrophages.	[34]
Clottocytes	These entities possess the biological attribute of 'instant' hemostatic action, commonly referred to as artificial mechanical platelets. In addition, they facilitate the transportation of chemicals that aid coagulation.	[35]
Chromallocyte	The initial action of the rehabilitation machine involves evaluating the state of the cellular substances and behaviors and working through a thorough inspection. The repair machines can perform a comprehensive overhaul of an entire cell.	[36]

Today, the majority of nanorobot investigations are carried out in circumstances that closely resemble the microenvironments found within the physical makeup of a person. It is necessary to optimize the efficacy of nanorobots in eradicating cancer cells within human corpulence, therefore researchers have established rigorous criteria for the foundational design components of nanorobots. It is crucial to acknowledge that the advancement in healthcare nanorobots is now in its early phases of advancement and has not yet been extensively integrated into medical interventions. These technologies' internal makeup and design might differ significantly depending on the purpose that they are designed to serve and on their unique criteria for reliability, efficiency, and sustainability.

4.3 Nanorobot propulsion systems for anticancer medicine delivery

Advancements at the nanoscale have resulted in the widespread use of nanorobots in malignancy therapy, particularly in the field of drug delivery. Nano-drug carriers have been produced, exhibiting notable characteristics such as diminutive dimensions, substantial specific surface area, inherent void volumes, as well as exceptional physicochemical qualities. In general, an ideal nanorobot exhibits numerous specialized skills, including controllable navigation, tissue penetration, propulsion, and the ability to transport and release cargo. In addition to the constraints imposed by passive mass transport, the majority of the current pharmaceutical nanocarriers depend on systemic circulation for their function. Furthermore, these nanocarriers possess the essential attributes of self-propulsion and navigation that are necessary for targeted administration and tissue penetration. Many research investigations have documented the efficacy of nanorobotics in facilitating the targeted drug delivery of therapeutic drugs to specific tumor regions [37–43]. Nanorobots have the potential to be utilized for the treatment of tumors by intravenous injection into the bloodstream or oral administration, which allow them to accumulate at the target site. This accumulation can lead to a substantial enhancement in anticancer efficacy while minimizing adverse effects on healthy normal cells. To achieve the precise targeting of therapeutic agents at tumor locations, various sophisticated technologies and developments have facilitated the delivery of nanorobots to the affected areas. In recent years, nanorobots have been categorized based on their propulsion mechanisms and the factors that drive them and enable their mobility.

4.3.1 Nanorobots propelled by magnets

Several investigations have employed the technique of magnetic propulsion to exemplify the transport functions and characteristics of nanorobotics [44–49]. Moreover, extensive investigation has led to significant advancements in the utilization of nanorobots for the diagnosis and management of malignancy, leading to a multitude of commendable results. To establish this driving pattern, it is necessary to ensure that the magnetic nanorobots possess a helical structure and may be propelled by rotational-to-translational motion. The propulsion mechanism depends upon the generation of torque through the application of an external magnetic field [50–53].

In their study, Andheri *et al* [54] developed a sophisticated magnetic nanorobot composed of many components. The nanorobot was constructed by incorporating the chemotherapy drug doxorubicin (DOX) and an anticancer antibody inside multiwalled carbon nanotubes (CNTs). The proposed magnetic nanorobot possessed the ability to maneuver itself through the application of an external magnetic field, even in complex biological fluids. Furthermore, it exhibited the capability to administer anticancer drug payloads within 3D spheroidal tumors, triggered by intracellular potassium H_2O_2 or localized pH alterations within the tumor microenvironment. The nanorobot consisted of magnetic iron oxide nanoparticles that were chemically conjugated and showed the ability to preferentially release DOX into the internal lysosomal compartments of cells affected by HCT116, a type of human colorectal cancer. The release was achieved by activating a gate mechanism located at the nanoscale interface of the ferric oxide.

A novel nickel–silver nanoscale swimmer demonstrated the ability to be propelled by an external magnetic field. The nanoscale swimmer was able to transport micron-sized fragments at impressive velocities exceeding 10 $\mu m\ s^{-1}$ [55]. Poly (D, L-lactic-co-glycolic acid) (PLGA) was utilized to produce polymeric microspheres that were afterward treated with DOX. The propulsion of the robotic device was facilitated by a variable magnetic field, enabling it to transport microspheres containing drugs through an elongated conduit made of polydimethylsiloxane (PDMS). Upon approaching human cervical carcinoma (HeLa) cells, the nano swimmer proceeded to discharge the drug-carrying microspheres to eliminate the cancerous cells that were present.

In another study, scientists employed a biological template approach to convert pine pollen into magnet-equipped microrobots. They successfully loaded docetaxel into the microrobot's inherent cavity using vacuum loading. Subsequently, they utilized the collective behavior of the microrobots to deliver pharmaceuticals through small channels made of PDMS. Magnetic rotors were used by the magnetized microrobot to achieve a quasi-natural state within a cancerous cell's interior to induce fluid flow and administer therapeutic chemical compounds, resulting in the eradication of cancerous cells [56]. The application of magnetically propelled nanorobotics is a common practice that emulates the motion of bacterial flagella by introducing external magnetic fields, hence facilitating the targeted delivery of anticancer medications [57, 58]. In a further study, investigators discovered that the application of biohybrid microrobots, namely those derived from the *Magnetococcus marinus* strain MC-1, proved effective in propelling drug-loaded nanoliposomes to hypoxic locations inside the tumor utilizing an electromagnetic field that was applied outside the body [59].

4.3.2 Nanorobots propelled by ultrasound

Establishing an acoustical state might be considered a reasonably straightforward task. Acoustic waves can propagate across several media, including solids, liquids, and air. This property enables them to permeate biological tissues to effectively externally energize nanorobots while minimizing any discernible adverse effects on

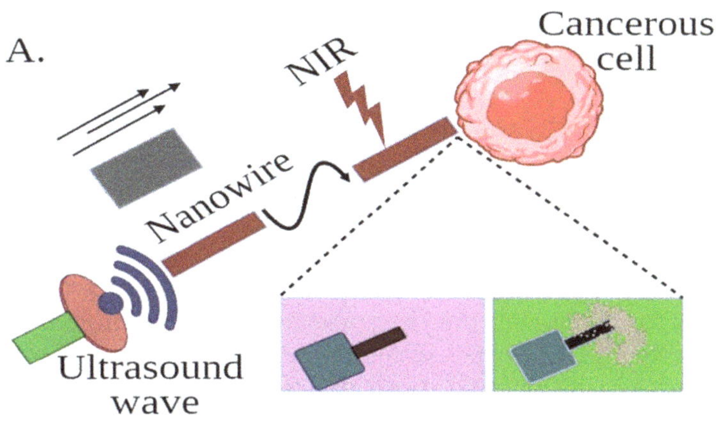

Figure 4.2. A diagram illustrating the nanowire motor propelled toward cancer cells by ultrasound, subsequently leading to the release of drugs activated by NIR light.

the human body. Nevertheless, the utilization of ultrasound has the potential to induce cellular oxidative stress, hence affecting both malignant tumor cells and healthy cells [60]. The fundamental method involves the application of ultrasonic waves to induce a localized phenomenon of auditory streams, thus inducing asymmetric strains on the outer layer. The resulting strain subsequently provides a propulsive force that facilitates the movement of the nanorobots. The application of high-intensity focused ultrasound has the potential to facilitate the rapid evaporation of chemical fuel and enable the propulsion of nanorobotics in the form of tubing that can move flexibly. Robots constructed entirely out of microtubes can achieve rapid movement and effectively enter tissues due to their great propulsive force [61]. In their study, Garcia *et al* [62] provided evidence of the effectiveness of their ultrasound-driven nanowire motors in facilitating effective medication administration to HeLa cancer cells, with the added benefit of NIR light-induced release of medication. In this instance, it was disclosed that 32%–40% of the DOX-loaded medicine was discharged into cancerous cells after 14–18-min of exposure to NIR irradiation, as seen in figure 4.2.

4.3.3 Biologically propelled nanorobots

The terms 'propelled microrobots' and 'nanorobotics' refer to miniature robotic systems that are propelled and controlled by biological mechanisms and those that operate at the nanoscale, respectively. These entities are formed by combining biological organisms (cells) with synthetic materials. Microorganisms such as sperm and bacteria, which are motile due to their use of flagella, possess the potential to serve as a propulsive mechanism for biohybrid micro- and nanorobots. However, the unique capacity of sperm to adhere to bodily cells raises notable concerns. The biological compatibility as well as reliability of micro- and nanorobots are important considerations in their development and utilization. According to one report, a biohybrid robot with a 3D-printed magnetic tube substructure and four appendages used a free-moving sperm as both its energy source and means of transporting drugs. In contrast to fully manufactured microrobots or other nanocarriers, these sperm-hybridized microrobots can encapsulate high-concentration pharmaceuticals within the male reproductive system membrane, therefore safeguarding their loaded medications against dilution by bodily fluids or enzymatic destruction [50].

4.3.4 Hybrid-drive nanorobots

Numerous research studies have provided evidence supporting the efficacy of nanorobots in accomplishing precise medicine delivery through the usage of a hybrid power source. One study demonstrated that nanorobots possess robust affinity towards viruses and toxins, which enables them to effectively carry out detoxification processes [63]. In another study, He *et al* [64] constructed a tubing microrobot with multiple layers utilizing the successive layer self-assembly technique. By employing a fusion of bubble-driven and magnetic field guiding mechanisms, these microrobots were able to efficiently transport DOX to cancerous cells, achieving impressive velocities of around 68 $\mu m\ s^{-1}$. In addition to various power generation techniques, the mobility of nanorobots may be controlled by applying a magnetic field [65]. As a case study, an investigation led by Wang from the University of California employed an electrodeposition technique to fabricate nanorobots with a perforated metallic rod-like structure [62]. The nanorobots possessed a porous framework that enabled them to accommodate an increased number of medicinal compounds, surpassing the capacity of their planar metal counterparts by a factor of 20. Drug release from the nanorobots was initiated by NIR light. The tumor cells were successfully eradicated by the administered medications, facilitated by the application of ultrasonic frequencies and the direction provided by an external magnetic field.

A hybrid magnetoelectric nanorobot has been shown to perform precise drug delivery, wherein the release of the medication was activated using an externally applied magnetic field [66]. In this device, nanoscale motors included three components in separate sections made from Au, Ni, and Au, respectively, which were directed by a magnetic field and pushed using ultrasonic energy [67]. Altering the orientation of the applied magnetic field enabled the particles driven by ultrasound to exhibit multidirectional motion. Recent studies have demonstrated the promising potential of bismuth (Bi) compounds in the field of biological applications [68, 69]. The authors introduced a study of the fabrication of self-propelled microrobots with tube-like components using bismuth (Bi) as the main material. They also conducted experimental tests to validate the feasibility of these microrobotic devices for smart drug delivery purposes. Biocompatible materials were employed in the development of microrobots to serve as drug carriers in clinical studies. The microrobots were fabricated using Bi and coated with DOX inhibitors, which are widely used as preliminary medications for chemotherapy for cancer. By harnessing the magnetic characteristics of the nickel coating, these robots were efficiently directed towards cancerous cells to provide precise administration. The microrobots, equipped with a significant amount of cargo, were guided by a magnet

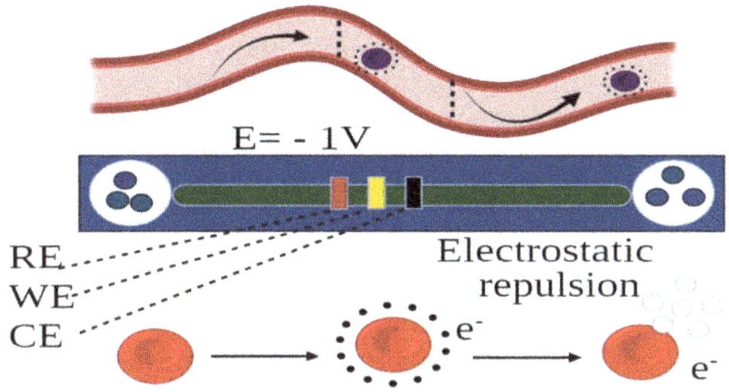

Figure 4.3. The figure depicts a tubular microrobot based on bismuth (Bi), which has demonstrated its efficacy in delivering smart pharmaceuticals or heavy metals via the veins using an electrochemical release mechanism.

into a tunnel that housed a piece of electromechanical equipment. The device facilitated the controlled and rapid discharge of the payloads within a short period [70] (figure 4.3).

4.3.5 Nanorobots propelled by other power sources

While the concept appears to have potential, it is essential to consider that the majority of the reported investigations have been performed *in vitro*. The efficacy of achieving directional movement of nanorobots in a complex internal biological environment, comparable to that shown in *in vitro* research, has yet to be substantiated. The research demonstrates the potential of a nanorobotic technology to manifest regulated locomotion in reaction to NIR light [71]. The authors found that when subjected to NIR irradiation, the presence of gold half-nanoshells within the nanorobot system generated a thermal gradient, enabling self-heating energy to counteract the effects of Brownian motion on the system. The system driven by NIR light was further enclosed within macrophages in the cell membranes. This additional coating gave the nanorobots the immunological ability to specifically adhere to cancerous cells. Recent advancements in research have demonstrated significant progress in the development and application of micro-/nanorobots for drug delivery purposes. These innovative micro-/nanorobots have tremendous potential for use as highly effective delivery agents in a wide range of therapeutic applications, particularly those that are currently difficult to achieve with conventional passive methods of delivery.

4.4 Precision cancer diagnosis and treatment with nanorobots

In contrast to conventional methods of combating cancer, targeted therapy can specifically engage with certain biomarkers implicated in tumor formation and hence impede the growth of tumors [72]. The utilization of targeted treatment offers distinct benefits in comparison to conventional therapy, such as chemotherapy, since it selectively focuses on biomarkers specifically associated with the proliferation of tumors [73]. In recent years, several studies have shown the effective application of nanorobots as a means of achieving targeted therapy in the context of antitumor treatments [74–77]. The application of nanorobots in targeted therapy has the potential to mitigate the adverse effects associated with the high levels of toxicity commonly observed in standard chemotherapy. This innovative approach offers a promising alternative for the therapeutic management of cancer [78]. However, it is worth noting that power-operated miniature robots have the potential to target specific lesions; carry out controlled movements; identify, position, and retrieve objects; as well as deliver therapeutic compounds in a precisely targeted approach [79, 80]. Table 4.2 presents a succinct summary of the prevailing therapeutic uses of miniature robots in potential malignancies and their treatment.

Nanorobotics is a multidisciplinary domain that integrates the fundamental concepts of robotics, nanotechnologies, and materials science to further the development of robots operating at the nanoscale. The application of nanorobots has the potential to promote substantial progress in several domains, including medicine, manufacture, energy generation, and environmental remediation. The field of nanorobotics has the potential to facilitate novel advances in science and enhance comprehension of the nanoscale realm.

Table 4.2. Common pathways that clinical applications of nanorobots will take in the detection and management of malignancies in the near future.

Application	Description
Targeted imaging	Nanorobots can be deliberately designed in a manner that enables them to specifically identify and engage with cancer cells and tumor tissues, hence enhancing their capabilities for tumor imaging and visualization.
Tumor biopsy	Nanorobots possess the potential to be engineered with the capability to conduct minimally invasive biopsy operations, hence facilitating the retrieval of tissue samples for diagnostic purposes.
Molecular diagnosis	Nanorobots possess the capability to be deliberately designed and programmed to conduct molecular diagnostics, hence facilitating the timely identification of certain cancer biomarkers and enhancing the process of diagnosing the disease.
Targeted administration	Nanorobots can be deliberately designed to specifically target cancer cells or tumor tissues, augmenting the effectiveness of immunotherapy while concurrently mitigating any potential negative consequences.
Continual monitoring	Nanorobots can consistently observe the localized alterations inside a tumor and provide immunotherapy drugs as necessary, offering a treatment approach that is both adaptable and dynamic.
Conjoint therapy	Nanorobots can be deliberately designed in a manner that enables the simultaneous administration of numerous immunotherapy drugs. This attribute therefore facilitates the provision of cancer therapies that are completer and more efficacious.
Tumor ablation	Nanorobots can selectively eliminate cancer cells using several mechanisms, including but not limited to thermal, optical, and mechanical ablation.

4.4.1 The identification and assessment of cancerous conditions

There is a pressing necessity for the early diagnosis of malignancies, as it has the potential to significantly enhance rates of patient survival [81]. The development of nanorobots designed to eliminate tumors continues to progress, and advancements in nanorobot design are resulting in improved efficacy and precision in the early detection of cancer throughout its clinical stages [82–85].

Nehru and colleagues designed a novel nanorobot for tumor detection [86]. The nanorobot was capable of *in vivo* examination of tumor cell proliferation by applying the technique of positron emission tomography (PET). Meanwhile, a system with embedded components was integrated to facilitate control of the nanorobot using preprogrammed processes on the Arduino programming platform [87]. To reduce any adverse effects on the human body, a nanorobot was constructed using a nano-carbon substance that was isotopically labeled. Upon introduction into the human body, nanorobots exhibit a commendable level of stability as well as security, hence ensuring the absence of any detrimental effects on human physiology. After a nanorobot has completed its predetermined objectives, it is expelled from the human body in the form of waste material. The nanorobot, like its macrorobot counterpart, consists of essential components such as sensors, power devices, and a camera. Furthermore, sophisticated algorithms are utilized to devise the most efficient route, while the integrated sensor aids the nanorobot in avoiding obstructions. The overexpression of biomarkers on the surface of cancer cell membranes presents promising opportunities for disease diagnostics, treatments, and advancements in the field of biomedical engineering.

Peng *et al* designed and constructed a three-dimensional DNA nanorobot [88]. They developed a nanomachine using three-dimensional DNA-based logic gates, which were specifically intended to selectively target cancerous cells with overexpressed biomarkers. The targeting mechanism involved bispecific recognition [89]. In addition, the DNA nanorobot was able to execute Boolean logic operations on the membranes of cancer cells and hence has significant theranostic prospects for its application in the medical management of cancer [90].

Deng *et al* produced natural killer (NK) cell-mimicking nanorobots by encapsulating an aggregation-induced emission (AIE)-active polymeric nano endoskeleton in the membrane of an NK cell [91]. After they were excited by light, the nanorobots exhibited a high level of biological compatibility and could emit highly intense fluorescence in the NIR-II range. In addition, they were able to migrate across the brain–blood barrier on their own by opening tight junction frameworks. They precisely accumulated at brain tumor locations in complex brain matrices to give tumor images with high contrast and skull penetration. Moreover, they did this in an independent way.

In another study, Shi *et al* [92] introduced a novel approach called the nanorobot-assisted multichannel cancer identification process (MCDP). Their technique incorporated the use of niche genetic algorithm (NGA) technology for multichannel cancer identification. The nanorobots, prompted by the NGA, exhibited the ability to detect tumors by navigating through particularly vulnerable tissue areas. Such functionality may be conceptualized as an autonomous search process, whereby the framework endeavors to identify the most favorable solutions for an arbitrary function inside the parameter space while adhering to certain limitations. The efficient localization of nanorobots to tumor locations, while considering actual *in vivo* propagation and control, can effectively address the multifunctional optimization challenge.

4.4.2 Gene therapy involving the precise administration of nucleic DNA

In addition to their role in delivering pharmaceutical medications, nanorobots can be used to precisely distribute other theranostic chemicals, offering a potential way to circumvent the adverse reactions commonly associated with traditional chemotherapeutics, such as elevated toxicity. This innovative approach presents a novel method that can be used to combat the progression of malignant tumors. The utilization of magnetic helical microswimmers enables the targeted transportation of plasmid genetic material to human fetus kidney cells. Motorized vehicles containing plasmid DNA (pDNA) are remotely directed toward the target cell, where they subsequently deliver their genetic payload into the cell upon exposure. Scientists have constructed a gold nanoscale device that moved like a snake. It was able to hybridize with siRNA (small interfering RNA) particles and thus become coated with amplified genetic material. This modified nanowire was designed to deliver siRNA molecules into the intracellular environment [92]. An ultrasound-induced pressure gradient facilitated rapid and forceful propulsion of the nanorobot, enabling efficient penetration into cancerous cells. Subsequently, the target mRNA was cleaved by the scissor-like structure of siRNA, resulting in a silencing efficiency of up to 94% within a brief processing time.

A further study presented a genetically engineered nanorobot that had a sorting capability. The DNA nanorobot was engineered to possess a pair of ambulatory appendages and manipulative limbs for transporting goods. The vehicle was able to collect a designated cargo and transport it to specified destinations. As demonstrated through experimental investigations, this nanorobot exhibited a delivery capability wherein goods may be successfully transported to a designated location with a success rate of 80%. When employed in the context of tumor therapy, this technology can administer medications within the body of an individual, resulting in the eradication of tumor cells with a success rate of 80%. Nevertheless, within the realm of therapeutic applications, a 20% level of ambiguity remains, indicating the potential for unidentified detrimental effects on the normal regular operation of cells inside the body of an individual. This nanorobot possesses the capacity to commence the medication offloading procedure upon receiving a directive from a control system. In the absence of such a directive, the nanorobot continues its movement without discharging the payload drug. DNA nanorobots can establish intercommunication through algorithmic processes, enabling them to locate concealed tumor cells and deliver targeted medication payloads for their eradication. The design of this nanorobot, which is capable of targeting and destroying tumors, primarily utilizes biological chemicals that naturally occur within the human body. This approach enables the nanorobot to effectively adapt to the complex physiological milieu within the human body.

4.4.3 Vascular infarction in tumors

The application of DNA-guided thrombin-inducing nanorobots has emerged as a potent therapeutic approach in the management of malignancies [93–96]. This method has demonstrated encouraging effectiveness against malignancy and caused little collateral harm in preclinical situations. The transformative investigations of this technology performed in clinical trials signify a significant progression in the implementation of nanotechnology based on genetically engineered material for anticancer treatment. In 2018, Li and colleagues [94] developed a nanorobot using a methodology based on genetically engineered material origami. Li *et al* proposed the utilization of genetically engineered origami technology to create a tailored tube-shaped DNA nanorobot capable of being flexed into a precise configuration [94]. Thrombin was contained and protected within the tube to prevent enzymatic degradation during shipment. In addition, a sophisticated intelligent system was integrated into the genetic material nanorobot, rendering it physiologically targeted and enabling it to accurately locate the concealed sites of tumor cells. The genetically engineered nanorobot successfully identified its intended target by binding to a specific receptor located on the surface of the tumor cell membrane. Upon encountering the receptor, a molecular switch that was inherently present was triggered, leading to the release of thrombin within the targeted blood artery. This process effectively obstructed the blood channel and denied nutrients to the tumor tissues.

The DNA-guided thrombin-inducing nanorobot has been shown to effectively produce the rapid and substantial death of tumor cells, surpassing the effectiveness of other alternative treatments. This nanorobot operates by causing an acute blood event. Moreover, this treatment option does not exhibit any detrimental impacts on cardiac health and does not induce discernible harm to essential organs, in contrast to alternative efficacious anticancer methods. Life-threatening cardiovascular toxicities resulting from recombinant antigen receptor T (chimeric antigen receptor T (CAR-T)) cell immunotherapy have been reported in previous studies [97–99]. However, several relevant therapeutic considerations have recently arisen because the nanorobot is designed to induce thromboembolism under the guidance of genetic material (DNA). Vasculogenic rebounds may manifest after tumor vascular infarction has been induced by the genetic material (DNA) nanorobot, alongside an elevated susceptibility to tumor lysis syndrome (TLS), leading to a severe metabolic crisis [100–105].

4.5 Nanorobots in cancer therapy: potential and clinical problems

Nanobots exhibit significant potential to transform cancer therapy by enhancing the precision with which cancerous tumor cells are targeted, mitigating adverse effects, and optimizing treatment results. Nevertheless, some obstacles must be overcome before nanorobots can be widely used in therapeutic cancer treatments [106, 107].

This section will analyze several obstacles to the development and implementation of nanorobotics in therapeutic cancer therapy. These variables include the complexity of technological innovation, accuracy, safety considerations, legislative complexities, financial constraints, and scalability.

4.5.1 The complexity and accuracy of the technology

The process of creating and managing nanorobots for therapeutic cancer therapies needs many technological challenges to be resolved. These challenges encompass the development of nanoscale components, the regulation of their motion, and the assurance of their stability. A significant concern is the exact manipulation of miniature robots made of magnetic materials that are driven by externally produced magnetic energies. The intricate nature of magnetic fields in confined areas and the potential disruption caused by other electromagnetic waves pose challenges in attaining precise and meticulous manipulation of nanorobot movements. This can lead to the imprecise localization of nanorobots in tumor locations and prospective damage to human tissues and organs [108, 109].

Moreover, the fluidic milieu within the human body, characterized by low Reynolds numbers, presents additional problems for the operational precision and velocities of nanorobotics. The operational precision and velocity of nanorobots can be significantly impacted by interference originating from biological surroundings [110]. Nanorobots' movement and functioning in the circulatory system may be hampered or eliminated due to their contact with circulating protein molecules, blood cells, and antibodies [111, 112]. To facilitate the movements and operations of nanorobots within living organisms, it is imperative to enhance energy conversion efficiency. In contrast to blood, urine and saliva are two distinct kinds of bodily fluids that require careful consideration. Catalytic motors propelled by diffusion and electrophoresis experience diminished effectiveness and metal corrosion in both environments.

4.5.2 Concerns regarding personal safety

The utilization of nanorobots in healthcare contexts, namely in the realm of cancer-related therapies, elicits legitimate apprehensions concerning their safety and the possible detrimental consequences they may have on individuals undergoing treatment. The potential negative consequences of malfunctioning nanorobots extend beyond patient injury, encompassing unanticipated side effects that might introduce additional complexities to the therapeutic procedure. If malignant tumors exhibit underdeveloped vasculature, the application of tubular DNA nanorobots that express thrombin may be ineffective, resulting in an inability to successfully attain the desired therapeutic objectives [113, 114].

To ensure the successful resolution of these issues and the assurance of nanorobots' efficacy and safety within the domain of malignant tumor treatment, it is crucial to embrace a meticulous strategy that incorporates thorough experimental and clinical studies. This methodology facilitates the assessment of the biocompatibility pharmacokinetics and pharmacodynamics of these nanoscale instruments across many biological environments. Furthermore, the application of rigorous quality control procedures throughout the manufacturing procedure is imperative to mitigate the potential for device malfunction and guarantee reliable operation across different batches of nanorobots [115, 116].

4.5.3 Regulatory concerns

The absence of comprehensive criteria for the development and application of nanorobots might hinder their widespread acceptance by both governmental and commercial entities. The effective integration of nanorobots in the context of therapeutic cancer therapy requires the establishment of suitable regulatory structures that can successfully tackle the unique issues associated with nanorobotics. These regulatory structures should also promote innovation and protect public health [10].

Regulatory bodies should prioritize the formulation of comprehensive rules that embrace the entirety of the nanorobot's lifespan, from the first stages of design and development through the latter phases of clinical studies and post-market surveillance. Regulations must have measures for fostering cooperation and facilitating data sharing among researchers, industry participants, and regulatory authorities. This inclusive approach is essential to enable all relevant parties to make a significant contribution to the advancement of nanorobotic treatments, ensuring their safety and efficacy [117].

4.5.4 Scalability

Augmenting the advancement and proliferation of a substantial volume of nanorobots for therapeutic cancer therapies is a significant hurdle, mostly attributable to the intricate and time-intensive characteristics of the manufacturing procedures. This scaling concern encompasses several crucial elements that need attention, such as manufacturing methodologies, cost analysis, quality assurance, and supply chain administration [118].

4.5.5 Cost

The exorbitant expenses associated with the development and production of nanorobots provide a substantial impediment to their widespread implementation. To achieve a reduction in production costs, it is imperative to make advancements in the field of nanomaterials, alongside enhancing manufacturing efficiency. For example, the identification of novel nanomaterials that are more economically efficient or the enhancement of currently available nanomaterials may contribute to a reduction in the overall expenditure associated with nanorobots. Furthermore, enhanced collaboration among academics, manufacturers, and funding agencies has the potential to facilitate the advancement of cost-effective manufacturing methods [119].

4.5.6 Quality control

Ensuring both the safety and effectiveness of nanorobots requires the implementation of rigorous quality control measures throughout their mass production process. This involves the formulation of comprehensive evaluation and validation procedures to detect any flaws and guarantee that nanorobots adhere to the requisite performance criteria [120, 121]. The integration of process monitors and real-time feedback systems can enhance quality control measures by facilitating the prompt identification and resolution of production-related problems.

4.5.7 Management of the supply chain and its components

The escalating manufacture of nanorobots will inevitably lead to commensurate growth in the intricacy of their supply chain. Effectively addressing this intricacy necessitates the formulation of proficient supply chain methods capable of effectively managing the acquisition, warehousing, and conveyance of nanoscale constituents and substances. This process may entail the formation of collaborations among the entities involved in the production and distribution of goods, namely producers, suppliers, and logistics firms to enhance the efficiency of the transportation of materials and guarantee the punctual distribution of nanorobots to healthcare professionals and patients [122–125].

4.6 Future perspectives and conclusions

As previously discussed, the field of nanorobotics in the context of cancer therapy is now undergoing significant advancements and research efforts. To completely utilize the possibilities for using nanorobotics in the field of chemotherapy for cancers, investigators of materials and artificial intelligence must establish close collaborations with medical researchers. This collaborative effort is necessary to conduct comprehensive investigations into the behaviors and functions of miniature robots in a range of applications including medication administration, individualized therapy, minimally invasive surgical procedures, cancer detection, early diagnostics, and other sophisticated therapies facilitated by nanorobot assistance. Given the significant advances observed in recent *in vivo* and *in vitro* studies, researchers must investigate the requirements of, and difficulties faced by oncologists. This will enable researchers to develop specialized medical micro/nanorobots with a focus on cancer-related diagnostic or therapeutic applications. Such efforts are crucial to expedite the transition of micro/nanorobotic cancer research from theoretical exploration to practical clinical implementation [126]. It is anticipated that the integration of nanorobots as a comprehensive platform to address various objectives in diverse anticancer areas will be achieved shortly.

The efficient delivery of therapeutic effects in cancer treatment through the employment of nanomedicines requires the effective traversal of a vascular barrier at the micron size. Although dynamically targeted nanomedicines have shown excellent targeting effectiveness on cancer cells *in vitro*, their efficacy *in vivo* is challenged by the diverse nature of the tumor microenvironment. On the other hand, a notable feature, namely the immediate exposure of vascular endothelial cells to the circulation, presents advantageous prospects for the specific identification and functionality of nanomedicines that are designed to target the blood vessels of tumors. However, it is crucial to prioritize the enhancement of the specificity of the pertinent targets and the responses of the tumor microenvironment. The clinical application of experimental micro/nanorobots is constrained by the intricate and diverse nature of tumor biology, our limited comprehension of interactions between nanomaterials and biology, and the absence of scalable synthesis and mass production techniques for micro/nanorobots. The application of DNA nanotechnology, specifically DNA origami, to deliver thrombin, demonstrates the promising prospects of achieving precise drug administration [127]. However, many obstacles need to be addressed before this approach can be successfully translated into clinical practice. These issues include the risk of unwanted immune responses, the behavior of the drug within the body, and the ability to produce these DNA-based drug delivery systems on a large scale. To advance scientific understanding and practical applications, it is imperative to conduct thorough investigations into the intricate mechanisms underlying the interactions that occur between micro/nanorobots and proteins, cells, tissues, and organs [128]. In addition, it is essential to maintain control over drug uptake by modulation. To optimize the use of nanomaterials in biomedical applications, it is crucial to identify relevant target molecules and prioritize the usage of nanomaterials with well-established biosafety profiles and defined *in vivo* metabolic characteristics. Furthermore, the application of sophisticated preparatory techniques and comprehensive characterization systems is crucial for the expansion of the therapeutic utility of nanorobots.

It is anticipated that in the future, medical micro/nanorobots with basic structures will undergo evolution, resulting in enhanced sophistication and the ability to carry out various medical activities and duties.

References

[1] Battistella C and Klok H A 2017 Controlling and monitoring intracellular delivery of anticancer polymer nanomedicines *Macromol. Biosci.* **17** 1700022.2

[2] Crosby D, Bhatia S, Brindle K M, Coussens L M, Dive C and Emberton M 2022 Early cancer detection *Science* **375** 9040

[3] Shao S, Zhou Q, Si J, Tang J, Liu X and Wang M 2017 A non-cytotoxic dendrimer with innate and potent anticancer and anti-metastatic activities *Nat. Biomed. Eng.* **17** 45–57

[4] Nanotechnology K T 1994 Basic concepts and definitions *Clin. Chem.* **40** 1797–9

[5] Medina-Sanchez M and Schmidt O G 2017 Medical microbots need better imaging and control *Nature* **545** 406–8

[6] Agrahari V, Agrahari V, Chou M L, Chew C H, Noll J and Burnouf T 2020 Intelligent micro-/nanorobots as drug and cell carrier devices for biomedical therapeutic advancement: promising development opportunities and translational challenges *Biomaterials* **260** 120163

[7] Ghosh A, Xu W, Gupta N and Gracias D H 2020 Active matter therapeutics *Nano Today* **31** 100836

[8] Sanchez S, Soler L and Katuri J 2015 Chemically powered micro- and nanomotors *Angew. Chem. Int. Ed. Engl.* **54** 1414–44

[9] Chen X Z, Jang B, Ahmed D, Hu C, De Marco C and Hoop M 2018 Small-scale machines driven by external power sources *Adv. Mater.* **30** 1705061
[10] Soto F, Wang J, Ahmed R and Demirci U 2020 Medical micro/nanorobots in precision medicine *Adv. Sci.* **7** 2002203
[11] Mei Y, Solovev A A, Sanchez S and Schmidt O G 2022 Rolled-up nanotech on polymers: from basic perception to self-propelled catalytic micro engines *Chem. Soc. Rev.* **40** 2109–19
[12] Wang J 2009 Can man-made nanomachines compete with natural bio motors? *ACS Nano* **3** 4–9
[13] Oldham K, Sun D and Sun Y 2018 Focused issue on micro-/nano-robotics *Int. J. Intell. Robot. Appl.* **2** 381–2
[14] Lenaghan S C, Wang Y, Xi N, Fukuda T, Tarn T and Hamel W R 2013 Grand challenges in bioengineered nanorobotics for cancer therapy *IEEE Trans. Biomed. Eng.* **60** 667–73
[15] Soto F and Chrostowski R 2018 Frontiers of medical micro/nanorobotics: *in vivo* applications and commercialization perspectives toward clinical uses *Front. Bioeng. Biotechnol.* **6** 170
[16] Fernandez-Leiro R and Scheres S H 2016 Unraveling biological macromolecules with cryo-electron microscopy *Nature* **537** 339–46
[17] Li M, Xi N, Wang Y and Liu L 2021 Progress in nanorobotics for advancing biomedicine *IEEE Trans. Biomed. Eng.* **68** 130–47
[18] Wang J, Dong Y, Ma P, Wang Y, Zhang F and Cai B 2022 Intelligent micro-/nanorobots for cancer theragnostic *Adv. Mater.* **34** 2201051
[19] Yang M, Guo X, Mou F and Guan J 2022 Lighting up micro-/nanorobots with fluorescence *Chem. Rev.* **123** 3944–75
[20] Li J, de Esteban-Fernandez A B, Gao W, Zhang L and Wang J 2017 Micro/nanorobots for biomedicine: delivery, surgery, sensing, and detoxification *Sci. Robot.* **2** eaam6431
[21] Martel S 2017 Beyond imaging: macro- and microscale medical robots actuated by clinical MRI scanners *Sci. Robot.* **2** 8119
[22] Nelson B J, Kaliakatsos I K and Abbott J J 2010 Microrobots for minimally invasive medicine *Annu. Rev. Biomed. Eng.* **12** 55–85
[23] Sitti M, Ceylan H, Hu W, Giltinan J, Turan M and Yim S 2015 Biomedical applications of untethered mobile milli/microrobots *Proc. IEEE Inst. Electr. Electron. Eng.* **103** 205–24
[24] Kim K, Guo J, Liang Z and Fan D 2018 Artificial micro/nanomachines for bio applications: biochemical delivery and diagnostic sensing *Adv. Func. Mater.* **28** 1705867
[25] Luo M, Feng Y, Wang T and Guan J 2018 Micro-/nanorobots at work in active drug delivery *Adv. Func. Mater.* **28** 1706100
[26] Kong L, Guan J and Pumera M 2018 Micro- and nanorobots-based sensing and biosensing *Curr. Opin. Electrochem.* **10** 174–82
[27] Halder A and Sun 2019 Biocompatible propulsion for biomedical micro/nanorobotics *Biosens. Bioelectron.* **139** 111334
[28] Peng F, Tu Y and Wilson D A 2017 Micro/nanomotors towards *in vivo* application: cell tissue and biofluid *Chem. Soc. Rev.* **46** 5289–310
[29] Safdar M, Khan S U and Janis J 2018 Progress toward catalytic micro- and nanomotors for biomedical and environmental applications *Adv. Mater.* **30** e1703660
[30] Suhail M, Khan A, Rahim M A, Naeem A, Fahad M and Badshah S F 2022 Micro and nanorobot-based drug delivery an overview *J. Drug. Target.* **30** 349–58
[31] Mani S A, Sachdeva S, Mani A, Vora H R and Sodhi J K 2021 Nano-robotics: the future of health and dental care *IP Int. J. Periodontal. Implantol.* **6** 6–10

[32] Žnidaršič A B, Alenka B and Werber B 2022 Attitudes toward microchip implant in groups pro and con its insertion for healthcare purposes *BLED 2020 Proceedings 33rd BLED eConference* 1 (Atlanta, GA: Association for Information Systems) 629–40
[33] Kumar J P S, Sankaranarayanan R, Sujana J A J and Hynes N R J 2021 Advantages and disadvantages of nanodevices *Nanomedicine Manufacturing and Applications* ed F Verpoort, I Ahmad, A Ahmad, A Khan and C Y Chee (Amsterdam: Elsevier) 10 163–71
[34] Gandhi M and Joshi P N 2020 Nanorobots for In Vivo Monitoring: The Future of Nano-Implantable Devices *Nano Biomaterial Engineering* ed P Chandra and R Prakash (Singapore: Springer) 227–52
[35] Javaid A 2021 Medical nanorobots: our new healthcare defense *Acad. Lett.* **2021** 1629
[36] Sapra V, Sapra L, Sandhu J K and Chhabra G 2021 Biomedical diagnostics through nanocomputing *Nanotechnology* (Singapore: Jenny Stanford Publishing) 443–60
[37] Tirgar Bahnamiri P and Bagheri-Khoulenjani S 2017 Biodegradable microrobots for targeting cell delivery *Med. Hypotheses* **102** 56–60
[38] Peng F, Tu Y, van Heist J C and Wilson D A 2015 Self-guided supramolecular cargo-loaded nanomotors with chemotactic behavior towards cells *Angew. Chem. Int. Ed. Engl.* **54** 11662–5
[39] Peters C, Hoop M, Pane S, Nelson B J and Hierold C 2016 Degradable magnetic composites for minimally invasive interventions: device fabrication, targeted drug delivery, and cytotoxicity tests *Adv. Mater.* **28** 533–8
[40] Medina-Sanchez M, Schwarz L, Meyer A K, Hebenstreit F and Schmidt O G 2016 Cellular cargo delivery: toward assisted fertilization by sperm-carrying micromotors *Nano Lett.* **16** 555–61
[41] Katuri J, Ma X, Stanton M M and Sanchez S 2017 Designing micro- and nano swimmers for specific applications *Acc. Chem. Res.* **50** 2–11
[42] Sindhu R K, Kaur H, Kumar M, Sofat M, Yapar E A and Esenturk I 2021 The ameliorating approach of nanorobotics in the novel drug delivery systems: a mechanistic review *J. Drug. Target.* **29** 822–33
[43] Wang W and Zhou C 2021 A journey of nanomotors for targeted cancer therapy: principles, challenges, and a critical review of the state-of-the-art *Adv. Healthc. Mater.* **10** e2001236
[44] Zhang D, Liu S, Guan J and Mou F 2022 Motile-targeting drug delivery platforms based on micro/nanorobots for tumor therapy *Front. Bioeng. Biotechnol.* **10** 1002171
[45] Qiu F, Mhanna R, Zhang L, Ding Y, Fujita S and Nelson B J 2014 Artificial bacterial flagella functionalized with temperature-sensitive liposomes for controlled release *Sens. Actuators B Chem.* **196** 676–81
[46] Jang B, Gutman E, Stucki N, Seitz B F, Wendel-Garcia P D and Newton T 2015 Undulatory locomotion of magnetic multilink nano swimmers *Nano Lett.* **15** 4829–33
[47] Gao W, Sattayasamitsathit S, Manesh K M, Weihs D and Wang J 2010 Magnetically powered flexible metal nanowire motors *J. Am. Chem. Soc.* **132** 14403–5
[48] Li T, Li J, Zhang H, Chang X, Song W and Hu Y 2016 Magnetically propelled fish-like nano swimmers *Small* **12** 6098–105
[49] Gutman E and Or Y 2016 Optimizing undulating magnetic microswimmers for cargo towing *Phys. Rev.* E **93** 063105
[50] Xu H, Medina-Sanchez M, Magdanz V, Schwarz L, Hebenstreit F and Schmidt O G 2018 Sperm-hybrid micromotor for targeted drug delivery *ACS Nano* **12** 327–37
[51] Alcanzare M M, Karttunen M and Ala-Nissila T 2019 Propulsion and controlled steering of magnetic nano helices *Soft Matter* **15** 1684–91

[52] Song X, Qian R, Li T, Fu W, Fang L and Cai Y 2022 Imaging-guided biomimetic M1 macrophage membrane-camouflaged magnetic nanorobots for photothermal immunotarget Ing cancer therapy *ACS Appl. Mater. Interfaces* **14** 56548–59
[53] Gong D, Celi N, Zhang D and Cai J 2022 Magnetic biohybrid microrobot multimers based on chlorella cells for enhanced targeted drug delivery *ACS Appl. Mater. Interfaces* **14** 6320–30
[54] Andhari S S, Wavhale R D, Dhobale K D, Tawade B V, Chate G P and Patil Y N 2020 Self-propelling targeted magneto-nanobots for deep tumor penetration and Ph-responsive intracellular drug delivery *Sci. Rep.* **10** 4703
[55] Gao W, Kagan D, Pak O S, Clawson C, Campuzano S and Chuluun-Erdene E *et al* 2012 Cargo-towing fuel-free magnetic nano swimmers for targeted drug delivery *Small* **8** 460–7
[56] Sun M, Fan X, Meng X, Song J, Chen W and Sun L 2019 Magnetic biohybrid micromotors with high maneuverability for efficient drug loading and targeted drug delivery *Nanoscale* **11** 18382–92
[57] Hu M, Ge X, Chen X, Mao W, Qian X and Yuan W E 2020 Micro/nanorobot: a promising targeted drug delivery system *Pharmaceutics* **12** 665
[58] Yu H, Tang W, Mu G, Wang H, Chang X and Dong H Micro-/nanorobots are propelled by oscillating magnetic fields *Micromachines* **9** 540
[59] Felfoul O, Mohammadi M, Taherkhani S, de Lanauze D, Zhong Xu Y and Loghin D 2016 Magneto-aerotactic bacteria deliver drug-containing nanoliposomes to tumor-hypoxic regions *Nat. Nanotechnol.* **11** 941–7
[60] Basta G, Venneri L, Lazzerini G, Pasanisi E, Pianelli M and Vesentini N 2003 *In vitro* modulation of intracellular oxidative stress of endothelial cells by diagnostic cardiac ultrasound *Cardiovasc. Res.* **58** 156–61
[61] Kagan D, Benchimol M J, Claussen J C, Chuluun-Erdene E, Esener S and Wang J 2012 Acoustic droplet vaporization and propulsion of perfluorocarbon-loaded micro bullets for targeted tissue penetration and deformation *Angew. Chem. Int. Ed. Engl.* **51** 7519–22
[62] Garcia-Gradilla V, Sattayasamitsathit S, Soto F, Kuralay F, Yardimci C and Wiitala D 2014 Ultrasound-propelled nanoporous gold wire for efficient drug loading and release *Small* **10** 4154–9
[63] de Esteban-Fernandez A B, Angsantikul P, Ramirez-Herrera D E, Soto F, Teymourian H and Dehaini D 2018 Hybrid biomembranes-functionalized nanorobots for concurrent removal of pathogenic bacteria and toxins *Sci. Robot.* **3** 0485
[64] Wu Z, Wu Y, He W, Lin X, Sun J and He Q 2013 Self-propelled polymer-based multilayer nano rockets for transportation and drug release *Angew. Chem. Int. Ed. Engl.* **52** 7000–3
[65] Li J, Li T, Xu T, Kiristi M, Liu W and Wu Z 2015 Magneto-acoustic hybrid nanomotor *Nano Lett.* **15** 4814–21
[66] Chen X Z, Hoop M, Shamsudhin N, Huang T, Özkale B and Li Q 2017 Hybrid magnetoelectric nanowires for nanorobotic applications: fabrication, magnetoelectric coupling, and magnetically assisted *in vitro* targeted drug delivery *Adv. Mater.* **29** 1605458
[67] Garcia-Gradilla V, Orozco J, Sattayasamitsathit S, Soto F, Kuralay F and Pourazary A 2013 Functionalized ultrasound-propelled magnetically guided nanomotors: toward practical biomedical applications *ACS Nano* **7** 9232–40
[68] Li Z, Hu Y, Howard K A, Jiang T, Fan X and Miao Z 2016 Multifunctional bismuth selenide nanocomposites for antitumor thermo-chemotherapy and imaging *ACS Nano* **10** 984–97
[69] Wang X, Cai J, Sun L, Zhang S, Gong D, Li X and Yue S 2019 Facile fabrication of magnetic microrobots based on spirulina templates for targeted delivery and synergistic chemo-photothermal therapy *ACS Appl. Mater. Interfaces* **11** 4745–56

[70] Beladi-Mousavi S M, Khezri B, Krejcova L, Heger Z, Sofer Z and Fisher A C 2019 Recoverable bismuth-based microrobots: capture, transport, and on-demand release of heavy metals and an anticancer drug in confined spaces *ACS Appl. Mater. Interfaces* **11** 13359–69
[71] Kong X, Gao P, Wang J, Fang Y and Hwang KC 2023 Advances of medical nanorobots for future cancer treatments *J. Hematol. Oncol.* **16** 74
[72] Khezri B, Beladi Mousavi S M, Krejčová L, Heger Z, Sofer Z and Pumera M 2019 Ultrafast electrochemical trigger drug delivery mechanism for nanographene micromachines *Adv. Funct. Mater.* **29** 1806696
[73] McGuire S 2016 World Cancer Report 2014 Geneva, Switzerland: World Health Organization, International Agency for Cancer Research, WHO Press *Adv. Nutr.* **7** 418–9
[74] Ali E S, Sharker S M, Islam M T, Khan I N, Shaw S and Rahman M 2021 A targeting cancer cells with nanotherapeutics and nano diagnostics: current status and future perspectives *Semin. Cancer Biol.* **69** 52–68
[75] Neuhouser T, L'Homme C, Beaulieu I, Mazurkiewicz S, Kuss S and Kraatz H B 2016 Ferrocene-modified phospholipid: an innovative precursor for redox-triggered drug delivery vesicles selective to cancer cells *Langmuir* **32** 4169–78
[76] Gullotti E and Yeo Y 2009 Extracellularly activated nanocarriers: a new paradigm of tumor-targeted drug delivery *Mol. Pharm.* **6** 1041–51
[77] Galvin P, Thompson D, Ryan K B, McCarthy A, Moore A C and Burke C S 2012 Nanoparticle-based drug delivery: case studies for cancer and cardiovascular applications *Cell. Mol. Life Sci.* **69** 389–404
[78] Balakrishnan D, Wilkens G D and Heddle J G 2019 Delivering DNA origami to cells *Nanomedicine* **14** 911–25
[79] Wicki A, Witzigmann D, Balasubramanian V and Huwyler J 2015 Nanomedicine in cancer therapy: challenges, opportunities, and clinical applications *J. Control. Release* **200** 138–57
[80] Ouyang C, Zhang S A-O, Xue CA-OX, Yu X, Xu H and Wang Z 2020 Precision-guided missile-like DNA nanostructure containing warhead and guidance control for aptamer-based targeted drug delivery into cancer cells *in vitro* and *in vivo* *J. Am. Chem. Soc.* **142** 1265–77
[81] Wang D, Peng Y, Deng Z, Tan Y, Su Y and Kuai H 2020 Modularly engineered solid-phase synthesis of aptamer-functionalized small molecule drugs for targeted cancer therapy *Adv. Ther.* **3** 2000074
[82] Bohunicky B and Mousa S A 2010 Biosensors: the new wave in cancer diagnosis *Nanotechnol. Sci. Appl.* **4** 1–10
[83] Erbas-Cakmak S, Leigh D A, McTernan C T and Nussbaumer A L 2015 Artificial molecular machines *Chem. Rev.* **115** 10081–206
[84] Zhang S, Wang K, Huang C, Li Z, Sun T and Han D M 2016 An enzyme-free and resettable platform for the construction of advanced molecular logic devices based on magnetic beads and DNA *Nanoscale* **8** 15681–8
[85] Meng H M, Liu H, Kuai H, Peng R, Mo L and Zhang X B 2016 Aptamer-integrated DNA nanostructures for biosensing, bioimaging, and cancer therapy *Chem. Soc. Rev.* **45** 2583–602
[86] Nehru S, Misra R and Bhaswant M 2022 Multifaceted engineered biomimetic nanorobots toward cancer management *ACS Biomater. Sci. Eng.* **8** 444–59
[87] Liu L, He H and Liu J 2019 Advances on non-genetic cell membrane engineering for biomedical applications *Polymers* **11** 2017

[88] Peng R, Zheng X, Liu Y, Xu L, Zhang X and Ke G 2018 Engineering a 3D DNA-logic gate nanomachine for bispecific recognition and computing on target cell surfaces *J. Am. Chem. Soc.* **140** 9793–6

[89] Ren K, Liu Y, Wu J, Zhang Y, Zhu J and Yang M 2016 A DNA dual lock-and-key strategy for cell-subtype-specific siRNA delivery *Nat. Commun.* **7** 13580

[90] Pedrero M, Gamella M and Serafín V 2022 Nanomachines and nanorobotics: improving cancer diagnosis and therapy *The Detection of Biomarkers* (London: Academic) 503–43

[91] Deng G, Peng X, Sun Z, Zheng W, Yu J and Du L 2020 Natural-killer-cell-inspired nanorobots with aggregation-induced emission characteristics for near-infrared-II fluorescence-guided glioma theranostics *ACS Nano* **14** 11452–62

[92] Shi S, Chen Y and Yao X Nga-inspired nanorobots-assisted detection of multifocal cancer *IEEE Trans. Cybern.* **52** 2787–97

[93] de Esteban-Fernandez A B, Angell C, Soto F, Lopez-Ramirez M A, Baez D F and Xie S 2016 Acoustically propelled nanomotors for intracellular siRNA delivery *ACS Nano* **10** 4997–5005

[94] Li S, Jiang Q, Ding B and Nie G 2019 Anticancer activities of tumor-killing nanorobots *Trends Biotechnol.* **37** 573–7

[95] Li S, Jiang Q, Liu S, Zhang Y, Tian Y and Song C A 2018 DNA nanorobot functions as a cancer therapeutic in response to a molecular trigger *in vivo Nat. Biotechnol.* **36** 258–64

[96] Li H, Liu J and Gu H 2019 Targeting nucleolin to obstruct vasculature feeding with an intelligent DNA nanorobot *J. Cell. Mol. Med.* **23** 2248–50

[97] Li Z, Di C, Li S, Yang X and Nie G 2019 Smart nanotherapeutic targeting of tumor vasculature *ACC. Chem. Res.* **52** 2703–12

[98] Zheng P P, Kros J M and Li J 2018 Approved car T cell therapies: ice bucket challenges on glaring safety risks and long-term impacts *Drug Discov. Today* **23** 1175–82

[99] Zheng P P, Kros J M and Wang G 2019 Elusive neurotoxicity in t cell-boosting anticancer therapies *Trends Immunol.* **40** 274–8

[100] Gill J H, Rockley K L, De Santis C and Mohamed A K 2019 Vascular disrupting agents in cancer treatment: cardiovascular toxicity and implications for co-administration with other cancer chemotherapeutics *Pharmacol. Ther.* **202** 18–31

[101] Zheng K, Kros J M, Li J and Zheng P P 2020 DNA-nanorobot-guided thrombin-inducing tumor infarction: raising new potential clinical concerns *Drug Discov. Today* **25** 951–5

[102] Liang W, Ni Y and Chen F 2016 Tumor resistance to vascular disrupting agents: mechanisms, imaging, and solutions *Oncotarget* **7** 15444–59

[103] Seidi K, Jahanban-Esfahlan R and Zarghami N 2017 Tumor rim cells: from resistance to vascular targeting agents to complete tumor ablation *Tumour. Biol.* **39** 1010428317691001

[104] Close A 2016 Antiangiogenesis and vascular disrupting agents in cancer: circumventing resistance and augmenting their therapeutic utility *Future Med. Chem.* **8** 443–62

[105] Higdon M L, Atkinson C J and Lawrence K V 2018 Oncologic emergencies: recognition and initial management *Am. Fam. Phys.* **97** 741–8 PMID: 30215936

[106] Williams S M and Killeen A Tumor lysis syndrome *Arch. Pathol. Lab Med.* **143** 386–93

[107] Klemencic S and Perkins J 2019 Diagnosis and management of oncologic emergencies *West J. Emerg. Med.* **20** 316–22

[108] Aggarwal M and Kumar S 2022 The use of nanorobotics in the treatment therapy of cancer and its future aspects: a review *Cureus* **14** e29366

[109] Manzari M T, Shamay Y, Kiguchi H, Rosen N, Scaltriti M and Heller D A 2021 Targeted drug delivery strategies for precision medicines *Nat. Rev. Mater.* **6** 351–70

[110] Zhu Y, Song Y, Cao Z, Dong L, Shen S and Lu Y 2023 A magnetically driven amoeba-like nanorobot for whole-process active drug transport *Adv. Sci.* **10** e2204793

[111] Wang X, Law J, Luo M, Gong Z, Yu J and Tang W 2020 Magnetic measurement and stimulation of cellular and intracellular structures *ACS Nano* **14** 3805–21

[112] Venugopalan P L, Sai R, Chandorkar Y, Basu B, Shivashankar S and Ghosh A 2014 Conformal cytocompatible ferrite coatings facilitate the realization of a nanovoyager in human blood *Nano Lett.* **14** 1968–75

[113] Lazarovits J, Chen Y Y, Sykes E A and Chan W C 2015 Nanoparticle-blood interactions: the implications on solid tumor targeting *Chem. Commun.* **51** 2756–67

[114] Zhao G, Viehrig M and Pumera M 2013 Challenges of the movement of catalytic micromotors in blood *Lab Chip* **13** 1930–6

[115] Zhang X, Liu N, Zhou M, Zhang T, Tian T and Li S 2019 DNA nanorobot delivers antisense oligonucleotides silencing C-Met gene expression for cancer therapy *J. Biomed. Nanotechnol.* **15** 1948–59

[116] Vujačić Nikezić A and Grbović Novaković J 2022 Nano/microcarriers in drug delivery: moving the timeline to contemporary *Curr. Med. Chem.* **30** 2996–3023

[117] Lai X, Jiang H and Wang X 2021 Biodegradable metal-organic frameworks for multimodal imaging and targeting theranostics *Biosensors* **11** 299

[118] Sohrabi Kashani A and Packirisamy M 2021 Cancer-nano-interaction: from cellular uptake to mechanobiological responses *Int. J. Mol. Sci.* **22** 9587

[119] Youden B, Jiang R, Carrier A J, Servos M R and Zhang X 2022 A nanomedicine structure-activity framework for research, development, and regulation of future cancer therapies *ACS Nano* **16** 17497–551

[120] Ullah R, Wazir J, Khan F U, Diallo M T, Ihsan A U and Mikrani R 2020 Factors influencing the delivery efficiency of cancer nanomedicines *AAPS PharmSciTech* **21** 132

[121] Germain M, Caputo F, Metcalfe S, Tosi G, Spring K and Åslund A K O 2020 Delivering the power of nanomedicine to patients today *J. Control Release Off. J. Control Release Soc.* **326** 164–71

[122] Koo K M, Mainwaring P N, Tomlins S A and Trau M 2019 Merging new-age biomarkers and nano diagnostics for precision prostate cancer management *Nat. Rev. Urol.* **16** 302–17

[123] Fu S, Li G, Zang W, Zhou X, Shi K and Zhai Y 2022 Pure drug nano-assemblies: a facile carrier-free nano platform for efficient cancer therapy *Acta Pharm. Sin.* B **12** 92–106

[124] Clack K, Soda N, Kasetsirikul S, Mahmudunnabi R G, Nguyen N T and Shiddiky M J A 2023 Toward personalized nanomedicine: the critical evaluation of micro and nanodevices for cancer biomarker analysis in liquid biopsy *Small* **19** e2205856

[125] Tyagi P and Subramony J A 2018 Nanotherapeutics in oral and parenteral drug delivery: key learnings and future outlooks as we think small *J. Control Release Off. J. Control Release Soc.* **272** 159–68

[126] Betz U A, Arora L, Assal R A, Azevedo H, Baldwin J, Becker M S and Zhao G 2023 Game changers in science and technology and beyond *Technol. Forecast. Soc. Change* **193** 122588

[127] Shen L, Wang P and Ke Y 2021 DNA nanotechnology-based biosensors and therapeutics *Adv. Healthcare Mater.* **10** e2002205

[128] Hu Q, Li H, Wang L, Gu H and Fan C 2018 DNA nanotechnology-enabled drug delivery systems *Chem. Rev.* **119** 6459–506

Rishabha Malviya, Deepika Yadav, Sonali Sundram, Seifedine Kadry and Gurvinder Singh Virk

Chapter 5

Magnetomechanical systems at the micro/nanoscale for cancer management

The aim of this chapter is to explore the potential applications of magnetomechanical robotic systems in cancer management. Magnetic nanoparticles (MNs) are being explored in sustainable development and healthcare engineering for applications in cancer diagnosis and therapy. They help to guide iron oxide transporters in tumor tissues, producing magnetic resonance (MR) signals for medical image processing. Magnetite (Fe_3O_4) MNs play a crucial role in tumor development, leading to oxidative stress. The magnetomechanical effect, which involves the application of magnetic forces to cells, may improve cancer diagnosis and therapy. Iron-oxide-based nanoparticles (IONPs) with magnetic characteristics are used in medical procedures as contrast materials and for iron supplementation.

5.1 Introduction

The utilization of MNs is increasingly being explored in the fields of sustainable development and healthcare engineering. The use of iron oxide MNs has extended well beyond recycling, ranging from cancer diagnosis to therapy [1]. The utilization of external magnetic fields, either fixed or alternating, in actively targeted delivery systems facilitates the precise guidance of iron oxide transporters. This approach enables MNs to accumulate in tumor tissues, which results in the production of MR signals. MNs can thus be used as contrast materials in medical image processing [2].

In the intricate web that connects iron and tumor development, magnetite (Fe_3O_4) MNs may prove to be of crucial importance. Although iron is required by all healthy cells, an excess of this element may be harmful. Fortunately, regulatory mechanisms keep the body in balance and prevent iron from becoming too unstable. The occurrence of cancer is associated with an elevation in the labile iron pool, leading to heightened oxidative stress due to the substantial iron demand imposed by tumor cells throughout their proliferation, expansion, and viability [3].

doi:10.1088/978-0-7503-6019-7ch5

Cancer cells may use redox signaling and oxidative stress to initiate the cell cycle and promote tumor development [4].

The magnetomechanical effect pertains to the effects of magnetic fields on MNs present in biological fluids, which results in the application of magnetic forces to cells [5, 6]. Recent investigations have prompted the utilization of specific MNs in rotating electromagnetic fields operating at an oscillation frequency of 100 Hz. Such fields initiate magnetomechanical phenomena, resulting in the perturbation of the cellular membranes and consequent facilitation of malignant cell apoptosis. The process by which tumors are killed is determined by the forces exerted on various cellular components, such as the cellular components surrounding the barrier, the nuclear envelope, the cytoskeleton, the nucleolus, and the cytoplasmic compartment, The utilization of magnetic targeting presents a potential avenue for the transportation of MNs to specific areas within the tumor and its surroundings [7]. Furthermore, MNs have magnetochemical properties in addition to the mechanical stresses they induce in their environments [8, 9].

The utilization of static electromagnetic fields in isolation is a prevalent method for the delivery of MNs and the regulation of tumor growth. Nevertheless, it is likely that the presence of an unmovable magnetic field in addition to the presence of MNs inside the tumor play an integral part in the formation of heterogeneous tissues through magnetomechanical mechanisms. Tumor cells demonstrate an increase in the activation of catenin signaling channels as a result of physiological stress [10, 11]. Static magnetic fields have been shown to cause iron oxide MNs to release reactive oxygen species (ROS) inside cells [12, 13]. Oxidative stress syndrome is widely recognized as a prominent factor in the pathogenesis of carcinoma of the breast. There has been an increased emphasis on the advancement of redox-focused methodologies in the management of carcinoma of the breast [14]. The presence of diverse redox signaling mechanisms contributes to the advancement and adaptability of tumors. Furthermore, the topic of controlling the generation and communication of iron-dependent ROS in the context of tumor uniqueness has been raised as a result of the contrasting attributes of ROS. The reconstitution rates of reactive oxygen species and the cellular redox state can be influenced by inhomogeneous static magnetic fields (ISMFs) due to a significant variation in the strength of the magnetic field gradient caused by the amount of space between electrons in radical pairs [15].

Tumors exhibit a higher susceptibility to the influence of ISMFs than that of normal cells, which leads to the propagation of malignancies by the subsequent transmission of mechanical and chemical communications [16]. The ability of a cell to divide is impacted by mechanical strains, which induce changes in intracellular tension, morphology, tumor growth factor signaling, and the matrix of extracellular protein (a complex of intervening proteins that offers morphological and pharmacological support). The impartment of mechanical stresses to the surrounding environment occurs as a consequence of the stimulation of several different cell types, including fibroblasts, smooth muscle cells, tumor-associated macrophages, and red blood cells, among others [17]. Prior research has linked mechanical force, namely interstitial or hyperproliferative pressure, to increased tumor development.

It is during necrosis that interactions between the tumor and its surroundings lead to neoangiogenesis [18, 19]. The volume of solid tumors is a clear indicator of the extent of necrosis [20, 21]. Overall, oxidative stress caused by mechanical means may promote cell proliferation and tumor development [10, 22, 23].

Clinical results for cancer diagnosis and therapy may be improved by magnetically targeting the delivery of MNs to the tumor location. The ability of magneto-mechanical effects to regulate ROS and tumor development *in vivo* is, however, still open to debate. One study aimed to examine the magnetomechanical impacts of magnetite nanoparticles and an alternating magnetic field (AMF), referred to as an isometric electromagnetic stimulation field (ISMF), on Walker-256 carcinosarcoma, which serves as a laboratory animal model for preclinical women's mammary gland malignancy [24].

IONPs have recently attracted researchers' attention due to their potential use in cancer prevention and treatment. This interest stems from the favorable characteristics of IONPs, such as their minimal toxicity and high biocompatibility in human subjects [1]. In the field of nanomedicine, the last few decades have seen the development of a broad variety of IONPs with carefully controlled dimensions, chemical makeups, and functionalities. These nanoparticles have been utilized in medical procedures for two main purposes: (i) as a contrast material for MRI scans or magnetic resonance imaging, and (ii) as a nutritional iron supplement to address anemia caused by inadequate iron consumption [2, 3]. IONPs can be used for a wide variety of medical applications, including but not limited to malignant cell elimination via magnetized high temperatures, regulated medication release, neurological stimulation, gene transcription, induction procedures, and disturbance of the matrix that surrounds cells inside the tumor environment. This involves subjecting the IONPs to a high-frequency alternating magnetic field, which results in the generation of heat and subsequent development of magnetic hyperthermia. This technique has seen a lot of attention from researchers over the last few decades, and the underlying science behind this potentially game-changing cancer therapy has been considerably developed [12–14]. The utilization of IONPs inside a charged field that alternates direction at a fast rate presents a promising approach for achieving remote control and manipulation. Consequently, the technique holds significant appeal as a potential method of tumor ablation within deep tissues. Nevertheless, the implementation of this innovation necessitates the utilization of electromagnetic fields spanning frequencies that range from tens of kilohertz to megahertz. This, in turn, induces the generation of eddy currents inside unaffected tissues, potentially leading to patient discomfort and significant ramifications. The application of loops and cores with magnetic properties on a considerable scale poses an operational obstacle owing to the substantial thermal effects they encounter when subjected to high-frequency signals and electromagnetic fields [15]. Hence, a smaller number of research studies have been conducted employing an electromagnetic field distinguished by a relatively low frequency of 100 kHz and a magnitude of 20 mT. These tests have identified several constraints, including the unequal dispersion of heat within the tumor due to the diffusion of heat into surrounding tissues [16, 17].

IONPs generate mechanical strain and torques when exposed to low-frequency magnetic fields. These forces are then transmitted to any object that interacts with the IONPs. Molecular manipulation, drug release stimulation, protein degradation induction, enzyme activation, and the destruction of cancer cells can all be achieved through the application of such torques [18–24]. It may even be possible to avoid using invasive intratumoral injections due to the IONPs' confirmed ability to target cancers *in vitro* and *in vivo* that overexpress surface receptors [25, 26]. The potential for this novel method to address the issues with magnetic hyperthermia outlined above is exciting news for the field of IONP-based anticancer treatment. Numerous studies have demonstrated that the apoptosis of cancerous cells can be induced by subjecting micrometric disks, spheres, or wires to low-frequency opposing or revolving magnetic fields (RMFs) [27–30]. The exposure of IONPs to either AMFs or RMFs has been shown to kill cancer cells in several studies [31]. Nevertheless, these studies did not conduct rigorous theoretical and experimental research to determine the optimum features of a magnetic field, including its type, magnitude, and timescale; all of these are important factors to consider in studying this phenomenon that can generate torque and hence cause cell damage.

A tumor's defenses may be divided into many distinct categories. Another contributory aspect is the tumor microenvironment, which creates a conducive environment for the proliferation of tumor cells and hinders the infiltration and dissemination of chemotherapy medications. The tumor microenvironment is influenced by various important factors, one of which is the presence of cancer-associated fibroblasts (CAFs). CAFs perform a crucial function in the surroundings by proactively taking part in the formation of a framework called the extracellular matrix (ECM). This is achieved through the generation and secretion of many ECM proteins, including type I and type III collagen [28]. Furthermore, it is imperative to acknowledge the significant contribution of CAFs in promoting the advancement of tumors and bestowing resistance to conventional cancer prevention therapies in cases of pancreatic malignancy. This is achieved through the secretion of several chemicals, including hormones, growth factors, and chemokines, into the extracellular environment [29]. The utilization of nano-agents for the therapeutic targeting of CAFs represents a promising and innovative approach in contrast to conventional research focused on cancer cells. This strategy, known as precision monotherapy, aims to deliver nanoparticles directly to the tumor site for effective cancer treatment.

This chapter discusses a strategy that aims to eradicate CAFs using magneto-mechanical annihilation provided from a remote location [29]. Although it is anticipated that the pressures induced by ultrasmall MNPs are insufficient to cause cell membrane rupture, this study illustrates the possibility of achieving the desired outcome by employing nanoparticles as small as 6 nm. By employing advanced magnetic simulations, researchers have elucidated the observed phenomenon and its correlation with the magnetic field; these studies thus contribute significantly to our understanding of the intricate processes involved in the apoptosis of cells. The findings of these studies demonstrate significant potential, suggesting that the utilization of ultrasmall nanoparticles that specifically target lysosomes could be

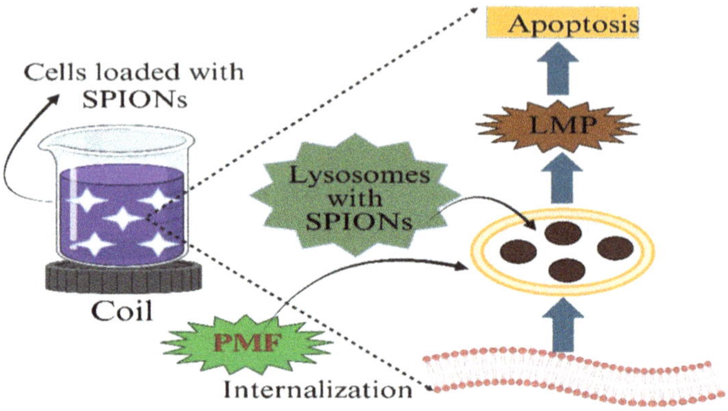

Figure 5.1. The method of use of emerging oncology nucleic acids (SIONPs) that have been documented as exhibiting encouraging potential in the field of cancer therapy.

employed to induce cell death using distant magnetomechanical means. This mechanism involves the disruption of lysosomes, so the study introduces a novel and pioneering therapeutic approach for addressing carcinogenic conditions. Figure 5.1 illustrates the emerging oncology nucleic acids (iron-oxide nanoparticles; IONPs) that have been reported to have promising new applications in cancer treatment.

5.2 Cancer therapy using magnetomechanical particles

5.2.1 Principle

This approach uses low-frequency magnetic particle vibrations to kill cancer cells or tumors while sparing nearby healthy cells. This approach is specific and safe because it induces physical qualities that match cancer cell and tissue species patterns. As in the cases of chemotherapies and targeted therapeutics, the species physics of the dysregulation of cancer cells explains how certain mechanical parameters affect cancer cells. This new method demands interdisciplinary skills. This chapter provides an overview of various types of therapeutic approach that involve the use of magnetic energy. The terms included within this category are magneto lysis, magnetomechanical actuation or stimulation for therapeutic therapy, magneto-actuation, the stimulation of cellular death without the use of chemotherapeutic agents, mechanical destruction of tumors, nonthermal implications, and vibrations or oscillations of magnetic particles. This therapeutic modality entails the administration of a nonthermal electromagnetic field which may exhibit rotational or alternating characteristics at low intensities. The implementation of electromagnetic stimulation and the subsequent mechanical response of particles on intracellular entities are both included in the therapeutic process known as the magnetomechanical effect of particles (treatment by magneto-mechanical effect of particle; TMMEP) approach [20].

The fundamental principle underlying the magnetomechanical effect referred to as TMMEP involves the utilization of the magnetomechanical phenomenon to induce the remote activation of magnetic materials in various arrangements [7, 20]. The average force of magnetism *M* acting on the particles, which is reliant on the strength and direction of the applied magnetic field *B*, creates a magnetic torque $M \times B$ and moves the particles toward alignment with the field when the uniformly applied magnetic field *B* penetrates the whole volume of the particles. When the magnetic anisotropy of a particle is sufficiently strong, it demonstrates significant dependency on particle composition, size, and shape. As a result, the magnetic moment *M* within the particle is predominantly aligned either (i) parallel to the axis of magnetization that offers the least resistance or (ii) within the surface of magnetization that offers the least resistance. Magnetomechanical forces exert their influence on particles that can move freely or are partially enveloped by fluids. The particle undergoes a process of reorientation in which its major axis or simple planes become aligned with the magnetic gradient that is being applied. This is similar to the way in which a compass needle becomes aligned with the electromagnetic field of the Earth. Therefore, TMMEP particles undergo rotation or vibration when subjected to homogenous rotating magnetic fields. Techniques that require the efficient application of magnetic torque necessitate the use of highly anisotropic particles, such as magnetic disks exhibiting either 'magnetic shape anisotropy' with a value of 24 or 'perpendicular magnetic anisotropy' [7, 20]. When exposed to an oscillating magnetic field, the particles transfer mechanical energy to biological cells, fluids, and tissues. The rotational or vibrational motion of particles is constrained to a narrow range of frequencies, often on the order of tens of hertz, due to the viscosity of the fluid. Conversely, mechanical vibrations experience a significant reduction in amplitude as the frequency increases. The morphological characteristics of the cellular environment can influence the efficacy of the treatment strategy. Nanoparticles subjected to a nonuniform magnetic field, specifically an electromagnetic gradient that is nonzero, experience magnetic forces that cause them to move towards regions with higher field amplitudes. These forces have the potential to guide particles toward certain naturally occurring regions [28]. The gradient of a nonuniform magnetic field may generate particle oscillations via temporal fluctuations in the field gradient, although this is less effective than the torque effect.

5.3 The magnetomechanical identification of telomerase and nuclear acids in cancerous cells

Considerable research efforts have been devoted to enhancing techniques for the recognition of nucleic acids. Enzymes have been utilized to facilitate genetic material recognition procedures that occurred on electrodes, leading to an enhanced and resilient electrical output for genetic material detection. The recognition procedures for the genetic material were facilitated through the utilization of biocatalytic amplifiers and electrochemical or photonic readout. Such amplifiers can stimulate ROS enzymes, which in turn precipitate an insoluble product on the electrode, or digestive enzymes that electrically generate chemical luminescence following genetic material hybridization [29]. The application of metallic or semiconductor nanoparticles customized with nucleic acids has led to an enhancement in DNA analysis

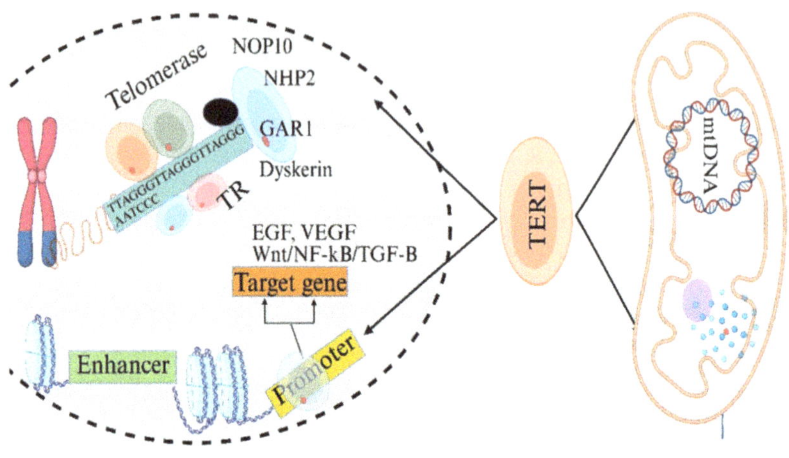

Figure 5.2. Modified cantilevers utilized for research, including the utilization of magnetomechanical techniques for identifying the presence of genetic material, the study of single-base mismatches within genetic material, and the identification of telomerase activity, specifically that of cancer cells.

through electronic transduction. The detection of genetically modified material using a microgravimetric quartz crystalline microbalance or electrical strategies was made possible by employing electroless catalysts that deposited metallic substances on micron-sized particles. A voltammetric assessment of the resultant ions could potentially be carried out by dissolving the metal or semiconductor nanomaterials. An augmentation in the recognition of genetic material was reported to take place as a result of incorporating specific materials, which included biotin labeled during digestion or redox-active components, within the procedure used to replicate the nucleic acid sequence under examination. The electrochemical identification of the pertinent genetic material was improved by activating additional biocatalytic mechanisms, which resulted in the precipitation of byproducts on electrodes or the activation of oxidative enzymes. In recent years, there has been a growing utilization of active matrices composed of magnetic particles functionalized with nucleic acids for DNA recombination and labeling. DNA amplification has been accomplished by rotating magnetic particles, utilizing the transmission capability of electrogenerated chemical luminescence [30]. The rotation of magnetic particles in this system facilitated the regulation of electrogenerated chemiluminescence through the generation of convection currents.

The production and insertion of microsatellite repetitions into the 3′ end of the chromosomal nucleotide has been carried out by the telomerase enzyme, which is a ribonucleoprotein complex [31]. Figure 5.2 illustrates the interest in the utilization of magnetomechanical methods for the detection of cancer cell nucleic acids and telomerase. The chromosomes' telomeres prevent them from being eroded too far in a cell and serve as a signal of when a cell's life cycle should finish. Cells with telomerase are protected from telomere degradation, making them eternal [13]. The presence of telomerase has been observed in nearly all cancer cells, and there is conclusive evidence linking the activities of telomerase to malignancy [32].

Numerous analytical approaches have been used to quantify and evaluate telomerase activity [15, 16]. To advance the field of biosensing, it will be imperative to develop miniature sensing devices at the nanoscale level and establish the capability to effectively process and analyze samples with low volumes. The investigation of recognition events at the molecular level involves the measurement of force interactions between antigen–antibody complexes or double-stranded DNA, as exemplified by previous studies [17, 18]. According to a separate study, the incorporation of functionalized nano-elements within pliable biomaterials, such as carbon nanotubes, has the potential to enable the detection of distinctive interactions between biomolecules; examples include biotin and avidin, or antigens and antibodies [19]. Cantilevers, which possess the ability to undergo chemical modifications and enable the optical monitoring of nanometric deflections, exhibit considerable potential as mechanical sensors [20]. According to certain studies, it has been proposed that the mechanical deflection of cantilevers can be attributed to stress interactions occurring on their surfaces. One illustrative instance involves the assertion that a slender polyaniline film, when combined with a lever, has the potential to operate as a mechanically reversible electrochemical device [21]. The phenomenon of polymeric film oxidization initiates electrostatic repulsion between the polymeric chains, leading to mechanical stress on the cantilever and consequent deformation of the cantilevered framework. Upon the reduction of the oxidized polymer, the surface tension is reduced and the lever reverts to its initial position. The phenomenon of cantilever mechanical deflection has been reported to be influenced by biorecognition events, such as the binding processes of antibody–antigen interactions or nucleic acid–DNA interactions. Prior study has indicated that electrostatic repulsion between surface-hybridized DNA fragments can result in the production of surface stress, subsequently leading to the electromechanical deflection of a lever [17]. The deflection of a cantilever may be influenced by the application of a magnetic field within its environment; a lever covered with magnetized particles experiences an impact. The utilization of magnetized particles affixed to a cantilever has facilitated the development of a sensor that exhibits unparalleled sensitivity toward magnetic fields [17]. The deflection of a cantilever has the potential to detect magnetic field variations as small as 10 nT [32]. It is feasible to improve the magnetomechanical detection of biorecognition operations, given the widespread use of particles with magnetic properties as a sustaining mechanism for biological sensing protocols. The applications of cantilevers have been changed by the use of functionalized magnetic particles. Such altered cantilevered structures are employed for the magnetomechanical recognition of genetic material, the study of single-base abnormalities in genetic material, and the recognition of telomerase activity within cancerous cells.

5.4 The therapeutic applications of telomerase studies in cancer

To prevent the occurrence and accumulation of harmful genetic defects, somatic superior eukaryotic cells have a limited capacity for reproduction; after a particular number of sections, they undergo senescence and eventually die [33]. Nevertheless, circumventing these protective measures frequently leads to the development of cells that possess enhanced abilities to proliferate and evade signals that inhibit growth and induce cell death. Several of these traits are defining features of cancer, which encompass mechanisms that aid in the spread of cancer cells of cancer cells and regulate the alteration of local immunological and angiogenic microenvironments [34]. The attainment of replicative permanence is an essential prerequisite for the propagation of the genetic abnormalities that promote tumor growth. Consequently, genomic instability might be regarded as a potential origin for several other distinctive features of cancer. Telomeres, which are the terminating components that can be identified on longitudinal chromosomes, play an important part in the aging process of cells and are critical components that determine the capacity of cells to replicate themselves [35, 36]. Cells that experience disrupted telomere homeostasis are thus granted replicative immortality [37]. Telomeres and their related variables have been implicated in a range of cellular events, including genetic instability [6, 7], perpetuated proliferation signaling [8, 9], the evasion of differentiation suppressor genes, susceptibility to cell death, the induction of angiogenesis, the regulation of the immune system, and the stimulation of metastatic growth and invasion, among other processes [10–15]. The structural characteristics and regulatory processes that safeguard telomeres play a significant role in determining their flexibility in operation.

Telomeres, being nucleoprotein frameworks, are comprised of sequential repetitions of nucleotides. In human beings, they have a mean length of around 10 kb [38]. In addition, an indispensable complex of proteins called shelterin, consisting of six distinct components, is associated with telomeres [39]. The inclusion of shelterin-bound chromosomes serves to resolve the challenges that arise during the organization of the genetic material in chromosomes with linear structures that undergo interrupted replication. The end-replication dilemma pertains to the progressive loss of genetic material that arises throughout the replication procedure for DNA as a result of unbalanced replication among multiple strands of DNA [40]. In addition, the end-protection problem involves the detection of unprotected chromosomal ends such as double-strand breakages (DSBs) and the subsequent occurrence of errors. Following the sequential procedure for shelterin assembly, the initial binding of the double-strand telomere DNA is facilitated by the homodimers of telomeric repeat-binding factors 1 and 2 (TRF1 and TRF2). The TRF1 protein plays a pivotal function in the process of DNA replication by promoting and enhancing the procedure of replication, specifically in G-rich telomeric regions [41]. Furthermore, the binding of TRF1 and TRF2 serves as a protective mechanism that prevents unauthorized DNA repair from occurring by inhibiting the detection of DNA damage at the ends of chromosomes [42]. In addition, it promotes the creation of telomere loops (t-loops), which conceal the required presence of 3′ single-strand telomerase extensions that have been seen in triplex genetic material constructions [39]. The amino acid designated as 'protection of telomeres 1' (POT1) operates as an antibody that binds to single-stranded DNA (ssDNA). The main function of this entity is to protect ssDNA found at telomeres by inhibiting the activation of the DNA damage response (DDR). This protective function is achieved by an interaction with the TPP1 component of the shelterin complex. Through this interaction, POT1 effectively hinders the activity of many DNA repair pathways. The POT1 protein plays a crucial role in the coordination of nucleolytic end-processing of chromosomes following DNA replication [40]. Upon encountering telomeric repeat sequences, TRF1 and TRF2 play a crucial role in recruiting other shelterin components. These components include POT1-TPP1, TIN2, and RAP1, as documented in previous studies [30, 31]. In addition, the binding of shelterin regulates the recruitment of several components involved with telomeres. The exonuclease Apollo, known for its role in processing telomere strand extensions, has been observed to have a role in the inhibition of aberrant recombination-based genetic material repair procedures [34, 35], This function is carried out in conjunction with NBS1 and Ku70/Ku80, forming an aggregate mechanism that detects DSBs and facilitates enzymatic DSB repair. NBS1, Ku70/Ku80, and TERB1/TERB2 [32, 33] are all instances of alternative proteins that bind to double-stranded DNA at telomeres. The histone proteins that establish distinct topologies on telomeric chromatin [42–47] or that serve as constituents of enzyme complexes involved in telomere processing [48] contribute to the characterization of the proteome landscape associated with telomeres. Shelterin, along with other telomere-binding proteins, facilitates processes that regulate telomere homeostasis by addressing challenges related to end-replication and end-protection.

Telomeres serve as a protective mechanism against chromosomal attrition, safeguarding genetic material during the processes of DNA recombination and cell division. Therefore, telomeres have the potential to address the challenge of terminating the replication procedure through the utilization of telomeres, which are specialized DNA sequences that protect the ends of chromosomes. Telomere-maintaining mechanisms (TMMs) play a crucial role in ensuring the accurate and complete replication of genetic material and the manufacture of additional telomerase repetitions. Telomeres undergo dynamic elongation during early embryonic growth, in postpartum germinal cells, and in embryonic stem cell populations. However, in many other kinds of cells, telomeres are not sustained [49–51]. However, if the telomere length in cancerous cells reaches a critically short level (with an average telomere measuring 12.8 repeats in length [52], a state known as telomere crisis), the reactivation of the TMM takes place. This reactivation leads to the occurrence of genomic unpredictability and enhances the dissemination of DNA damage lesions, thereby promoting the development of cancer [53–55]. It is noteworthy that a considerable number of cancerous growths exhibit telomeres that are regularly preserved at or near their essential length [56, 57]. This observation implies that the components responsible for telomerase homeostasis act in conjunction with DDR proteins to prevent apoptosis resulting from telomere crisis. Therefore, the processes of telomere reduction and telomere extension are both of the utmost importance in the context of telomerase-dependent malignancies. At present, two further distinct methodologies are employed for telomere elongation: the telomerase pathway and the other lengthened telomeres pathway. The process of the Ranas-dependent synthesis of DNA necessitates the presence of templates. Telomerase, a ribonucleoprotein (RNP), consists of a core dimer that includes a reverse transcriptase (RT) protein component known as telomerase reverse transcriptase (TERT), as well as an RNA-based component referred to as TR or telomerase RNA component (TERC) [48]. On the other hand, it should be noted that the alternative lengthening of telomeres (ALT) bears a resemblance to break-induced replication (BIR) in terms of its utilization of homology recombination-mediated invasions of neighboring telomeres to commence the template-based synthesis of DNA [58]. The enzymatic process known as the telomerase mechanism is commonly utilized by a significant proportion of cancerous cells to extend the length of telomeres. The cooperative interaction between the cellular components of telomerase transcription and shelterin, as well as other crucial telomere-binding proteins, plays a substantial role in modulating the replicative and protective capabilities of telomeres. In addition, telomerase exhibits multiple extratelomeric activities that are not dependent on telomeres. These activities have implications for telomere homeostasis, signal transduction, cellular energy regulation, and the control of gene expression through transcriptional mechanisms [59]. In this study, researchers investigated the mechanisms by which telomerase is associated with malignancy hallmarks, focusing on both telomeric and extratelomeric activities. In addition, the investigators provided a comprehensive analysis of the mechanisms that govern the synthesis, assembly, and functionality of telomeres. These fundamental understandings may potentially contribute to the development of cancer treatments that target telomeres.

5.5 The clinical applications of telomeres and telomerase in oncology

Although significant mechanistic knowledge has been gained from molecular examinations of telomerase, further study is required to effectively translate these results into therapeutic applications. The investigation of the mechanisms by which malignancies sustain the length of their telomeres is a promising avenue for enhancing cancer detection, prognosis, and treatment strategies. In biopsies, the telomeres of tumor cells are typically observed to be shorter in comparison to the telomeres of their corresponding normally developing counterparts [60]. A wide variety of malignant subtypes demonstrate a beneficial relationship between telomere length and disease stage, even though an inverse association has also been noted in certain instances [61–63]. This implies that the association between telomere length and the advancement of disease is more complex than previously believed. The observed inconsistencies may arise due to changes in telomerase dynamics specific to different tissues or due to an atypical relationship between telomeres and cellular homeostasis mechanisms within certain tumor types. Furthermore, the assessment of telomerase lengths in cancerous cells and mimic tissues might serve as a valuable indicator of an individual's response to therapy and provide prognostic insights into their survival outcomes [64]. The identification of TMMs, along with telomere length, is associated with several pathological and clinical features, such as survival rates and the occurrence of metastasis [65, 66]. There is a correlation between decreased telomeric repeat-containing RNA

(TERRA) expression and unfavorable survival outcomes as well as heightened metastatic progression across numerous types of cancer. In addition, similar methodologies can be utilized to assess the manifestation of TERRA [67–69]. Likewise, the occurrence of alterations, reorganizations, or duplicates that unduly activate telomerase transcription is suggestive of several kinds of cancers. These modifications increase the expression of the TERT gene via various genomic and epigenetic pathways [70, 71]. The prospective utilization of medicinal vulnerability can be supported by the presence of certain therapeutic molecular markers (tissue-mimicking materials; TMMs) and their related variants in the genome. To enhance our understanding of the fundamental processes that regulate telomerase homeostasis in various tumor classifications and to build a framework for personalized diagnostics and prognosis methodologies based on telomerase dynamics, further investigation is warranted. Forthcoming investigations must systematically document the associations between telomere length, TMM identity, and the advancement of disease across various cancer types [72].

Recent advancements in the therapeutic targeting of telomerase have included the inhibition of enzymes, carcinogenic substrate inclusion, chromosomal unpredictability, and anti-telomerase immunotherapy [72]. In a range of preclinical cancer models, both small-molecule inhibitors of enzymes and TR template antagonists have demonstrated anticancer effects [73–75]. Furthermore, several clinical trials have assessed the efficacy of the antagonists BIBR1532 and GRN163L (often referred to as Imetelstat) in various cancer types, including cases of recurrent and metastatic disease [76]. To date, the trials conducted have demonstrated a moderate advantage compared to conventional treatment. However, a limited number of trials have indicated a possible therapeutic effect that is contingent upon telomere length, an effect that can be attributed to the intricate correlation between the measured length of telomeres and the advancement of tumors [77]. According to previous research conducted on the experimental inhibition of telomerase [78–80], there is a suggestion that malignancies that are driven by telomerase may exhibit adaptive activation of ALT as a response to therapy. The apparent lack of therapeutic outcomes may be explained by this phenomenon that has been effectively observed in the use of telomerase inhibitors thus far. Furthermore, if this were the case, it would establish a basis for conducting experiments to assess the effectiveness of combination medications that target multiple TMMs [80]. As previously indicated, the development of metastatic phenotypes necessitates telomere crises in addition to TMM reactivation and carcinogenesis [81, 82]. Therefore, the concurrent utilization of telomerase inhibitors alongside. There is a growing interest in the development of small chemical inhibitors that concentrate on certain telomeric protein molecules, including tankyrase 1. Such inhibitors have the potential to reduce resistance, leading to enhanced telomere degeneration and subsequent cell demise [83]. The observed outcomes appear to be influenced not only by a reduction in the observed increase in the telomerase activity but also a concomitant decrease in Wnt signaling. This provides an additional route for anti-telomerase treatment that is not dependent on telomere length [84].

The utilization of small molecules as substrates with a strong affinity for telomerase, while also triggering cytotoxic DNA damage response pathways upon integration into telomere DNA, presents an additional approach for suppressing telomerase activity [85]. Medications based on this approach exhibit a high degree of selectivity towards cells that possess functional telomerase, hence diminishing the probability of undesired side effects. This strategy offers a significant advantage compared to the prevailing pharmaceutical approach of telomerase inhibition, as it leads to a more rapid occurrence of therapy-induced cell death, hence diminishing the probability of the development of resistance. As a result, experimental investigations have exhibited significant effectiveness against malignant telomere substrates in several preliminary models of pulmonary, breast, intestine, and pancreatic malignancy [86]. Additional research is necessary to assess the safety and efficacy of these medications in human subjects and to gain a more comprehensive understanding of their *in vivo* pharmacokinetic and pharmacodynamic characteristics. The introduction of mutant-template TR has been observed to potentially disrupt telomeres by inducing misincorporation during the process of telomere DNA synthesis. This disruption might result in adverse effects such as cell death or heightened vulnerability to various anticancer treatments. Furthermore, it is worth noting that this approach can also be employed to influence telomere length [87, 88]. Although laboratory investigations have examined the effects of telomere instability, the practical implementation of these findings on a human level presents challenges. Therefore, additional research is necessary to ascertain the optimal methods for the transportation, production, and integration of mutant TR templates within the human body.

Telomerase also can be seen as a neoantigen that is associated with tumors and has the potential to elicit robust immune responses against tumors when utilized in medical therapies. Peptide and dendritic cell (DC) vaccinations represent two distinct categories of telomere immunotherapeutic approaches that are now undergoing research and assessment in a wide range of experimental and healthcare settings with varying degrees of diversity [89]. Peptide vaccinations have the potential to be utilized either independently or in conjunction with immunological modulatory medicines or additional medications that target malignancy. These vaccinations consist of short chains of amino acids derived from the whole TERT sequence. Antigen-presenting cells (APCs) contain a complex of major histocompatibility class II (MHCII) proteins, which facilitate the presentation of TERT peptide vaccines such as GV1001, GX301, and Vx-001. The procedure used to present an antigen is of the utmost importance in eliciting potent allergic reactions that are unique to the antigen and involves the activation of both cellular and humoral immune responses. More precisely, the stimulation of CD4+ T lymphocytes and B-cell lymphocytes is orchestrated by MHCII proteins, leading to the development of these immune responses [90]. Multiple clinical trials have demonstrated the reliability and acceptability of these vaccinations. Furthermore, these vaccinations have been found to enhance rates of survival in patients with different tumor types, with the efficacy of their immune responses to tumors [91]. Nevertheless, these DC vaccines provide a limited group of genetically modified dendritic cell types that can generate, process, and present tumor-associated antigens. DCs are of paramount importance in the initiation and coordination of an immune system response that adapts to the presence of cancerous cells by activating naïve T lymphocytes [92]. The activation of cytotoxic T-cell responses and the establishment of immunological recollection have been demonstrated in both preclinical and clinical trials involving TERT DC vaccines [93]. Furthermore, clinical trials have demonstrated that patients have shown an immune system reaction across many forms of cancer [94]. Subsequent analyses have indicated potential disease stability and improved disease-free survival [95]. It is important to highlight that peptides and DC vaccinations have been evaluated in the context of metastatic conditions, and both demonstrated promise, notwithstanding persistent concerns regarding their general effectiveness in metastatic scenarios [96]. Recent studies have investigated the viability of utilizing the progressive transfer of anti-telomerase chimera antigen receptors (CAR) T lymphocytes and evaluating the efficacy of telomere DNA vaccinations [97]. Although the expression of telomerase is not observed in all cell types, it is maintained and functional in specific populations of tissue-resident stem cells, such as those found in the hematopoietic, intestinal, and germline systems [98, 99]. The effectiveness of therapeutic interventions directed toward cancer cells that express telomerase may have implications for the survival and regeneration potential of stem cell populations associated with these groups. Notwithstanding the constraints linked to these methodologies, the targeting of telomerase continues to be an attractive area of study that merits further exploration.

An alternate, interesting approach to telomere-directed treatment is to focus on telomerase's non-telomeric activities, although this is fraught with difficulty. First and foremost, our inability to rationally develop targeted medicines is hampered by our poor understanding of the molecular processes underpinning these pathways. Yet, typical telomerase-targeting medicines may trigger resistance mechanisms that allow cancer cells not only to continue to survive but also to acquire extremely aggressive traits [100, 101]. These results indicate that a multimodal approach may be the most effective method of addressing TMM plasticity. Hence, combining telomeric and extratelomeric strategies to successfully eliminate telomerase-driven malignancies and reduce their propensity to develop resistance and recurrence [82, 97] is a promising direction to pursue. In future investigations, it is recommended that researchers prioritize the enhancement of techniques employed in the measurement and comprehension of patient telomere length and TMM status, both at the point of diagnosis and over an extended period. In addition, there is a need to explore and examine more effective treatments that specifically attempt to achieve a balance between telomerase's canonical and extratelomeric roles. Finally, efforts should be made to expedite the implementation of these therapeutic approaches in clinical trials.

5.6 Conclusions

In summary, ultra-hollow mesoporous magnetites (UHMMs) exhibiting robust electromagnetic strength and low cytotoxicity have been synthesized with the intention of applying them in the field of cancer therapy. Ultrahigh-frequency magnetic fields have been observed to exhibit a significant cytotoxic effect on laryngeal carcinoma cells, leading to their destruction. In addition, research has indicated that individuals who are exposed to dynamic low-frequency magnetic fields also experience some effects. Due to their inherent dark pigmentation and porous structure, UHMMs demonstrate exceptional suitability as photothermal reagents and drug delivery vehicles. The integration of chlorin e6 (Ce6) molecules into UHMMs resulted in an increased ability of light to destroy tumor cells (photodynamic cytotoxicity) and more efficient prevention of tumor development. This effect was observed after irradiation with an 808 nm laser, resulting in the formation of UHMMs@Ce6. The simultaneous use of both a dynamic electromagnetic field and a laser led to the almost total eradication of cancerous cells in the vicinity of UHMMs@Ce6. Furthermore, the amalgamation of mechanical pressure, photothermal, and photodynamic effects led to the comprehensive elimination of tumors in mice, rendering them indiscernible. This study presented innovative findings on the application of magnetic microspheres with a unique structure in cancer therapy. The utilization of this combination has significant potential as a versatile approach for treating many types of tumors, particularly superficial solid tumors. Moreover, throughout the anticipated time frame for the discovery of receptors or a combination of ligands that can be effectively employed for the precise target of pro-tumoral malignancy-associated fibroblasts in particular populations and/or cancerous cells, another studies demonstrated that ultrasmall superparamagnetic iron oxide nanoparticles (USPIONs) coated with gastrin peptide were effectively internalized and accumulated within the lysosomes of pancreatic CAFs expressing the cholecystokinin 2 receptor (CCK2R), which was selected as a representative model. To achieve successful tumor targeting and treatment response, future preclinical and clinical investigations will likely require the multifunctionalization of MNs. To selectively interact with a variety of receptors present on both the microenvironment surrounding the tumor and cancerous cells, a multifaceted approach was employed. This illustrated the impact of magnetic field rotation on CCK2-targeting nanoparticles, leading to the generation of internal torque. This torque, in turn, induced localized mechanical damage to the lysosomal membrane, ultimately culminating in effective cell death. The apoptosis of malignant fibroblasts resulted from the destruction of lysosomes by the consistent application of mechanical stress. This was used to investigate the phenomenon of mechanosensitive ion channel stimulation on the outermost layer of lysosomes in response to rotating magnetic fields. The cellular uptake of magnetic materials is more pronounced for their nanoscale variants compared to their counterparts at the microscale due to their smaller size. Moreover, in contrast to the disruption of the plasma membrane, the destruction of intracellular cell membranes has been demonstrated to be a viable method for inducing cellular apoptosis. The utilization of low-frequency rotating magnetic fields in this remote magnetomechanical actuation strategy is deemed safe, as they can penetrate the human body without inducing any adverse effects. Moreover, this approach has the potential to substantially decrease the expense associated with instrumentation, rendering it an appealing technique. The objective of this technique is to specifically and strategically focus on cancerous cells and the cells present in the surroundings of the tumor. The utilization of magnetomechanical methods to reduce the fibrocytes that have been associated with malignancy (the population within tumors) represents a compelling supplementary approach in the field of anticancer treatment. The future promise of this approach lies in its ability to augment the effectiveness of established therapeutic modalities such as radiation therapy and chemotherapy, given the substantial influence exerted by the tumor milieu on the origin, progression, and metastasis of tumors. Recent studies offer promising prospects for the application of magnetic nanomedicines in the non-invasive therapy of malignancies, particularly those characterized by a dense tumor microenvironment.

Funding

This chapter did not receive any specific monetary support from governments, businesses, or nonprofit financing entities.

Conflict of interest

The authors declare that there are no conflicts of interest.

References

[1] Miller K D, Nogueira L, Mariotto A B, Rowland J H, Yabroff K R and Alfano C M 2019 Cancer treatment and survivorship statistics *CA Cancer J. Clin.* **69** 363–85

[2] Pujo K, Philouze P, Scalabre A, Cérusea P, Poupartd M and Buiret G 2018 Salvage surgery for recurrence of laryngeal and hypopharyngeal squamous cell carcinoma: a retrospective study from 2005 to 2013 *Eur. Ann. Otorhinol.* **135** 111–7

[3] Čoček A, Ambruš M, Dohnalová A, Chovanec M, Kubecová M and Licková K 2018 Locally advanced laryngeal cancer: total laryngectomy or primary non-surgical treatment? *Oncol. Lett.* **15** 6701–8

[4] Karabulut B, Deveci I, Surmeli M, Şahin-Yilmaz A and Oysu Ç 2018 Comparison of functional and oncological treatment outcomes after transoral robotic surgery and open surgery for supraglottic laryngeal cancer *J. Laryngol. Otol.* **132** 832–6

[5] Rajan A and Sahu N K 2020 Review on magnetic nanoparticle-mediated hyperthermia for cancer therapy *J. Nanopart. Res.* **22** 319

[6] Pavese I, Collon T, Chait Y, Cherait A, Bisseux L, MBarek B and Miette C 2018 Impact on treatment adherence, side effects control, patients QoL, and rehospitalization rate through new management of oral chemotherapy *J. Clin. Oncol.* **36** e18533

[7] Das P, Colombo M and Prosperi D 2019 Recent advances in magnetic fluid hyperthermia for cancer therapy *Colloids Surf.* B **174** 42–55

[8] Perevedentseva E, Karmenyan A, Lin Y C, Song C Y, Lin Z R and Ahmed A I 2018 Multifunctional biomedical applications of magnetic nanodiamond (vol 23, 091404, 2018) *J. Biomed. Opt.* **23** 091404

[9] Liu Z Y, Liu Y C, Shen S H and Wu D C 2018 Progress of recyclable magnetic particles for biomedical applications *J. Mater. Chem.* B **6** 366–80

[10] Stafford S, Garcia R S and Gun'ko Y K 2018 Multimodal magnetic-plasmonic nanoparticles for biomedical applications *Appl. Sci.* **8** 97

[11] Sun C R, Du K, Fang C, Veiseh O, Kievit F and Stephen 2010 PEG-mediated synthesis of highly dispersive multifunctional superparamagnetic nanoparticles: their physicochemical properties and function *in vivo* *ACS Nano* **4** 2402–10

[12] Stephen Z R, Kievit F M and Zhang M Q 2011 Magnetite nanoparticles for medical MR imaging *Mater. Today* **14** 330–8

[13] Gossuin Y, Gillis P, Hocq A, Vuong Q L and Roch A 2009 Magnetic resonance relaxation properties of superparamagnetic particles *WIREs Nanomed. Nanobiotechnol.* **1** 299–310

[14] Krishnan K M 2010 Biomedical nanomagnetics: a spin through possibilities in imaging, diagnostics, and therapy *IEEE Trans. Magn.* **46** 2523–58

[15] Estelrich J M and Busquets A 2018 Iron oxide nanoparticles in photothermal therapy *Molecules* **23** 1567

[16] Nikitin A, Khramtsov M, Garanina A, Mogilnikov P, Sviridenkova N and Shchetinin I 2019 Synthesis of iron oxide nanorods for enhanced magnetic hyperthermia *J. Magn. Magn. Mater.* **469** 443–9

[17] Espinosa A, Corato R D, Kolosnjaj-Tabi J, Flaud P, Pellegrino T and Wilhelm C 2016 Duality of iron oxide nanoparticles in cancer therapy: amplification of heating efficiency by magnetic hyperthermia and photothermal bimodal treatment *ACS Nano* **10** 2436–46

[18] Zhou Z G, Sun Y A, Shen J C, Wei J, Yu C and Kong B 2014 Iron/iron oxide core/shell nanoparticles for magnetic targeting MRI and near-infrared photothermal therapy *Biomaterials* **35** 7470–8

[19] Kashevsky B E, Kashevsky S B, Terpinskaya T I and Ulashchik V S 2019 Magnetic hyperthermia with hard-magnetic nanoparticles: in vivo feasibility of clinically relevant chemically enhanced tumor ablation *J. Magn. Magn. Mater.* **475** 216–22

[20] Ma X X, Tao H Q, Yang K, Feng L Z, Cheng L and Shi X Z 2012 A functionalized graphene oxide-iron oxide nanocomposite for magnetically targeted drug delivery, photothermal therapy, and magnetic resonance imaging *Nano Res.* **5** 199–212

[21] Mousavi S J and Doweidar M H 2016 Numerical modeling of cell differentiation and proliferation in force-induced substrates via encapsulated magnetic nanoparticles *Comput. Methods Programs Biomed.* **130** 106–17

[22] Li S T, Zhang P, Zhang M, Fu C H, Zhao C F and Dong Y S 2012 Transcriptional profile of taxus chinensis cells in response to methyl jasmonate *BMC Genom* **13** 295

[23] Gao J H, Gu H W and Xu B 2009 Multifunctional magnetic nanoparticles: design, synthesis, and biomedical applications *Acc. Chem. Res.* **42** 1097–107

[24] Wahsner J, Gale E M, Rodríguez-Rodríguez A and Caravan P 2019 Chemistry of MRI contrast agents: current challenges and new frontiers *Chem. Rev.* **119** 957–1057

[25] Corato R D, Béalle G, Kolosnjaj-Tabi J, Espinosa A, Clément O and Silva A K A 2015 Combining magnetic hyperthermia and photodynamic therapy for tumor ablation with photo-responsive magnetic liposomes *ACS Nano* **9** 2904–16

[26] Burachaloo H R, Gurr P A, Dunstan D E and Qiao G G 2018 Cancer treatment through nanoparticle-facilitated Fenton reaction *ACS Nano* **12** 11819–37

[27] Nie X, Xia L, Wang H L, Chen G, Wu B and Zeng T Y 2019 Photothermal therapy nanomaterials boost the transformation of Fe (III) into Fe (II) in tumor cells for highly improving chemodynamic therapy *ACS Appl. Mater. Interfaces* **11** 31735–42

[28] Liu Y, Zhen W Y, Jin L H, Zhang S T, Sun G Y and Zhang T Q 2018 All-in-one theranostic nano agent with enhanced reactive oxygen species generation and modulating tumor microenvironment ability for effective tumor eradication *ACS Nano* **12** 4886–93

[29] Feng W, Han X G, Wang R Y, Gao X, Hu P and Yue W W 2019 Nanocatalysts-augmented and photothermal-enhanced tumor-specific sequential nanocatalytic therapy in both NIR-I and NIR-II bio windows *Adv. Mater.* **31** 1805919
[30] Di Z H, Zhao J, Chu H Q, Xue W T, Zhao Y L and Li L L 2019 An acidic-microenvironment-driven DNA nanomachine enables specific ATP imaging in the extracellular milieu of the tumor *Adv. Mater.* **31** 1901885
[31] Liu Y, Wu J D, Jin Y H, Zhen W Y, Wang Y H and Liu J H 2019 Copper(I) phosphide nanocrystals for *in situ* self-generation magnetic resonance imaging-guided photothermal-enhanced chemodynamic synergetic therapy resisting deep-seated tumor *Adv. Funct. Mater.* **29** 1904678
[32] Ying W W, Zhang Y, Gao W, Cai X J, Wang G and Wu X F 2020 Hollow magnetic nanocatalysts drive starvation–chemodynamic–hyperthermia synergistic therapy for tumor *ACS Nano* **14** 9662–74
[33] Chu M Q, Shao Y X, Peng J L, Dai X Y, Li H K and Wu Q S 2013 Near-infrared laser light-mediated cancer therapy by photothermal effect of Fe3O4 magnetic nanoparticles *Biomaterials* **34** 4078–88
[34] Wu X Z, Suo Y K, Shi H, Liu R Q, Wu F X and Wang T Z 2020 Deep-tissue photothermal therapy using laser illumination at NIR-IIa window *Nanomicro Lett.* **12** 38
[35] Barbora A, Bohar O, Sivan A A, Magory E, Nause A and Minnes R 2021 Higher pulse frequency of near-infrared laser irradiation increases penetration depth for novel biomedical applications *PLoS One* **16** e0245350
[36] Sun A H, Guo H, Gan Q, Yang L, Liu Q and Xi L 2020 Evaluation of visible NIR-I and NIR-II light penetration for photoacoustic imaging in rat organs *Opt. Express* **28** 9002–13
[37] Lammertyn J, Peirs A, Baerdemaeker J D and Nicolaï B 2000 Light penetration properties of NIR radiation in fruit concerning non-destructive quality assessment *Postharvest Biol. Tec.* **18** 121–32
[38] Shen Y, Wu C, Uyeda T Q P, Plaza G R, Liu B, Han Y, Lesniak M S and Cheng Y 2017 Elongated nanoparticle aggregates in cancer cells for mechanical destruction with low-frequency rotating magnetic field *Theranostic* **7** 1735–48
[39] Wong W, Gan W L, Teo Y K and Lew W S 2018 Interplay of cell death signaling pathways mediated by alternating magnetic field gradient *Cell Death Discov.* **4** 49
[40] Spyridopoulou K, Makridis A, Maniotis N, Karypidou N, Myrovali E, Samaras T, Angelakeris M, Chlichlia K and Kalogirou O 2018 Effect of low-frequency magnetic fields on the growth of MNP-treated HT29 colon cancer cells *Nanotechnology* **29** 175101
[41] Chiriac H, Radu E, Tibu M, Stoian G, Ababei G, Labusca L, Herea D D and Lupu N 2018 Fe-Cr-Nb-B ferromagnetic particles with shape anisotropy for cancer cell destruction by magneto-mechanical actuation *Sci. Rep.* **8** 11538
[42] Olive K P *et al* 2009 Inhibition of Hedgehog signaling enhances delivery of chemotherapy in a mouse model of pancreatic cancer *Science* **324** 1457–61
[43] Hwang R F, Moore T, Arumugam T, Ramachandran V, Amos K D, Rivera A, Ji B, Evans D B and Logsdon C D 2008 Cancer-associated stromal fibroblasts promote pancreatic tumor progression *Cancer Res.* **68** 918–26
[44] Duluc C *et al* 2015 Pharmacological targeting of the protein synthesis mTOR/4E-BP1 pathway in cancer-associated fibroblasts abrogates pancreatic tumor chemoresistance *EMBO Mol. Med.* **7** 735–53

[45] Richard S *et al* 2016 USPIO size control through microwave nonaqueous sol-gel method for neoangiogenesis T_2 MRI contrast agent *Nanomedicine* **11** 2769–79
[46] Berna M J, Seiz O, Nast J F, Benten D, Blaker M, Koch J, Lohse A W and Pace A 2010 CCK1 and CCK2 receptors are expressed on pancreatic stellate cells and induce collagen production *J. Biol. Chem.* **285** 38905–14
[47] Smith J P, Cooper T K, McGovern C O, Gilius E L, Zhong Q, Liao J, Molinolo A A, Gutkind J S and Matters G L 2014 Cholecystokinin receptor antagonist halts the progression of pancreatic cancer precursor lesions and fibrosis in mice *Pancreas* **43** 1050–9
[48] Mohammed A, Janakiram N B, Suen C, Stratton N, Lightfoot S, Singh A, Pathuri G, Ritchie R, Madka V and Rao C V 2019 Targeting cholecystokinin-2 receptor for pancreatic cancer chemoprevention *Mol. Carcinog* **58** 1908–18
[49] Carrey J and Hallali N 2016 Torque undergone by assemblies of single-domain magnetic nanoparticles Unpublished to a rotating magnetic field *Phys. Rev.* B **94** 184420
[50] Afrin R, Yamada T and Ikai A 2004 Analysis of force curves obtained on the live cell membrane using chemically modified AFM probes *Ultramicroscopy* **100** 187–95
[51] Nikitin A A, Yurenya A Y, Zatsepin T S, Aparin I O, Chekhonin V P, Majouga A G, Farle M, Wiedwald U and Abakumov M A 2021 Magnetic nanoparticles as a tool for remote DNA manipulations at a single-molecule level *ACS Appl. Mater. Interfaces* **13** 14458–69
[52] Knecht L D, Ali N, Wei Y, Hilt J Z and Daunert S 2012 Nanoparticle-mediated remote control of enzymatic activity *ACS Nano* **6** 9079–86
[53] Zamay T N *et al* 2017 Noninvasive microsurgery using aptamer-functionalized magnetic microdisks for tumor cell eradication *Nucleic Acid Ther.* **27** 105–14
[54] Xu M and Dong X P 2021 Endo lysosomal TRPMLs in Cancer *Biomolecules* **11** 65
[55] Chen C C, Krogsaeter E and Grimm C 2021 Two-pore and TRP cation channels in Endo lysosomal osmo-/mechanosensation and volume regulation *Biochim. Biophys. Acta, Mol. Cell. Res.* **1868** 118921
[56] Zhang X, Hu M, Yang Y and Xu H 2018 Organellar TRP channels *Nat. Struct. Mol. Biol.* **25** 1009–18
[57] Morelli M B, Amantini C, Tomassoni D, Nabissi M, Arcella A and Santoni G 2019 Transient receptor potential mucolipin-1 channels in glioblastoma: role in patient's survival *Cancers* **11** 525
[58] Colletti G A, Miedel M T, Quinn J, Andharia N, Weisz O A and Kiselyov K 2012 Loss of lysosomal ion channel transient receptor potential channel mucolipin-1 (TRPML1) leads to cathepsin B-dependent apoptosis *J. Biol. Chem.* **287** 8082–91
[59] Serrano-Puebla A and Boya P 2016 Lysosomal membrane permeabilization in cell death: new evidence and implications for health and disease *Ann. N. Y. Acad. Sci.* **1371** 30–44
[60] Rhyu M S 1995 Telomeres, telomerase, and immortality *JNCI: J. Natl. Cancer Inst.* **87** 884–94
[61] Kordinas V, Ioannidis A and Chatzipanagiotou S 2016 The telomere/telomerase system in chronic inflammatory diseases. Cause or effect? *Genes* **7** 60
[62] Ochi S, Roy B, Prall K, Shelton R C and Dwivedi Y 2023 Strong associations of telomere length and mitochondrial copy number with suicidality and abuse history in adolescent depressed individuals *Mol. Psychiatry* **21** 1–0
[63] Wu K D, Orme L M, Shaughnessy Jr J, Jacobson J, Barlogie B and Moore M A 2003 Telomerase and telomere length in multiple myeloma: correlations with disease heterogeneity, cytogenetic status, and overall survival *Blood* **101** 4982–9

[64] Samavat H, Xun X, Jin A, Wang R, Koh W P and Yuan J M 2019 Association between prediagnostic leukocyte telomere length and breast cancer risk: the Singapore Chinese Health Study *Breast Cancer Res.* **21** 1–0
[65] Robinson N J and Schiemann P 2022 Telomerase in cancer: function, regulation, and clinical translation *Cancers* **14** 808
[66] Nath A R and Natarajan J 2023 Identification of effect of gene mutations related to telomere maintenance in gastric cancer patients *Med. Omics* **10** 100025
[67] Cosgrove N *et al* 2022 Mapping molecular subtype-specific alterations in breast cancer brain metastases identifies clinically relevant vulnerabilities *Nat. Commun.* **13** 514
[68] Gutschner T and Diederichs S The hallmarks of cancer: a long non-coding RNA point of view *RNA Biol.* **9** 703–19
[69] Parra E R *et al* 2020 Variants in epithelial-mesenchymal transition and immune checkpoint genes are associated with immune cell profiles and predict survival in non–small cell lung cancer *Arch. Pathol. Lab. Med.* **144** 1234–44
[70] Saxe C and Phelps W C 2018 The principles and drivers of cancer *Am. Cancer Soc. Princip. Oncol.: Preven. Survivor.* **20** 137–52
[71] Griewank K G, Murali R and Wiesner T 2020 Molecular pathology and genomics of melanoma *Cutaneous Melanoma* (Cham: Springer) 381–422
[72] Jain K K 2021 Personalized management of cancers of various organs/systems *Textbook of Personalized Medicine* (Cham: Springer) 509–602
[73] Chauhan D *et al* 2012 A small molecule inhibitor of ubiquitin-specific protease-7 induces apoptosis in multiple myeloma cells and overcomes bortezomib resistance *Cancer Cell* **22** 345–58
[74] Scozzafava A, Owa T, Mastrolorenzo A and Supuran C T 2003 Anticancer and antiviral sulphonamides *Curr. Med. Chem.* **10** 925–53
[75] Singh S, Sadanandam A, Nannuru K C, Varney M L, Mayer-Ezell R, Bond R and Singh R K 2009 Small-molecule antagonists for CXCR2 and CXCR1 inhibit human melanoma growth by decreasing tumor cell proliferation, survival, and angiogenesis *Clin. Cancer Res.* **15** 2380–6
[76] Kelland L R 2005 Overcoming the immortality of tumor cells by telomere and telomerase-based cancer therapeutics–current status and prospects *Eur. J. Cancer* **41** 971–9
[77] Ruden M and Puri N 2013 Novel anticancer therapeutics targeting telomerase *Cancer Treat. Rev.* **39** 444–56
[78] Raghunandan M, Geelen D, Majerova E and Decottignies A 2021 NHP2 downregulation counteracts h TR-mediated activation of the DNA damage response at ALT telomeres *EMBO J.* **40** e106336
[79] Recagni M, Bidzinska J, Zaffaroni N and Folini M 2020 The role of alternative lengthening of telomeres mechanism in cancer: translational and therapeutic implications *Cancers* **12** 949
[80] Viswanath P, Batsios G, Mukherjee J, Gillespie A M, Larson P E, Luchman H A, Phillips J J, Costello J F, Pieper R O and Ronen S M 2021 Non-invasive assessment of telomere maintenance mechanisms in brain tumors *Nat. Commun.* **12** 92
[81] Chu T W 2016 *Mutations in the Insertion in the Finger's Domain of Human Telomerase Reverse Transcriptase Impair Recruitment to Telomeres, Lead to Growth Defects, and Potentially Contribute to Premature Aging Disease Phenotypes* McGill University document number pc289m728

[82] Robinson N J 2020 *Uncovering the Dynamic Regulation of Telomeres in Cancer by SLX4IP* Case Western Reserve University document number case1594212703749698

[83] Seimiya H, Muramatsu Y, Ohishi T and Tsuru T 2005 Tankyrase 1 as a target for telomere-directed molecular cancer therapeutics *Cancer Cell* **7** 25–37

[84] Thompson C A and Wong J M 2020 Non-canonical functions of telomerase reverse transcriptase: emerging roles and biological relevance *Curr. Top. Med. Chem.* **20** 498–507

[85] Rosen J, Jakobs P, Ale-Agha N, Altschmied J and Haendeler J 2020 Non-canonical functions of telomerase reverse transcriptase–impact on redox homeostasis *Redox Biol.* **34** 101543

[86] Guo L, Zhang D, Wang Y, Malmberg R L, McEachern M and Cai L 2011 TRFolder: computational prediction of novel telomerase RNA structures in yeast genomes *Int. J. Bioinf. Res. Appl.* **7** 63–81

[87] Zhang D, Xue X, Malmberg R L and Cai L TRFolder-W: a web server for telomerase RNA structure prediction in yeast genomes *Bioinformatics* **28** 2696–7

[88] Brown Y, Abraham M, Pearl S, Kabaha M M, Elboher E and Tzfati Y 2007 A critical three-way junction is conserved in budding yeast and vertebrate telomerase RNAs *Nucleic Acids Res.* **35** 6280–9

[89] Nicolette C A, Healey D, Tcherepanova I, Whelton P, Monesmith T, Coombs L, Finke L H, Whiteside T and Miesowicz F 2007 Dendritic cells for active immunotherapy: optimizing design and manufacture to develop commercially and clinically viable products *Vaccine* **25** B47–60

[90] Delfi M *et al* 2021 Self-assembled peptide and protein nanostructures for anti-cancer therapy: targeted delivery, stimuli-responsive devices and immunotherapy *Nano Today* **38** 101119

[91] Caro J J, Salas M, Ward A and Goss G Anemia as an independent prognostic factor for survival in patients with cancer: a systematic, quantitative review *Cancer* **91** 2214–21

[92] Dumitriu I E, Dunbar D R, Howie S E, Sethi T and Gregory C D 2009 Human dendritic cells produce TGF-β1 under the influence of lung carcinoma cells and prime the differentiation of CD4+ CD25+ Foxp3+ regulatory T cells *J. Immunol.* **182** 2795–807

[93] Su Z *et al* 2005 Telomerase mRNA-transfected dendritic cells stimulate antigen-specific CD8+ and CD4+ T cell responses in patients with metastatic prostate cancer *J. Immunol.* **174** 3798–807

[94] Heiser A, Maurice M A, Yancey D R, Coleman D M, Dahm P and Vieweg J 2001 Human dendritic cells transfected with renal tumor RNA stimulate polyclonal T-cell responses against antigens expressed by primary and metastatic tumors *Cancer Res.* **61** 3388–93 PMID: 11309297

[95] Tay R E, Richardson E K and Toh H C 2021 Revisiting the role of CD4+ T cells in cancer immunotherapy—new insights into old paradigms *Cancer Gene Ther.* **28** 5–17

[96] Sondak V K, Sabel M S and Mule J J 2006 Allogeneic and autologous melanoma vaccines: where have we been and where are we going? *Clin. Cancer Res.* **12** 2337s–41s

[97] Romaniuk A, Kopczynski P, Ksiazek K and Rubis B 2014 Telomerase modulation in therapeutic approach *Curr. Pharm. Design* **20** 6438–51

[98] Alt E U, Senst C, Murthy S N, Slakey D P, Dupin C L, Chaffin A E, Kadowitz P J and Izadpanah R 2012 Aging alters tissue resident mesenchymal stem cell properties *Stem Cell Res.* **8** 215–25

[99] Grenier G, Scimè A, Le Grand F, Asakura A, Perez-Iratxeta C, Andrade-Navarro M A, Labosky P A and Rudnicki M A 2007 Resident endothelial precursors in muscle, adipose, and dermis contribute to postnatal vasculogenic *Stem Cells* **25** 3101–10

[100] Gao J and Pickett H A 2022 Targeting telomeres: advances in telomere maintenance mechanism-specific cancer therapies *Nat. Rev. Cancer* **22** 515–32

[101] Faraoni I, Bonmassar E and Graziani G 2000 Clinical applications of telomerase in cancer treatment *Drug Resist. Updat.* **3** 161–70

Rishabha Malviya, Deepika Yadav, Sonali Sundram, Seifedine Kadry and Gurvinder Singh Virk

Chapter 6

The role of micro/nanorobotics in personalized healthcare

The development of healthcare robotics holds the potential to enhance contemporary healthcare practices and improve overall wellbeing. The diminution in the size of these advanced robotic systems has resulted in a wide range of uses that exploit the potential of personalized healthcare. This chapter delves into contemporary patterns in healthcare micro- and nanorobotics, specifically focusing on their applications in treatment, surgical procedures, diagnostics, and healthcare imaging. The application of micro- and nanorobots in personalized healthcare continues to encounter several technological, governance, and commercial hurdles that hinder their extensive implementation within clinical environments. However, recent advancements in translating proofs of concept into *in vivo* studies have demonstrated the prospective benefits of these interventions in the field of personalized healthcare.

6.1 Introduction

The miniaturization of robotic systems offers the promise of improving patient healthcare and diagnostics. The application of miniature robotic surgeons has the potential to facilitate exploration and intervention in anatomical regions that are remote or hard to access, hence enabling the execution of a wide range of healthcare treatments. In contrast to the advancements made in the realm of healthcare micro/nanorobotics over the last decade, a key area that remains unaddressed and poses considerable difficulties pertains to the translation of these technologies for widespread clinical use [1–5]. This chapter endeavors to elucidate current developments in micro/nanorobotics studies, with a specific emphasis on their application in personalized healthcare to facilitate their integration into healthcare practice (figure 6.1). In the context of this chapter, a healthcare micro/nanorobot is characterized as an autonomous micro/nanostructure with a propulsion system that can convert various forms of energy into mechanical forces to execute a

doi:10.1088/978-0-7503-6019-7ch6

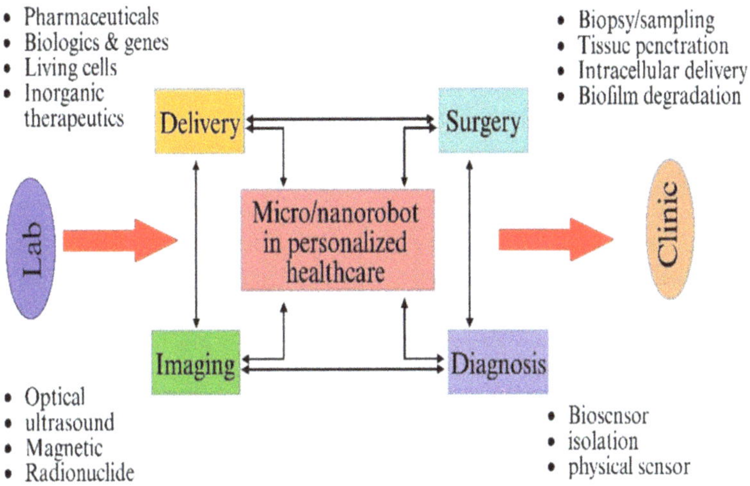

Figure 6.1. Contemporary patterns in micro- and nanorobotics research, with a specific emphasis on their application in personalized healthcare to facilitate clinical integration [14] John Wiley & Sons. [© 2020 The Authors. Published by Wiley-VCH GmbH.]

healthcare procedure [6–10]. While previous assessments have discussed various aspects of healthcare applications in personalized healthcare, this chapter seeks to provide a broad examination of the latest advancements in micro/nanorobotics, specifically those deployed in the field of personalized healthcare [11–13].

The objective of this chapter is to identify the most promising academic possibilities that have the potential to significantly improve the wellbeing of humans within the next decade. These domains encompass therapeutic interventions, surgical procedures, diagnostic techniques, and healthcare imaging modalities. Each of these domains seeks to tackle distinct difficulties within the field of healthcare. One potential application is the application of mobile micro/nanorobots, which possess the ability to navigate through bodily fluids and reach specific anatomical locations, enabling the targeted delivery of medicinal agents in exact quantities [7]. Therefore, by employing an active delivery technique with highly effective localization, it is possible to maintain the therapeutic efficacy of the treatment while mitigating the adverse effects which frequently arise when passive delivery methods are employed. In contrast, the application of micro/nanorobots in surgical procedures has the potential to access anatomical areas that are otherwise inaccessible by catheterization or invasive surgical techniques [8]. This capability enables the sampling of tissues or the targeted delivery of therapeutic payloads to deeper layers of afflicted tissue. The utilization of miniature robotic surgeons has the potential to mitigate the need for invasive processes and surgical interventions, hence minimizing patient discomfort and expediting postoperative recuperation [11]. Micro- and nanorobots provide substantial opportunities in the field of healthcare diagnostics. These miniature robotic devices possess the capability to isolate pathogenic organisms and measure the physiological characteristics of tissues in the real time. They permit accurate disease diagnoses to be made and important signals to be monitored [2–6]. The incorporation of micro/nanorobots into healthcare imaging techniques could result in precise intra-body localization. The roles of micro- and nanorobotics in personalized healthcare are discussed below.

6.2 Surgical operations

The absence of micro/nanoscale equivalents for substantial surgical equipment is a significant obstacle in performing operations at minuscule scales, leading to limited tissue penetration. The potential benefits of miniaturizing surgical instruments lie in their reduced dimensions, which enable them to access anatomical regions that are inaccessible to conventional catheterization and blades. Micro/nanorobotics have the potential to function as surgical instruments to directly access and extract biological tissues. The application of untethered minimally invasive instruments would enable the exploration of anatomical areas that are beyond the comprehension of their larger-scale robotic equivalents. Moreover, these interventions possess the capacity to reduce the likelihood of getting infected and expedite the process of recuperation. Micro/nanorobots have the potential to enhance existing surgical robotic devices by augmenting the accuracy and control capabilities of human surgeons.

6.2.1 Biopsy and sample collection

Studies have shown that micro/nanorobotic instruments can gather specimens of tissue and microorganisms, thereby reducing injuries to tissues, surgical intervention, and diagnostics. Untethered microscale robots mostly fall within the centimeter to millimeter length scales. This dimensional range allows mobile robotic pills to have communications circuitry [11, 12]. However, the additional miniaturization of these instruments would enable sampling to take place in smaller locations. Star-shaped gripping devices can shut and grasp tissues in response to various environmental factors [13]. Animal experiments have shown that small surgical instruments can remove tissues from a pig's bile ducts [14]. Magnetically guided biocompatible hydrogels with magnetic alginate microbeads can be gripped by infrared light [15–18]. The use of micro/nanorobotics to capture bodily microorganisms has also been investigated. Motile robotic collection might improve biome comprehension. Deployable microtraps have been used to capture liquid-borne mobile microbes. These gadgets confined microorganisms in subdivided trap chambers with micro-engineered funnels [19]. Recently, onion-inspired multilayer mobile microtraps were employed to gather mobile pathogenic organisms. The depletion of the magnesium engine's core created a hollow trap. The inner layer also produced serine, which is a chemoattractant that attracts motile bacteria and traps *Escherichia coli* in the microtrap [20]. These examples demonstrate the possibilities of microrobotic biopsies and specimen gathering; however, they struggle the most with sample preservation and contamination. Motile micro/nanorobots can also gather biological markers and exosomes [21–25].

6.2.2 The invasion or penetration of tissues

Robotic technologies serve as valuable instruments for accessing deeply embedded tissue regions that are beyond the reaches of the blood's vascular uptake. Robotic tools with dimensions in the centimeter range have been extensively employed in the field of intestinal-aided administration. In this context, these robots are utilized for tissue penetration or collecting specimens [26, 27]. The potential for improved accessibility to very inaccessible regions within the human corpus might be significantly enhanced by miniaturizing robotic instruments. The majority of the existing research related to tissue penetration has focused on the application of externally stimulated micro/nanorobots, as external fields have demonstrated the capability to effectively penetrate dense biological tissues. The intentional use of external sources facilitates uninterrupted functioning in various situations and enables a significant level of control. Magnetic nano/microrobots have been utilized to traverse the neural tissue of a deceased mouse specimen. Microdriller robots were introduced through the nose into the brain of the mouse and propelled using several modes of movement, which were regulated by adjusting the magnetic field that had been applied [28]. The use of rotating motion in the microdrillers resulted in improved penetrative capabilities compared to those produced by conventional magnetic gradients [29]. Furthermore, the scope of the study was broadened to showcase the capacity to elicit alterations in the behavior of diminutive animals by activating magnetized microrobotic devices that were surgically implanted into brain tissues. The application of low-intensity external stimuli led to a heightened degree of masticatory activity in comparison to the control trials. These experiments have demonstrated the possibility of mechanically stimulating neuronal tissue using unthreaded micro/nanorobots. Furthermore, the application of revolving micro-robot drillers propelled by an external rotating magnetic field has exhibited the capability to effectively traverse the depths of several organs. To establish the viability of operative implementation, tubular microdrillers featuring pointed tips were employed. The microdriller was operated using an external magnetic field, which facilitated the execution of various forms of movement by manipulating the intensity of the applied field. This modification allowed for the attainment of either horizontal or vertical alignment, while concurrently permitting the rotation of the framework around its axis. The microdriller was compelled to traverse pig hepatocytes while positioned vertically and immobilized by its contact with the coarse tissue surfaces. After 10 min of operation, the microdriller had penetrated to a depth of 25 μm [30]. The microstructure was retrieved with a permanent magnet, resulting in the drilling of a hole in the hepatocyte tissue. The resultant space had the potential to serve as a site for cell implantation or a site for the implantation of sustained medication dispensing patches. Researchers have employed enzyme-activated biomimetic or micro propellers to facilitate the penetration of mucin gels. The objective of this study was to address the constraint associated with the retrieval of pathogens situated inside a mucus layer. It was achieved by employing a magnetized microdriller that was modified with the urease enzyme on its external surface. The interaction between the exogenous catalytic surface and the mucus layer led to a localized rise in pH, causing the mucous to undergo liquefaction [31]. This enabled the micro/nanorobot to effectively navigate across the biopolymeric layer. Magnetically driven microrobots have also been employed for intraocular navigation, demonstrating a notable level of precision and compliance with biological systems. Micro/nanorobots were introduced into the vitreous humor via a surgical incision in the ocular region. Researchers employed a magnetized coil system to guide the micro/nanorobots into the posterior section of a rabbit eye. The application of polypyrrole coatings was found to improve the biological compatibility of the micro/nanorobots, resulting in a significantly reduced inflammatory reaction compared to the reaction to uncoated counterparts [32]. In a recent study, researchers employed submicrometer magnet-driven robots that were covered with an aqueous perfluorocarbon protective layer [33]. The purpose of the coating was to reduce the occurrence of biofouling and limit the contact of the robotics with biopolymeric networks present within the vitreous humor of the eye. The microrobots demonstrated effective movement within a pig eye, exhibiting the capability to traverse its anatomical framework without hindrance. The results of this investigation provided empirical data that supported the notion that robotics with dimensions of less than 500 nm are capable of unrestricted movement within the eye because they are smaller than the mesh size of the biopolymeric mesh network [34]. The application of microrobots in optometry has demonstrated promising prospects in the realms of medication administration for retinal blood vessel blockage as well as surgical procedures involving surgical manipulation and peeling of the epiretinal membrane. An additional category of miniature surgical robotics encompasses microrobots that are propelled by ultrasound. These appliances utilize a high-power acoustical droplet vaporization–ignition process. The droplet, resembling a micro bullet, was composed of a cylindrical tube with a dimension of 5 μm, which had been filled with perfluorocarbon emulsions that exhibited electrostatic interactions with the inner surface of the tube. The application of a high-intensity focused ultrasonic pulse targeted at the micro bullet resulted in the vaporization of the perfluorocarbon emulsion, producing an instantaneous change from a liquid to a gaseous state. This transformation served the purpose of functioning as a propellant. The impressive velocity exhibited by the object produced sufficient force to penetrate deep tissue, induce ablation, and cause annihilation [35]. A functional very small cannon was produced by modifying the design. The original hollowed cylindrical framework was filled with a hydrogel that included 1 μm nano bullets or fluorescent microspheres as well as a perfluorocarbon emulsion. Utilization of a focused ultrasonic pulse led to the spontaneous vaporization of the perfluorocarbon emulsion, expeditiously expelling the nano bullets at a considerable velocity measured in meters per second. Ultrasound ballistic microrobots possess the capability to exert increased mechanical force within biological tissues, hence enabling enhanced deep penetration and the autonomous delivery of medicinal substances, regardless of the microscopic structure of the robot. However, their applications are restricted and need an additional magnetic field for precise navigation toward the intended destination. In contrast, the majority of magnetically actuated robotic microsurgeons have a prolonged operational lifespan and possess integrated guidance facilitated by an external magnetic field.

6.2.3 The breakdown of biofilms

Biofilms and bacterial infections cause significant problems in the field of medical therapy because of the ability of various microorganisms to rapidly multiply and establish colonies in various parts of the human body, thereby leading to the development of several diseases [36]. Furthermore, it has been shown that biofilms commonly exhibit resistance to antimicrobial therapies, which underscores the necessity for the application of physical therapy modalities in combating disease [37]. Various micro/nanorobotic systems have been utilized to mechanically dislodge bacterial infections in this particular context. Magnetic spinning nanowires have been employed to mechanically disrupt a biofilm formed by *Aspergillus fumigatus*. The efficiency of microbial eradication was enhanced by the utilization of spinning nanorobots in conjunction with an antibacterial treatment substance [38]. In an alternative scenario, the application of a biohybrid micro/nanorobot was investigated. The biohybrid entity consisted of magnetotactic bacteria (MSR-1) combined with mesoporous silica that contained an antibiotic. The objective of this investigation was to exert mechanical forces on *E. coli* biofilms [39]. The study employed urease-powered micro/nanorobots to provide targeted, penetrative, and therapeutic interventions for bladder cancer. The micro/nanorobot was equipped with an anti-FGFR3 antibody, which was designed to specifically attach to the outermost layer of the three-dimensional malignant spheroids (as shown in figure 6.2).

Upon entering the system, the locally generated ammonium byproducts facilitated the degradation of the engine's urea, leading to a significant inhibition in spheroid growth [40]. The treatment of other biofilms might potentially benefit from the implementation of a comparable method. In addition, catalytic antimicrobial robots were employed to facilitate the degradation and eradication of various types

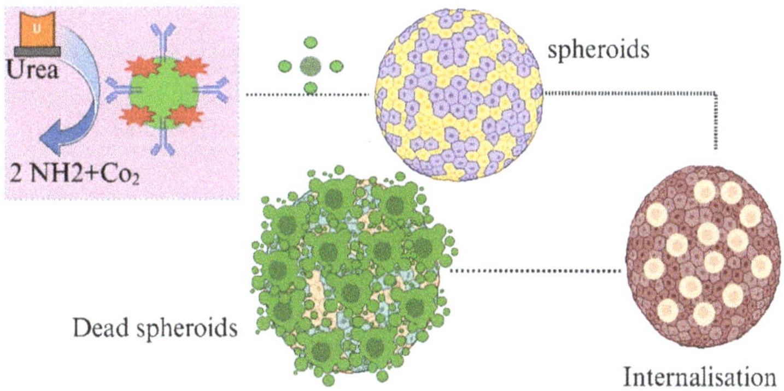

Figure 6.2. Micro/nanorobots equipped with anti-FGFR3 antibodies, which were designed to specifically target and bind to the external surface of three-dimensional cancer spheroids [14] John Wiley & Sons. [© 2020 The Authors. Published by Wiley-VCH GmbH.]

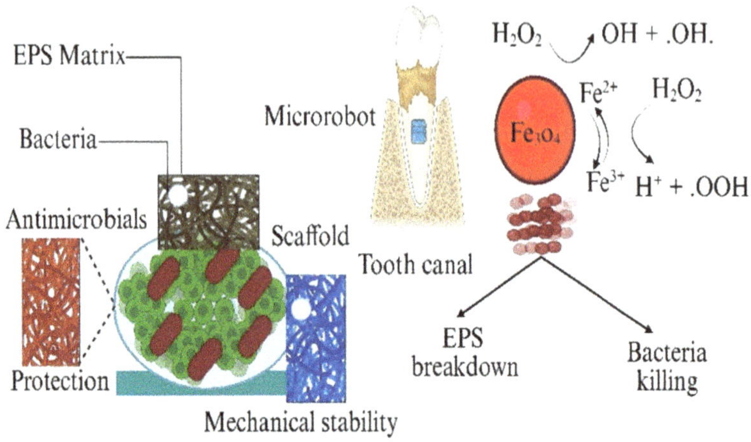

Figure 6.3. The purpose of the robotic platform was to effectively eliminate biofilms on a level surface, clear obstructions in a capillary tube, and cleanse biofilms within a simulated dental model. From [42]. Reprinted with permission from the AAAS.

of biofilms. The microrobots were comprised of a hydrogel structure containing iron oxide nanoparticles, which had two main functions: propulsion through the application of an external magnetic field, and the ability to act as antimicrobial agents. The purpose of this robotic framework was to effectively eliminate biofilms on a level surface as well as within a confined capillary tube and an internal tooth model (figure 6.3) [41].

Therefore, the potential application of microrobots in the mechanical eradication of biofilms might be extended to encompass the removal of blood clots and the cleansing of arteries.

6.2.4 Deliveries conducted within cells

Recent advancements have focused on reducing the size of the robotic platforms employed in surgical procedures, specifically targeting the cellular level [43–46]. The potential to externally operate and actively manipulate micro/nanorobots within living tissues has provided an unparalleled opportunity to investigate the biophysical approaches and principles underlying numerous cellular activities, ranging from the transcription of genes and the dynamical mechanical modeling of intracellular environments to medication administration and perception [47]. The application of ultrasound radiation has been shown to enable microrobots to effectively enter and navigate within particular live cells. This capacity has been employed to transport genetic material into cellular entities. Magnetically driven micromotors have been employed to enhance cellular control and hence enable subcellular surgical procedures to take place. The application of microrobotic platforms in innovative surgical applications holds promise, as they possess the ability to serve as important instruments for tasks such as collecting specimens, unclogging arteries, and transferring genes. The initial documentation of the incorporation of nanomotors within cellular frameworks and the subsequent control of these synthetic devices within the internal milieu described the use of sound-propelled nanomotors within viable HeLa cells [48]. Subsequently, nanorobots were internalized into malignant cells and employed for recognition applications as well as the delivery of nucleotides, proteins, and payloads. Sensing applications within functional cells have successfully identified the presence of miRNA-21, a microRNA often observed in cancerous cell lineages, including MCF-7. A sensing device for miRNA-21 was constructed using a gold-based nanorobot that was covered with a fluorescent single-strand DNA/graphene oxide composite. This sensor was enabled to function through the application of ultrasonic fields. The fluorescence of the single-stranded DNA (ssDNA) was first suppressed by the presence of the graphene oxide as it was being carried by the nanomotor. Nevertheless, following the process of hybridization based on the specific miRNA or messenger, the dye-labeled single-stranded DNA (ssDNA) probes relocated away from the nanomachine's surface, resulting in the restoration of fluorescence and enabling the detection of the miRNA [49]. Regarding the transportation of goods, subsequent studies have utilized gold nanorobot frameworks to achieve effective intracellular delivery and application. These frameworks have been improved by incorporating a rolling loop-amplifying DNA strand, which serves as an anchor for the siRNA and allows for gene silencing. In addition, they have been equipped with the protein caspase-3 to induce cell death in acidic environments, enabling active intracellular oxygen delivery [50–53]. Furthermore, nanoshells were successfully internalized and acoustically driven within live MCF-7 malignancies, employing a distinct and expanded framework. The motion of the shell nanomotors was driven by acoustic streaming stress exerted on their asymmetrical surfaces [54]. These frameworks exhibited enhanced cargo-hauling capability in comparison to the nanowires employed for cellular internalization. A subsequent idea involved the use of hollowed gold shells with cutting edges which were driven using ultrasonic technology [55]. The internalization of the microrobot was improved by the utilization of a near-infrared (NIR) field, which facilitated the invasion of the cell membrane via photomechanical perforation. The application of stimuli-responsive intracellular nanorobots was also observed in the transportation of the payload within HeLa cell membranes. The miniature robots were composed of mesoporous silicon dioxide nanoparticles, which included urease-based chemical engines powered by the presence of urea found in the surrounding environment. In addition, they had pH-responsive supramolecular nano valves that facilitated the release of their cargoes. The caps containing benzimidazole/cyclodextrin-urease were exclusively unsealed under acidic conditions, facilitating the intracellular release of chemotherapeutic cargo within the lysosomal compartments of HeLa cells [56]. In this study, researchers employed mesoporous Janus microrobots to achieve thermomechanical percolation within a cellular membrane subjected to NIR irradiation. This process had the objective of facilitating the controlled release of doxorubicin. In contrast to approaches that utilize ultrasonic sound or chemical-based power, which disturb the entirety of the experimental volume, surgical procedures employing magnetic motors only disturb the robot and the micro-environments of the cells.

In a comparable vein, microrobots with a pollen grain morphology characterized by spiky protrusions (resembling sea urchins) were employed for a cellular drilling process. The pointed configuration administered chemotherapy to HeLa cells by direct contact with the cellular membrane. The cutting edges disengaged from the cell while the main framework maintained a parallel rotation with the substrates [57]. Simultaneously, the cutting edges penetrated the membrane. In a separate study, researchers employed magnetically driven micro/nanorobots coated with titanium and nickel to facilitate the transfection of human embryonic kidney cells. The microrobots were equipped with lipoplexes that contained plasmid genetic material. The effective delivery of genetic materials into mammalian cells was facilitated by the external cationic lipid lipofectamine, which underwent a fusion with the negatively charged cell membrane and subsequent endocytosis [58]. However, certain magnetic materials have a low magnetism remanence, such as iron oxide, or lack biocompatibility, as is the case with nickel. A microhelix consisting of iron-based platinum exhibited enhanced biological compatibility and retained robust ferromagnetic properties, as documented in the study. A technique based on the intracellular transfection of plasmids was employed to specifically target cancer cells and induce the production of green fluorescent protein within the cells [59]. Intracellular surface-enhanced Raman spectroscopy has also been facilitated by employing magnetized nanorobots [60]. The development and fabrication of biocompatible magnetic materials have significant relevance for risk reduction and improved performance.

6.3 Diagnosis

Motile micro/nanorobots have distinctive prospects for diagnostic purposes, since they facilitate enhanced targeted receptor contact and fluid mixing. A selective approach based on recognition agents, such as those capable of identifying target molecules of genetic material, proteins, tissues, or genetic information, can be utilized in the process of assessment. These compounds play a crucial role in detecting and diagnosing many biological targets under varying conditions.

6.3.1 Biological sensors

Micro/nanorobots have exhibited their potential in the field of monitoring by successfully detecting various biological targets through the observation of alterations in their movement or the inhibition of fluorescence [61]. As an illustration, a study presented a pH-dependent nano switch composed of triplex DNA labeled with Förster resonance energy transfer to observe microenvironments' pH balance. The ammonium generated as a result of the decomposition of urea produced by the microrobot's engines was identified by the DNA sensors [62]. In that study, a sandwiched double-stranded DNA tag was employed in conjunction with silver nanoparticles to facilitate the detection of ions containing silver. The presence of the electrons resulted from the acceleration of a chemically driven nanorobot. The DNA-sensing approach based on motion detection was predicated on the quantification of alterations in the velocity of the nanorobot. An optical visualization of distance signals was produced, taking into account the correlation with the concentration of the signals. The nanorobot successfully identified genetic material and bacterial RNA targets, specifically at a level as low as 40 moles, without requiring isolation or purification procedures [63]. Microrobots equipped with probes composed of oligonucleotides were utilized to identify the complementary nucleic acids strand of the targeted DNA or RNA molecule. After a nucleic acid of interest was acquired through the process of double-stranded DNA hybridization, an additional fluorescent antibody tag was utilized to deliver a signal that allowed for quantitative evaluation. The microrobots demonstrated the ability to extract specimens in various settings, such as a buffered solution, saliva, and feces [64]. An alternative method based on mobility was developed for genome recognition; it employed a microrobot propelled by catalytic activity. This microrobot was equipped with single-stranded genetic material, which enabled the capture of a rather large particle that had been functionalized with a double-stranded DNA strand. The microrobot and the cargo nucleotide strand exhibited noncomplementary sequences, but their respective ends included complementary sequences that enabled their connection through an additional strand that functioned as a bridge [65]. Hence, the presence of a specific strain in a solution allowed cargo particle movement to be detected using an optical microscope. In the same manner, microscopic robots were integrated with loop-mediated isothermal replication of an initial HIV infection. The introduction of HIV-1 RNA strands into a remedy microbot resulted in the initiation of a loop-mediated adiabatic amplifier, leading to the formation of extensive stem-looped amplicons. Consequently, the existence of these amplifiers caused a decrease in the velocity of the nanorobots. The alteration in velocity was quantified using a microscopy setup that was fabricated using three-dimensional printing technology and afterward affixed to the mobile device. This accessible platform demonstrated the ability to accurately identify the HIV-1 virus in patient specimens, exhibiting favorable levels of precision and sensitivity [66].

The double-stranded DNA sandwiched hybrid approach was further developed through the functionalization of nucleic probing within the framework of chemically propelled rockets. This was achieved by including complementary DNA strands that were linked to platinum nanoparticles and catalase-loaded DNA strands. A correlation was found to exist between the velocity of the microrobot and the degree of concentration of the genetic material (DNA) target [67–70]. The microrobots were equipped with aptamer antibody receptors that could attach, transport, and isolate fibrinogen. These studies demonstrated a significant level of specificity by effectively differentiating the targets from non-target proteins that were present in substantial amounts. The subsequent liberation of the protein was accomplished by the introduction of an adenosine triphosphate (ATP) molecule, which formed a complex with the aptamer, thus displacing the previously trapped fibrinogen. A quantitative assessment of protein capture was conducted by introducing an additional fluorescent tag [71]. A novel detection method for the Zika virus was showcased that utilized the movement of a nano/microrobot. The robotic sensor utilized the sandwich assay methodology, employing nanorobots coated with anti-Zika monoclonal antibodies (mAb) and small beads coated with anti-Zika mAb.

Differential concentrations of the virus were discovered by utilizing a cellular device to measure variations in the velocity of the microbeads. The motion-based technique demonstrated notable levels of specificity when confronted with various viruses, such as dengue fever, herpes simplex virus type 1, and human cytomegalovirus. In addition, other micro/nanorobots have been developed that served as sensors for the detection of ricin B toxin using an 'off–on' fluorescent process [72]. The microrobots had an exterior layer made of graphene oxide, which was able to bind to an aptamer labeled with fluorescein–amidine dye. The quiescent state of the probe's fluorescent emission was a consequence of the target loading and was caused by π–π interactions. The enhanced affinity of the aptamer for ricin led to a corresponding elevation in fluorescent intensity, enabling the ricin content to be quantified using optical detection [73]. A study showcased the utilization of tubular nanorobots that were functionalized with reduced graphene oxide (rGO); these were used to swiftly and economically detecting mycotoxins (namely fumonisin B1 and ochratoxin A) in real time, while also effectively isolating them. The operating premise of the method relied on the preferential behavior of aptamers, which isolate targeted mycotoxins and allow them to be quantified by measurement of the quenched fluorescence intensity. Ultimately, the utilization of rGO functionalized nanomotors has shown notable levels of sensitivity and selectivity, indicating promising prospects for their use in the field of biosensing [74]. A further study showcased the application of a Janus microrobot that was equipped with quantum dots as its sensor [75]. This microrobot demonstrated the ability to employ an 'on–off' fluorescence detection method which relied on the utilization of phenylboronic acid as a recognized receptor for bacterial endotoxins [75]. In addition, a fluorescence-based method employing an 'on–off' mechanism was utilized to identify the presence of a parasite and its associated released toxins. This detection system was designed to be portable and efficient, making it suitable for use on a mobile platform. The surface was coated with carbon dots that were functionalized and exhibited changes in their fluorescence in response to the presence of the specific toxin being targeted. The approach based on the use of quantum-dot-based microrobots has been expanded to separate toxins produced by *Clostridium difficile* from the fecal matter of patients. The mobility of the nanorobot was regulated by the use of an external magnetic field, thus enhancing the contact between the toxins and the nanorobot's interface. Quenching of a quantum dot fluorescent material occurred as a consequence of the absorption of the toxin onto the outermost layer of the microrobot. This phenomenon was utilized as an optical method to accurately measure the concentrations of *C. difficile* toxin in liquid solutions, which ranged from 0.38 to 17.80 ng mL^{-1} [76].

6.3.2 Isolation

The existing methods employed for the separation and purification of biotargets need extended periods of incubation and include many iterations of scrubbing [77]. Functionalized micro/nanorobots have recently been characterized as dynamic frameworks that enable the rapid differentiation of biological targets and pathogenic organisms. [78]. An illustration in figure 13(b) demonstrates the application of nanorobots that have been customized with the biological receptor concanavalin (conA) as a means of isolating *E. coli* bacteria in real time. ConA is a protein that has unique binding properties toward the polysaccharide surface found in gram-negative microbes, primarily targeting the enzyme mannose and sugar moieties [79, 80]. The liberation of trapped microorganisms was initiated by a reduction in pH achieved using a dissociation solution based on glycine. In the same manner, microrobots customized with anti-ProtA antibodies demonstrated the ability to selectively isolate *Staphylococcus aureus*, a bacterium that presents a complementary protA antibody on its external membrane. The cell separation approach exhibited a high degree of sensitivity toward the target, even when yeast cells were abundant in the solution [81]. In their study, Garcia *et al* used microrobots functionalized with anti-*Bacillus globilli* antibodies to isolate individual and numerous globilli spores inside intricate biological microenvironments [82].

E. coli was recovered from polluted water specimens using a non-specific isolation method [83]. This method involved the application of a chitosan hydrogel-surface coating which exhibited adhesive properties and facilitated the entrapment and eradication of the pathogenic organisms. Microrobots customized with anti-carcinoembryonic antigen antibodies have been shown to possess the capability to isolate malignancies in complex media. The isolation procedures employed in this study were predicated on the targeted identification of the anti-CEA antibody using the outermost antigens that are overexpressed by malignant pancreatic cells [84]. Cancer cells have also been identified through the use of physical stimuli. For instance, microrobots with chemical [85] and magnetic [86] properties demonstrated the capability to manipulate cells by a 'picking and dropping' mechanism involving the application of pushing forces. A separate study documented the utilization of peanut-shaped colloids for the noncontact manipulation and transportation of cells. This was achieved by generating localized microstreaming flows that effectively trapped the cells. This approach was investigated to effectively separate and convey many cells within microhydrodynamic environments [87]. Acoustic streaming has also been successfully employed to achieve comparable nanomanipulation of live cells [88, 89].

The application of red blood cell-based coatings has been documented as a method for the fast separation of infections and toxins. The use of ultrasound [90] and chemically [91] propelled small robots, which are enveloped by red blood cell membranes, has been successfully showcased as a means of effectively extracting toxins in various biological product settings. This strategy functioned as a prophylactic tactic aimed at sequestering harmful substances that typically exhibit an affinity for and induce lysis of erythrocytes. In addition, magnetic helical nanorobots that included plasma membranes derived from human platelets have been seen to exhibit characteristics resembling those of platelets. Like platelets, these nanorobots have demonstrated the ability to adhere to pathogenic organisms, such as *S. aureus* [92]. The addition of a hybrid cellular membrane coating to the nanorobots' surface led to a mutually beneficial separation between the pathogen and the toxin. The pathogen *S. aureus* was effectively separated by the platelet's membrane; however, the α-toxin released by the captured pathogens was absorbed by the red blood cell membrane [93].

6.3.3 Physical sensors

Micro/nanorobots have considerable promise for use as label-free biomechanical probes. A study examined the application of helical nanorobots propelled by rotating magnetic fields to investigate the mechanical environment within live cells. The nanomotors encountered the disadvantage of limited adhesion to their cellular surroundings, which, in some instances, might result in reduced biomechanical responsiveness. An investigation of the movement of spiral-shaped magnetic nanorobots was effectively conducted within the cellular environment, specifically within HeLa, renal, and endothelial cells, following the processes of incubation and internalization [94]. The authors of this investigation also showcased the application of the robotic intracellular probe technique in measuring viscous [95, 96] and adhesive forces within malignant cancerous cells. Piezoelectric microrobots have been documented as mobile probes and utilized for cerebral stimulus mapping. The differentiation of individual cells has been achieved through the application of a piezoelectric effect generated by an external ultrasonic field [97]. As an example, microrobots supplied with electricity were employed as mobile electrodes and demonstrated the ability to induce cell deformation. This deformation of the cell nucleus was shown to be associated with observable dielectrophoretic potential wells [98].

The property of viscosity is extremely important in the context of healthcare applications. However, the assessment of rheological parameters in biological fluids poses difficulties because they consist of many biocomponents. An investigation used spinning nanorobot coils as mechanical sensors to measure the rheological characteristics of a small volume. The consistency of the solution was assessed by the spinning nanorobot by measuring the time at which the nanorobot reached a position and the magnetic field oscillation that it was subjected to. Thus, the calculation of the torque exerted on the particle by the surrounding medium was established. Due to their reduced size relative to the suspended red blood cells, the nanorobots were only able to selectively investigate the fluid phase. The application of chemically propelled microrobots as viscometers was also investigated [99]. The acceleration of the microrobots enabled the fluid viscosity of a given solution to be estimated [100]. In the same way, distinct physical characteristics, namely pressure and flow rate, were measured by propelling a microrobot [101].

The investigation of macrophage pursuit behavior and immunological host defense inside the microscopic environment is very difficult due to the lack of physical probes capable of engaging with phagocytes in a manner akin to that of pathogens [102, 103]. These studies focused on investigating magnetic microrobots with five degrees of freedom to replicate the interactions observed in predator–prey relationships, foraging, and phagocytic behavior found in larger biological species. Specifically, the aim was to understand these behaviors within the context of the immunological host defense in small-scale environments. These studies involved the application of dynamic translation resistance and rotational forces as well as magnetic torque to position microrobots in proximity to macrophages. The purpose of the study was to detect the exerted force and rotational torques by observing optical displacements [104].

6.4 Imaging and diagnostic medicine

The integration of miniature robots with imaging systems for healthcare has been addressed through transitioning from *in vitro* to *in vivo* research [105–107]. The successful translation of healthcare micro/nanorobotics into clinical settings will heavily depend on the continual tracking of individuals or populations, using the underlying signals given off by human tissues [107]. Micro/nanorobots have the potential to enhance existing healthcare imaging methods by facilitating easy localization and guidance within the human body and by enabling transmitted signals to trigger releases. Contemporary traditional diagnostic imaging methodologies are employed to investigate the physiological aspects of organs and tissues. Furthermore, there has been a new focus on monitoring the dispersion of molecular visualization agents and nanoparticles inside the anatomical structures of a patient. The capability to monitor and guide individual and collective nanomotors within the human body will be imperative to facilitate their extensive use [108]. Hence, it is important to consider the distinct merits associated with individual imaging platforms and processing techniques, given that each imaging modality is more suitable for certain organ compositions and depths of focus inside the human body. The primary obstacle in the field of untethered micro/nanorobotic research is the difficulty of effectively differentiating between the framework of micro/nanorobots and their surrounding environment (background subtraction) while ensuring that the resolution of the acquired image is adequate to precisely record their movement in a three-dimensional setting. Given the intricate nature of the gathered data, it has become necessary to employ computer algorithms, rather than relying solely on healthcare professionals, to discern and track the motion of microrobots within the human body. In this context, it is important to contemplate the methodology of tagging individual micromotors by integrating contrasting imaging materials into them or employing uniquely designed forms. These approaches enable us to mitigate the impact of background noise. Various imaging modalities are employed in conjunction with micro/nanorobots, including optics, magnetic, acoustic, and radioactive imaging techniques.

6.4.1 Optical imaging

Medical professionals and researchers continue to have difficulties in diagnosing medical conditions, as the majority of patients do not exhibit symptoms until after they have reached a more advanced state of disease. This is mostly due to the limited sensitivity and specificity of current diagnostic methods in properly identifying premalignant lesions. Given this scenario, the use of micro/nanorobots has the potential to augment existing diagnostic capabilities. Early research in the field of micro/nanorobots utilized optical techniques, such as catheter recording devices and laser irradiation due to their cost-effectiveness and reliable imaging capabilities. Optical cameras have been utilized to determine the precise location of micromotors within the retina of a rabbit eye [32, 109, 110]. In addition, a microgripper situated within a pig bile duct has been successfully visualized using an endoscopic webcam. Despite their convenience, ingestible cameras have some limitations when it comes to accessing the internal regions of the human body. They may potentially induce distress in patients and, in certain instances, may not possess the capability to identify frameworks at the nano/micrometer scale. Noninvasive fluorescence scanning has the potential to precisely measure and localize microrobots at high resolutions. The fluorescence released by organic molecules or inorganic fluorescent nanoparticles within a living organism has been observed using a charge-coupled sensor camera, as depicted. The fluorescence signal was superimposed onto an authentic image of a living thing, enabling the precise determination of the spatial distribution of the molecule that served as the imaging agent. Hence, the broad implementation of intracorporeal imaging microrobots may be readily accomplished by the surface modification of these microrobots with fluorescent molecular visualization reagents.

Fluorescent imaging methods have conventionally been employed to view the spatial distribution of micromotors within live organisms. Whole-body fluorescent imaging was employed to monitor the presence of magnetically actuated helices that were customized with near-IR probes within the abdominal cavity of a mouse [111]. The study utilized *Spirulina* phytoplankton that were coated with iron oxide (Fe_3O_4) nanoparticles [112]. This coating of phytoplankton was employed to monitor a group of micromotors present inside the subcutaneous layer and abdominal cavity of naked mice utilizing fluorescence-based *in vivo* imaging [112]. One of the initial instances of biohybrid microrobots serving as carriers for imaging compounds is exemplified by a pioneering case of micromotor imaging. This case included the utilization of a biohybrid microrobot, specifically a bacteria-based one, which was equipped with 40 nm nanoparticles encapsulating the enzyme luciferase gene. The micromotors were administered through the abdomen to a murine subject to facilitate the transportation of the luciferase gene plasmid into neighboring cells. Subsequently, the luciferase protein was synthesized inside these cells, leading to luminescence in several organs [113]. In the same vein, the imaging of the movement of biohybrid microrobot bacteria containing small coated polystyrene beads was conducted within a tumor site using the signal emitted by a fluorescent dye [114]. In addition, the application of fluorescence generated by live cells has facilitated the imaging of microrobots that transported these cells [87, 115]. In these studies, the utilization of the fluorescence imaging capabilities was crucial in visually demonstrating the effective and precise transportation of microrobots to their intended destination.

6.4.2 Imaging using ultrasound

Ultrasound imaging presents itself as an appropriate choice for the real–time visualization of micro/nanorobots, offering biologically compatible as well as economical alternatives. The ultrasonic pulse's interaction with tissues exhibiting varying reflective characteristics results in discernible echoes, which are then captured and converted into a picture. While the utilization of ultrasonic external fields to power micro/nanorobots has seen significant advancements, its application as a means of image acquisition remains rather restricted [116]. The capacity to track the location of a micro/nanorobot as it moves through liquids by catalyzing hydrogen peroxide into a trail of oxygen microbubbles has been demonstrated in *in vitro* experiments [117]. One primary constraint of this technology is the detection capability of the imaging system, which can identify the tiny particles employed for propulsion, but not the micromotors. Consequently, it is necessary to analyze the acquired data points to determine the precise position of the micro/nanorobot. The primary obstacle associated with ultrasound imaging is its constrained resolution capabilities and the restricted array of contrast molecules available, which predominantly consists of stabilized microbubbles. To address this constraint, optoacoustic imaging systems combine the resolution and penetrative depth of ultrasound with the specificity offered by optical techniques. The fundamental mechanism underlying photoacoustic imaging involves the release of optical pulses which are subsequently absorbed by tissues. This absorption leads to thermoelastic expansion, generating ultrasound waves. Subsequently, a transducer can gather this data and convert it into visual representations of the molecular image-capture compounds present within biological tissues. Recent research demonstrated the capacity to visually perceive micromotors that were coated with biological imaging agents within an *ex vivo* chicken breast model; the resulting images exhibited a notable level of contrast and specificity [118]. In a separate instance, the capability to accurately determine the position of micro/nanorobots equipped with chemically powered engines within a live mouse was successfully demonstrated by the use of photoacoustic imaging. Furthermore, the propulsion of the microrobot was activated by disintegrating a protective layer using additional NIR light irradiation [118]. In recent years, there have been reports of the application of magnetotactic biohybrids coated with a polydopamine layer. This coating has been shown to boost signals for photoacoustic detection and enable more efficient photothermal therapy. This work demonstrated the feasibility of treating infections using an *in vivo* model, therefore serving as an illustration of the principle [119].

6.4.3 Imaging using radionuclides

Radionuclide imaging technologies provide a formidable instrument within the field of healthcare imaging. One of the notable features of these entities is their distinctiveness, which stems from their ability to provide molecular information and exhibit heightened sensitivity. Proton emission tomography (PET) is a medical imaging technique that involves the release of positive ions that induce the decay of radioactive materials. This process releases gamma radiation, which can be detected by a scanning device and utilized to produce a detailed map of the region under investigation. Various nuclides can be utilized to specifically target particular organs or biological processes. While radiation does have the capability to penetrate deeply into tissues, its prolonged usage may lead to negative consequences for health, which restricts the duration over which it can be used for imaging purposes. In a study, a PET system was employed to monitor the movement of a substantial population of Au/poly(3,4-ethylene dioxythiophene)/Pt chemically powered microrobots that were encapsulated in iodine isotopes [120]. The study employed thermoresponsive magnetic microrobots and emission computed tomography (CT) imaging. Few examples of the application of x-ray imaging have been seen in the field of microrobotics. The application of x-ray radiation has been experimentally proven to provide the necessary energy for the operation of Janus microparticles [121–123]. In addition, x-ray imaging radiation has been successfully employed for the detection of round microgrippers within the gastrointestinal tract. In conveying a broad perspective of the healthcare imaging domain, it is important to acknowledge that each modality possesses distinct advantages. Optical and ultrasonic imaging techniques are characterized by their comparatively affordable prices but exhibit a limited depth of penetration in comparison to magnetic and radionucleotide imaging techniques.

6.5 Prospective view

In brief, the use of microrobots in the field of personalized healthcare has been demonstrated to have a wide range of applications across various domains (see table 6.1). These applications include the transportation of medications, biological products, genetic material, and living organisms; the deployment of surgical instruments for purposes such as biopsies, connective tissue penetration, intracellular delivery, and biofilm degradation; and the development of diagnostic instruments, including both chemical and physical biosensors and isolation devices. The application that has achieved the most advanced stage of development is targeted delivery, and the current endeavors in this field are mostly concentrated on animal testing. However, the application of imaging techniques is necessary in conjunction with delivery, surgical procedures, or diagnostic methods to comprehend the intricate workings of micro/nanorobots and exploit their effectiveness and functionalities. The ongoing investigation of nano/microtools reflects the progressive convergence of personalized healthcare and micro/nanorobotics.

However, every application encounters distinct obstacles in its journey toward eventual clinical application. In the contexts of drug or substance delivery and surgical applications, the utilization of micro/nanorobots necessitates their operation inside anatomical areas that are difficult to access. Consequently, the development of recovery and deterioration procedures assumes paramount importance to mitigate potential risks to the wellbeing of patients [124]. *In vitro* diagnostic procedures are often employed, hence the main obstacles for microrobots as diagnostic instruments are to enhance their scalability and facilitate high-throughput detection. The primary obstacle encountered in healthcare imaging applications is the capacity of every type of imaging to effectively differentiate between an individual micro/nanorobot and huge clusters of micro/nanorobots within the surrounding tissue, all in real time [105]. This particular operation necessitates the application of high-frame-rate acquisition techniques at significant magnification levels, resulting in the generation of substantial volumes of data. The application of artificial intelligence (AI) algorithms has the potential to facilitate the rapid assessment of data, thus achieving closed-loop functionality in microrobots operating within living organisms.

Table 6.1. An overview of the prevailing trends in the field of micro/nanorobotics within the domain of precision medicine. The discussion encompasses various applications such as drug administration, surgical interventions, diagnostic procedures, and medical imaging techniques.

Application	Description	Examples	Challenges and prospects
Drug delivery system	The application of micro/nanorobots to deliver particular payloads with enhanced spatiotemporal precision in comparison to passive dissemination.	Medicines and pharmaceuticals Biological substances Cellular life Medications made with inorganic compounds	Dosage Deliberate dispersal Recovery of materials degraded by biological processes
Surgery/operations	The utilization of micro/nanorobots as surgical instruments to access distant anatomical sites, thus minimizing the need for invasive surgical interventions.	Taking a biopsy/sample Invasion of tissues Distribution within cells Disintegration of biofilms	The production of force Recovery of materials degraded by biological processes Restoration of samples
Imaging	The implementation of an adaptive feedback technique can facilitate the integration of numerous treatments and research into the human body.	Visual imaging, ultrasonic imaging, magnetic imaging, and radiological imaging.	Better definition or resolution More frames per second Handling of informational data
Diagnosis	The application of micro/nanorobots to augment the mixture of fluids and enhance mechanical force to improve sensory characteristics.	Biologically based sensors Separation Tactile sensors	The high volume of work performed Capacity for growth or expansion Cost

6.6 Regulatory challenges in personalized healthcare

The incorporation of micro- and nanorobots into personalized healthcare presents a range of complex regulatory obstacles that need meticulous evaluation. Ensuring the safety and efficacy of these small devices is considered to be one of the most crucial factors. Regulatory bodies must develop stringent criteria and testing methods to assess the interaction between these robots and the human body as well as their overall effectiveness. The limitations of conventional evaluation methods, stemming from their distinct dimensions and mechanisms, may render them inadequate, hence prompting the need for the creation of novel assessment procedures.

The challenge of manufacturing standards is also a matter of considerable importance. To ensure uniformity and excellence, regulatory entities are required to establish stringent quality assurance protocols and adhere to good manufacturing practices specifically designed for the fabrication of micro- and nanorobots [125]. The implementation of these standards is crucial in ensuring that these intricate gadgets adhere to particular requirements and do not pose any risks to patients. The question of biological compatibility is an essential factor that regulators must take into account. In consideration of the fact that micro- and nanorobots frequently engage in intimate relationships with biological systems, it is imperative to define a set of rules that allow their biocompatibility to be evaluated. This entails the need to ensure that these gadgets do not elicit detrimental immune responses or unfavorable reactions upon their introduction into the human body. Risk assessment is a significant concern that requires attention. Micro- and nanorobots exhibit a wide range of configurations and have the potential to be employed in a wide variety of healthcare contexts. The categorization and risk assessment of these robots should be conducted by the regulatory authorities, taking into consideration various aspects, such as their level of invasiveness and intended purpose [126]. This categorization system would serve as a framework that determined the degree of inspection and the set of obligations that manufacturers would be subject to.

The validation of the safety and efficacy of micro- and nanorobots using clinical studies presents distinct obstacles. Regulatory bodies have to adapt standard clinical trial techniques and endpoints to address the complexities associated with this novel technology. This may entail the development of experimental protocols that are specially designed to evaluate the efficacy and safety of these miniature robots in practical healthcare settings. Furthermore, it is important to consider the ethical and societal ramifications, since they should not be disregarded. The use of micro- and nanorobots may give rise to apprehensions about issues of permission, patient autonomy, and discrepancies in the accessibility of innovative healthcare technology [127]. Regulators are obligated to take account of the ethical elements associated with their decision-making processes and ensure that the rules they enact are aligned with wider social norms and expectations. The imperative for the international harmonization of rules is paramount, considering the worldwide scope of the healthcare industry. The facilitation of collaborative initiatives among regulatory bodies on a global scale has the potential to optimize the process of approving and implementing micro and nanorobotics in the context of personalized healthcare while concurrently mitigating the emergence of trade barriers. In addition, the safeguarding of intellectual property rights and the resolution of possible patent conflicts are of the utmost importance in promoting innovation within this domain [128]. Regulatory bodies ought to assume the responsibility for settling intellectual property conflicts and upholding the rights of innovators. Post-market surveillance systems play a crucial role in the monitoring of the ongoing safety and performance of micro- and nanorobots. Regulators must develop comprehensive mechanisms to monitor and address any developing safety concerns or performance difficulties to ensure the protection of patient welfare.

Resolving these regulatory difficulties necessitates a collective endeavor including researchers, industry stakeholders, and regulatory entities. Ensuring the harmonious integration of micro and nanorobotics into personalized healthcare necessitates a careful equilibrium between innovation, patient safety, and ethical issues.

6.7 Conclusions

The field of personalized healthcare has witnessed the emergence of micro- and nanorobotics as highly innovative technologies. The application of miniaturized robots, often operating at the micrometer or nanometer scales, possesses the significant potential to fundamentally transform the delivery of healthcare and the customization of treatments for particular patients. In summary, the application of micro- and nanorobotics in the context of personalized healthcare holds great potential for driving notable progress in several domains, such as diagnostics, medication administration, surgical procedures, and patient monitoring. This can consequently enhance patient results and overall quality of life. These little robots possess the ability to explore the human anatomy with exceptional accuracy, enabling them to gain access to regions that were formerly impassable or posed challenges for targeted intervention. This particular capacity facilitates diagnostic methods that are more precise and less intrusive. Micro- and nanorobots have the potential to transport sensors and imaging equipment, enabling the identification of illnesses in their early stages. This facilitates prompt intervention and the development of tailored treatment strategies. Furthermore, the application of micro- and nanorobotics in medication delivery presents a promising opportunity to augment the effectiveness and precision of drug administrations. Medication delivery can be targeted specifically to affected cells or tissues, therefore reducing adverse effects and enhancing therapeutic efficacy. The use of this specific drug delivery strategy results in a decrease in the total dosage, hence enhancing the safety and efficacy of therapies. Micro- and nanorobots have the potential to aid doctors in performing surgeries through their ability to offer precise control and enhance dexterity. The utilization of these robotic systems enables the exploration of distant or fragile anatomical regions, hence mitigating the invasive nature of surgical procedures and minimizing potential harm to surrounding healthy tissues. Such interventions not only accelerate the process of healing but also mitigate the likelihood of problems.

Furthermore, the field of micro- and nanorobotics is of paramount importance in the context of ongoing patient surveillance. These robotic systems may be engineered to continuously monitor a range of physiological indicators, including but not limited to glucose levels, oxygen saturation, and medication concentrations in real time. The availability of these data facilitates prompt modifications to treatment strategies, guaranteeing that patients receive individualized care specifically adapted to their distinct requirements. In conclusion, the incorporation of micro- and nanorobotics into personalized healthcare has significant potential. The technologies mentioned above possess the capacity to revolutionize diagnostics, drug administration, surgical interventions, and patient surveillance and thus represent more efficient, minimally intrusive, and exceptionally tailored healthcare remedies. With the ongoing progress in scientific and technological advancement, it is foreseeable that micro and nanorobots will assume a progressively more prominent position in enhancing the health and wellbeing of persons on a global scale.

References and further reading

[1] Soto F and Chrostowski R 2018 Frontiers of medical micro/nanorobotics: *in vivo* applications and commercialization perspectives toward clinical uses *Front. Bioeng. Biotechnol.* **14** 6–170

[2] Medina-Sánchez M and Schmidt O G 2017 Medical microbots need better imaging and control *Nature* **545** 406–8

[3] Sitti M 2018 Miniature soft robots—road to the clinic *Nat. Rev. Mater.* **3** 74–5

[4] Agrahari V, Agrahari V, Chou M L, Chew C H, Noll J and Burnouf T 2020 Intelligent micro-/nanorobots as drug and cell carrier devices for biomedical therapeutic advancement: promising development opportunities and translational challenges *Biomaterials* **260** 120163

[5] Ghosh A, Xu W, Gupta N and Gracias D H 2020 Active matter therapeutics *Nano Today* **31** 100836

[6] Wang J 2013 *Nanomachines: Fundamentals and Applications* (New York: Wiley) 4

[7] Wang W, Duan W, Ahmed S, Mallouk T E and Sen A 2013 Small power: autonomous nano-and micromotors propelled by self-generated gradients *Nano Today* **8** 531–54

[8] Sanchez S, Soler L and Katuri J 2015 Chemically powered micro-and nanomotors *Angew. Chem. Int. Ed.* **54** 1414–44

[9] Chen X Z, Jang B, Ahmed D, Hu C, De Marco C, Hoop M, Mushtaq F, Nelson B J and Pané S 2018 Small-scale machines driven by external power sources *Adv. Mater.* **30** 1705061

[10] Chen C, Soto F, Karshalev E, Li J and Wang J 2019 Hybrid nano vehicles: one machine, two engines *Adv. Funct. Mater.* **29** 1806290

[11] Rezaei Nejad H, Oliveira B C, Sadeqi A, Dehkharghani A, Kondova I, Langermans J A, Guasto J S, Tzipori S, Widmer G and Sonkusale S R 2019 Ingestible osmotic pill for *in vivo* sampling of gut microbiomes *Adv. Intell. Syst.* **1** 1900053

[12] Min J, Yang Y, Wu Z and Gao W 2020 Robotics in the gut *Adv. Therap.* **3** 1900125

[13] Breger J C, Yoon C, Xiao R, Kwag H R, Wang M O, Fisher J P, Nguyen T D and Gracias D H 2015 Self-folding thermo-magnetically responsive soft microgrippers *ACS Appl. Mater. Interfaces* **7** 3398–405

[14] Soto F, Wang J, Ahmed R and Demirci U 2020 Medical micro/nanorobots in precision medicine *Adv. Sci.* **7** 2002203

[15] Fusco S *et al* 2014 An integrated micro-robotic platform for on-demand, targeted therapeutic interventions *Adv. Mater.* **26** 952–7

[16] Jin Q, Yang Y, Jackson J A, Yoon C and Gracias D H 2020 Untethered single-cell grippers for active biopsy *Nano Lett.* **20** 5383–90

[17] Bassik N, Brafman A, Zarafshar A M, Jamal M, Luvsanjav D, Selaru F M and Gracias D H 2010 Enzymatically triggered actuation of miniaturized tools *JACS* **132** 16314–7

[18] Hui X, Luo J, Wang X, Wang R and Sun H 2022 Bimorph electrothermal micro-gripper with large deformation, precise and rapid response, and low operating voltage *Appl. Phys. Lett.* **11** 121

[19] Di Giacomo R, Krödel S, Maresca B, Benzoni P, Rusconi R, Stocker R and Daraio C 2017 Deployable micro-traps to sequester motile bacteria *Sci. Rep.* **7** 45897

[20] Soto F, Kupor D, Lopez-Ramirez M A, Wei F, Karshalev E, Tang S, Tehrani F and Wang J 2020 Onion-like multifunctional microtrap vehicles for attraction–trapping–destruction of biological threats *Angew. Chem. Int. Ed.* **59** 3480–5

[21] Yu L M *et al* 2019 Hypoxia-induced ROS contributes to myoblast pyroptosis during obstructive sleep apnea via the NF-κB/HIF-1α signaling pathway *Oxid. Med. Cell. Longev.* **11** 2019

[22] Ozen M O, Sridhar K, Ogut M G, Shanmugam A, Avadhani A S, Kobayashi Y, Wu J C, Haddad F and Demirci U 2020 Total microfluidic chip for multiplexed diagnostics (ToMMx) *Biosens. Bioelectron.* **150** 111930

[23] Liu F *et al* 2017 The exosome total isolation chip *ACS Nano* **11** 10712–23

[24] Mayeux R 2004 Biomarkers: potential uses and limitations *NeuroRx* **1** 182–8

[25] Broza Y Y, Zhou X, Yuan M, Qu D, Zheng Y, Vishinkin R, Khatib M, Wu W and Haick H 2019 Disease detection with molecular biomarkers: from the chemistry of body fluids to nature-inspired chemical sensors *Chem. Rev.* **119** 11761–817

[26] Abramson A *et al* 2019 An ingestible self-orienting system for oral delivery of macromolecules *Science* **363** 611–5

[27] Abramson A *et al* 2019 A luminal unfolding microneedle injector for oral delivery of macromolecules *Nat. Med.* **25** 1512–8

[28] Jafari S *et al* 2019 Magnetic drilling enhances intra-nasal transport of particles into rodent brain *J. Magn. Magn. Mater.* **469** 302–5

[29] Mair L O, Weinberg I O, Teceno D N, Jafari S and Sun D 2019 *2019 9th International IEEE/EMBS Conference on Neural Engineering (NER) Rat Behavioral Changes Due to Implanted Magnetic Particles Activated with Externally-Applied Magnetic Fields* (Piscataway, NJ: IEEE) 977

[30] Xi W, Solovev A A, Ananth A N, Gracias D H, Sanchez S and Schmidt O G 2013 Rolled-up magnetic microdriller: towards remotely controlled minimally invasive surgery *Nanoscale* **5** 1294–7

[31] Walker D, Käsdorf B T, Jeong H H, Lieleg O and Fischer P 2015 Enzymatically active biomimetic micro propellers for the penetration of mucin gels *Sci. Adv.* **1** e1500501

[32] Ullrich F, Bergeles C, Pokki J, Ergeneman O, Erni S, Chatzipirpiridis G, Pané S, Framme C and Nelson B J 2013 Mobility experiments with microrobots for minimally invasive intraocular surgery *Invest. Ophthalmol. Vis. Sci.* **54** 2853–63

[33] Pokki J, Ergeneman O, Chatzipirpiridis G, Lühmann T, Sort J, Pellicer E, Pot S A, Spiess B M, Pané S and Nelson B J 2017 Protective coatings for intraocular wirelessly controlled microrobots for implantation: corrosion, cell culture, and *in vivo* animal tests *J. Biomed. Mater. Res. Part B: Appl. Biomater.* **105** 836–45

[34] Wu Z *et al* 2018 A swarm of slippery micropropellers penetrates the vitreous body of the eye *Sci. Adv.* **4** eaat4388

[35] Kagan D, Benchimol M J, Claussen J C, Chuluun-Erdene E, Esener S and Wang J 2012 Acoustic droplet vaporization and propulsion of perfluorocarbon-loaded microbullets for targeted tissue penetration and deformation *Angew. Chem. Int. Ed.* **51** 7519–22

[36] Jernigan J A *et al* 2020 Multidrug-resistant bacterial infections in US hospitalized patients *New Engl. J. Med.* **382** 1309–19

[37] Rigo S, Cai C, Gunkel-Grabole G, Maurizi L, Zhang X, Xu J and Palivan C G 2018 Nanoscience-based strategies to engineer antimicrobial surfaces *Adv. Sci.* **5** 1700892
[38] Mair L O *et al* 2017 Biofilm disruption with rotating micro rods enhances antimicrobial efficacy *J. Magn. Magn. Mater.* **427** 81–4
[39] Stanton M M, Park B W, Vilela D, Bente K, Faivre D, Sitti M and Sánchez S 2017 Magnetotactic bacteria powered biohybrids target *E. coli* biofilms *Nano* **11** 9968–78
[40] Hortelao A C, Carrascosa R, Murillo-Cremaes N, Patino T and Sanchez S 2018 Targeting 3D bladder cancer spheroids with urease-powered nanomotors *ACS Nano* **13** 429–39
[41] Oh M J *et al* 2023 Nanozyme-based robotics approach for targeting fungal infection *Adv. Mater.* **4** 2300320
[42] Hwang Geelsu, Paula Amauri J., Hunter Elizabeth E., Liu Yuan and Babeer Alaa *et al* 2019 Catalytic antimicrobial robots for biofilm eradication *Sci. Robot.* **4** eaaw2388
[43] Zhang P, Wu G, Zhao C, Zhou L, Wang X and Wei S 2020 Magnetic somatotype-like nanomotor as photosensitizer carrier for photodynamic therapy-based cancer treatment *Colloids Surf.* **B 194** 111204
[44] Wang D, Gao C, Zhou C, Lin Z and He Q 2020 Leukocyte membrane-coated liquid metal nano swimmers for actively targeted delivery and synergistic chemo photothermal therapy *Research* **24** 3676954
[45] Vyskocil J, Mayorga-Martinez C C, Jablonska E, Novotny F, Ruml T and Pumera M 2020 Cancer cells microsurgery via asymmetric bent surface Au/Ag/Ni micro robotic scalpels through a transversal rotating magnetic field *ACS Nano* **14** 8247–56
[46] Wang W, Wu Z and He Q 2020 Swimming nanorobots for opening a cell membrane mechanically *View* **1** 20200005
[47] Venugopalan P L, Esteban-Fernández de Ávila B, Pal M, Ghosh A and Wang J L 2020 Fantastic voyage of nanomotors into the cell *ACS nanob* **14** 9423–39
[48] Wang W, Li S, Mair L, Ahmed S, Huang T J and Mallouk T E 2014 Acoustic propulsion of nanorod motors inside living cells *Angew. Chem. Int. Ed.* **53** 3201–4
[49] Esteban-Fernández de Ávila B, Martín A, Soto F, Lopez-Ramirez M A, Campuzano S, Vasquez-Machado G M, Gao W, Zhang L and Wang J 2015 Single cell real-time miRNAs sensing based on nanomotors *ACS Nano* **9** 6756–64
[50] Esteban-Fernández de Ávila B, Angell C, Soto F, Lopez-Ramirez M A, Báez D F, Xie S, Wang J and Chen Y 2016 Acoustically propelled nanomotors for intracellular siRNA delivery *ACS Nano* **24** 4997–5005
[51] Esteban-Fernández de Ávila B, Ramírez-Herrera D E, Campuzano S, Angsantikul P, Zhang L and Wang J 2017 Nanomotor-enabled pH-responsive intracellular delivery of caspase-3: toward rapid cell apoptosis *ACS Nano* **27** 5367–74
[52] Zhang F, Zhuang J, Esteban Fernández de Ávila B, Tang S, Zhang Q, Fang R H, Zhang L and Wang J 2019 A nanomotor-based active delivery system for intracellular oxygen transport *ACS Nano 26* 11996–2005
[53] Hansen-Bruhn M, de Ávila B E, Beltrán-Gastélum M, Zhao J, Ramírez-Herrera D E, Angsantikul P, Vesterager Gothelf K, Zhang L and Wang J 2018 Inside cover: active intracellular delivery of a Cas9/sgRNA complex using ultrasound-propelled nanomotors *Angew. Chem. Int. Ed.* **1** 2506
[54] Soto F, Wagner G L, Garcia-Gradilla V, Gillespie K T, Lakshmipathy D R, Karshalev E, Angell C, Chen Y and Wang J 2016 Acoustically propelled nanoshells *Nanoscale* **8** 17788–93

[55] Wang W, Wu Z, Lin X, Si T and He Q 2019 Gold-nanoshell-functionalized polymer nano swimmer for a photomechanical portion of the single-cell membrane *JACS* **3** 6601–8
[56] Llopis-Lorente A, Garcia-Fernandez A, Murillo-Cremaes N, Hortelao A C, Patino T, Villalonga R, Sancenon F, Martinez-Manez R and Sanchez S 2019 Enzyme-powered gated mesoporous silica nanomotors for on-command intracellular payload delivery *ACS Nano* **3** 12171–83
[57] Sun M, Liu Q, Fan X, Wang Y, Chen W, Tian C, Sun L and Xie H 2020 Autonomous biohybrid urchin-like microperforator for intracellular payload delivery *Small* **16** 1906701
[58] Qiu F, Fujita S, Mhanna R, Zhang L, Simona B R and Nelson B J 2015 Magnetic helical microswimmers functionalized with lipoplexes for targeted gene delivery *Adva. Funct. Mater.* **25** 1666–71
[59] Kadiri V M, Bussi C, Holle A W, Son K, Kwon H, Schütz G, Gutierrez M G and Fischer P 2020 Biocompatible magnetic micro-and nanodevices: fabrication of FePt nano propellers and cell transfection *Adv. Mater.* **32** 2001114
[60] Wang Y, Liu Y, Li Y, Xu D, Pan X, Chen Y, Zhou D, Wang B, Feng H and Ma X 2020 Magnetic nanomotor-based maneuverable SERS probe *Research* **5** 7962024
[61] Kim K, Guo J, Liang Z and Fan D 2018 Artificial micro/nanomachines for bio applications: biochemical delivery and diagnostic sensing *Adv. Funct. Mater.* **28** 1705867
[62] Patino T, Porchetta A, Jannasch A, Lladó A, Stumpp T, Schäffer E, Ricci F and Sánchez S 2019 Self-sensing enzyme-powered micromotors equipped with pH-responsive DNA nano switches *Nano Lett.* **1** 3440–7
[63] Wu J, Balasubramanian S, Kagan D, Manesh K M, Campuzano S and Wang J 2010 Motion-based DNA detection using catalytic nanomotors *Nat. Commun.* **13** 36
[64] Kagan D, Campuzano S, Balasubramanian S, Kuralay F, Flechsig G U and Wang J 2011 Functionalized micromachines for selective and rapid isolation of nucleic acid targets from complex samples *Nano Lett.* **11** 2083–7
[65] Simmchen J, Baeza A, Ruiz D, Esplandiu M J and Vallet-Regí M 2012 Asymmetric hybrid silica nanomotors for capture and cargo transport: towards a novel motion-based DNA sensor *Small* **9** 2053–9
[66] Draz M S, Kochehbyoki K M, Vasan A, Battalapalli D, Sreeram A, Kanakasabapathy M K, Kallakuri S, Tsibris A, Kuritzkes D R and Shafiee H 2018 DNA engineered micromotors powered by metal nanoparticles for motion-based cellphone diagnostics *Nat. Commun.* **16** 4282
[67] Van Nguyen K and Minteer S D 2015 DNA-functionalized Pt nanoparticles as catalysts for chemically powered micromotors: toward signal-on motion-based DNA biosensor *Chem. Commun.* **51** 4782–4
[68] Fu S, Zhang X, Xie Y, Wu J and Ju H 2019 An efficient enzyme-powered micromotor device fabricated by cyclic alternate hybridization assembly for DNA detection *Nanoscale* **9** 9026–33
[69] Xie Y, Fu S, Wu J, Lei J and Ju H 2017 Motor-based microprobe powered by bio-assembled catalase for motion detection of DNA *Biosens. Bioelectron.* **15** 31–7
[70] Zhang X, Chen C, Wu J and Ju H 2019 Bubble-propelled jellyfish-like micromotors for DNA sensing *ACS Appl. Mater. Interfaces* **19** 13581–8
[71] Orozco J, Campuzano S, Kagan D, Zhou M, Gao W and Wang J 2011 Dynamic isolation and unloading of target proteins by aptamer-modified micro transporters *Anal. Chem.* **15** 7962–9

[72] Draz M S *et al* 2018 Motion-based immunological detection of Zika virus using Pt-nanomotors and a cellphone *ACS Nano* **16** 5709–18
[73] Esteban-Fernández de Ávila B, Lopez-Ramirez M A, Báez D F, Jodra A, Singh V V, Kaufmann K and Wang J 2016 Aptamer-modified graphene-based catalytic micromotors: off–on fluorescent detection of ricin *ACS Sens.* **25** 217–21
[74] Molinero-Fernandez A, Moreno-Guzman M, López M A and Escarpa A 2017 Biosensing strategy for simultaneous and accurate quantitative analysis of mycotoxins in food samples using unmodified graphene micromotors *Anal. Chem.* **17** 10850–7
[75] Jurado-Sánchez B, Pacheco M, Rojo J and Escarpa A 2017 Magneto catalytic graphene quantum dots Janus micromotors for bacterial endotoxin detection *Angew. Chem. Int. Ed.* **6** 6957–61
[76] Zhang Y *et al* 2019 Real-time tracking of fluorescent magnetic spore–based microrobots for remote detection of C. diff toxins *Sci. Adv.* **11** eaau9650
[77] Weinberger S R, Morris T S and Pawlak M 2000 Recent trends in protein biochip technology *Pharmacogenomics* **1** 395–416
[78] Banerjee S S, Jalota-Badhwar A, Zope K R, Todkar K J, Mascarenhas R R, Chate G P, Khutale G V, Bharde A, Calderon M and Khandare J J 2015 Self-propelled carbon nanotube-based Microrocket for rapid capture and isolation of circulating tumor cells *Nanoscale* **7** 8684–8
[79] Chałupniak A, Morales-Narváez E and Merkoçi A 2015 Micro and nanomotors in diagnostics *Adv. Drug Deliv. Rev.* **95** 104–16
[80] Garcia-Gradilla V, Orozco J, Sattayasamitsathit S, Soto F, Kuralay F, Pourazary A, Katzenberg A, Gao W, Shen Y and Wang J 2013 Functionalized ultrasound-propelled magnetically guided nanomotors: toward practical biomedical applications *ACS Nano* **7** 9232–40
[81] Campuzano S, Orozco J, Kagan D, Guix M, Gao W, Sattayasamitsathit S, Claussen J C, Merkoçi A and Wang J 2012 Bacterial isolation by lectin-modified micro engines *Nano Lett.* **12** 396–401
[82] Garcia M, Orozco J, Guix M, Gao W, Sattayasamitsathit S, Escarpa A, Merkoçi A and Wang J 2013 Micromotor-based lab-on-chip immunoassays *Nanoscale* **5** 1325–31
[83] Orozco J, Pan G, Sattayasamitsathit S, Galarnyk M and Wang J 2015 Micromotors to capture and destroy anthrax simulant spores *Analyst* **140** 1421–7
[84] Delezuk J A, Ramírez-Herrera D E, de Ávila B E and Wang J 2017 Chitosan-based water-propelled micromotors with strong antibacterial activity *Nanoscale* **9** 2195–200
[85] Balasubramanian S, Kagan D, Jack Hu C M, Campuzano S, Lobo-Castañon M J, Lim N, Kang D Y, Zimmerman M, Zhang L and Wang J 2011 Cover picture: micromachine-enabled capture and isolation of cancer cells in complex media *Angew. Chem. Int. Ed.* **50** 4023
[86] Sanchez S, Solovev A A, Schulze S and Schmidt O G 2011 Controlled manipulation of multiple cells using catalytic microbots *Chem. Commun.* **47** 698–700
[87] Jeon S *et al* 2019 Magnetically actuated microrobots as a platform for stem cell transplantation *Sci. Robot.* **4** 4317
[88] Lin Z, Fan X, Sun M, Gao C, He Q and Xie H 2018 Magnetically actuated peanut colloid motors for cell manipulation and patterning *ACS Nano* **12** 2539–45

[89] Läubli N F, Shamsudhin N, Vogler H, Munglani G, Grossniklaus U, Ahmed D and Nelson B J 2019 3D manipulation and imaging of plant cells using acoustically activated microbubbles *Small Methods* **3** 1800527
[90] Lu X, Zhao K, Liu W, Yang D, Shen H, Peng H, Guo X, Li J and Wang J 2019 A human microrobot interface based on acoustic manipulation *ACS Nano* **13** 11443–52
[91] Wu Z, Li T, Gao W, Xu T, Jurado-Sánchez B, Li J, Gao W, He Q, Zhang L and Wang J 2015 Cell-membrane-coated synthetic nanomotors for effective biodetoxification *Adv. Funct. Mater.* **25** 3881–7
[92] Wu Z, Li J, de Ávila B E, Li T, Gao W, He Q, Zhang L and Wang J 2015 Water-powered cell-mimicking Janus micromotor *Adv. Funct. Mater.* **25** 7497–501
[93] Li J *et al* 2018 Biomimetic platelet-camouflaged nanorobots for binding and isolation of biological threats *Adv. Mater.* **30** 1704800
[94] Wang B, Handschuh-Wang S, Shen J, Zhou X, Guo Z, Liu W, Pumera M and Zhang L 2023 Small-scale robotics with tailored wettability *Adv. Mater.* **335** 2205732
[95] Pal M, Somalwar N, Singh A, Bhat R, Eswarappa S M, Saini D K and Ghosh A 2018 Maneuverability of magnetic nanomotors inside living cells *Adv. Mater.* **30** 1800429
[96] Pal M *et al* 2020 Helical nanobots as mechanical probes of intra-and extracellular environments *J. Phys. Condens. Matter* **32** 224001
[97] Dasgupta D, Pally D, Saini D K, Bhat R and Ghosh A 2020 Nanorobots sense local physiochemical heterogeneities of tumor matrisome *Angew Chem. Int. Ed. Engl.* **59** 23690–6
[98] Liu L, Chen B, Liu K, Gao J, Ye Y, Wang Z, Qin N, Wilson D A, Tu Y and Peng F 2020 Wireless manipulation of magnetic/piezoelectric micromotors for precise neural stem-like cell stimulation *Adv. Funct.* **30** 1910108
[99] Wu Y, Fu A and Yossifon G 2020 Active particle-based selective transport and release of cell organelles and mechanical probing of a single nucleus *Small* **16** 1906682
[100] Wang L, Li T, Li L, Wang J, Song W and Zhang G 2015 Microrocket-based viscometer *ECS J. Solid-State Sci. Technol.* **4** S3020
[101] Zizzari A, Cesaria M, Bianco M, del Mercato L L, Carraro M, Bonchio M, Rella R and Arima V 2020 Mixing enhancement induced by viscoelastic micromotors in microfluidic platforms *Chem. Eng. J.* **1** 391–123572
[102] Schoen I, Pruitt B L and Vogel V 2013 The Yin–Yang of rigidity sensing: how forces and mechanical properties regulate the cellular response to materials *Annu. Rev. Mater. Res.* **43** 589–618
[103] Vogel V and Sheetz M 2006 Local force and geometry sensing regulate cell functions *Nat. Rev. Mol. Cell Biol.* **7** 265–75
[104] Wang X *et al* 2022 microrobotic swarms for intracellular measurement with enhanced signal-to-noise ratio *ACS Nano* **16** 10824–39
[105] Wang B, Zhang Y and Zhang L 2018 Recent progress on micro- and nano-robots: towards *in vivo* tracking and localization *Quant. Imaging. Med. Surg.* **8** 461
[106] Alarcón-Correa M, Walker D, Qiu T and Fischer P 2016 Nanomotors *Eur. Phys. J. Spec. Top.* **225** 2241–54
[107] Gao C, Wang Y, Ye Z, Lin Z, Ma X and He Q 2021 Biomedical micro-/nanomotors: from overcoming biological barriers to *in vivo* imaging *Adv. Mater.* **33** 2000512
[108] van Moolenbroek G T, Patiño T, Llop J and Sánchez S 2020 Engineering intelligent nanosystem for enhanced medical imaging *Adv. Intell. Syst.* **2** 2000087

[109] Gultepe E, Randhawa J S, Kadam S, Yamanaka S, Selaru F M, Shin E J, Kalloo A N and Gracias D H 2013 Biopsy with thermally-responsive untethered micro tools *Adv. Mater.* **25** 514–9

[110] Chatzipirpiridis G, Ergeneman O, Pokki J, Ullrich F, Fusco S, Ortega J A, Sivaraman K M, Nelson B J and Pané S 2015 Microrobotics: electroforming of implantable tubular magnetic microrobots for wireless ophthalmologic applications *Adv. Healthcare Mater.* **4** 208

[111] Servant A, Qiu F, Mazza M, Kostarelos K and Nelson B J 2015 Controlled *in vivo* swimming of a swarm of bacteria-like micro robotic flagella *Adv. Mater.* **27** 2981–8

[112] Yan X *et al* 2017 Multifunctional biohybrid magnetite microrobots for imaging-guided therapy *Scie. Robot.* **2** eaaq1155

[113] Akin D, Sturgis J, Ragheb K, Sherman D, Burkholder K, Robinson P J, Bhunia A K, Mohammed S and Bashir R 2007 Bacteria-mediated delivery of nanoparticles and cargo into cells at *Nanotechnol* **2** 441

[114] Yanagida T, Nagashima K, Oka K, Kanai M, Klamchuen A, Park B H and Kawai T 2013 Scaling effect on unipolar and bipolar resistive switching of metal oxides *Sci. Rep.* **3** 1657

[115] Gao Y, Xiong Z, Wang J, Tang J and Li D 2022 Light hybrid micro/nano-robots: from propulsion to functional signals *Nano Res.* **15** 5355–75

[116] Li D, Jeong M, Oren E, Yu T and Qiu T 2019 A helical microrobot with an optimized propeller-shape for propulsion in viscoelastic biological media *Robotics* **8** 87

[117] Olson E S, Orozco J, Wu Z, Malone C D, Yi B, Gao W, Eghtedari M, Wang J and Mattrey R F 2013 Toward *in vivo* detection of hydrogen peroxide with ultrasound molecular imaging *Biomaterials* **34** 8918–24

[118] Aziz A, Medina-Sánchez M, Koukourakis N, Wang J, Kuschmierz R, Radner H, Czarske J W and Schmidt O G 2019 Real-time IR tracking of single reflective micromotors through scattering tissues *Adv. Funct. Mater.* **29** 1905272

[119] Xie L *et al* 2020 Photoacoustic imaging-trackable magnetic microswimmers for pathogenic bacterial infection treatment *ACS Nano* **14** 2880–93

[120] Vilela D, Cossío U, Parmar J, Martínez-Villacorta A M, Gómez-Vallejo V, Llop J and Sánchez S 2018 Medical imaging for the tracking of micromotors *ACS Nano* **12** 1220–7

[121] Iacovacci V, Blanc A, Huang H, Ricotti L, Schibli R, Menciassi A, Behe M, Pané S and Nelson B J 2019 High-resolution SPECT imaging of stimuli-responsive soft microrobots *Small* **15** 1900709

[122] Nguyen P B, Kang B, Bappy D M, Choi S, Park S Y, Ko J O, Park C S and Kim J T 2018 *Int. Comput. Assist. Radiol. Surg* **13** 1843

[123] Xu Z, Chen M, Lee H, Feng S P, Park J Y, Lee S and Kim J T 2019 X-ray-powered micromotors *ACS Appl. Mater. Interfaces* **11** 15727–32

[124] Bauer G F, Hämmig O, Schaufeli W B and Taris T W 2014 A critical review of the job demands-resources model: implications for improving work and health *Bridging Occupational, Organizational and Public Health: A Transdisciplinary Approach* (Dordrecht: Springer) 43–68

[125] Singh A V, Rosenkranz D, Ansari M H D, Singh R, Kanase A, Singh S P and Luch A 2020 Artificial intelligence and machine learning empower advanced biomedical material design for toxicity prediction *Adv. Intell. Syst.* **2** 2000084

[126] Holder C, Khurana V, Harrison F and Jacobs L 2016 Robotics and law: key legal and regulatory implications of the robotics age (part I of II) *Comput. Law Secur. Rev.* **32** 383–402

[127] Singh A V, Ansari M H D, Laux P and Luch A 2019 Micro-nanorobots: important considerations when developing novel drug delivery platforms *Exp. Opinion Drug Deliv.* **16** 1259–75

[128] McManis C R 2003 Intellectual property, genetic resources, and traditional knowledge protection: thinking globally, acting locally *Cardozo J. Int'l Comp.* L **11** 547

[129] Jiao X, Wang Z, Xiu J, Dai W, Zhao L, Xu T, Du X, Wen Y and Zhang X 2020 NIR powered Janus nanocarrier for deep tumor penetration *Appl. Mater. Today* **1** 100504

[130] Pané S, Puigmartí-Luis J, Bergeles C, Chen X Z, Pellicer E, Sort J, Počepcová V, Ferreira A and Nelson B J 2019 Imaging technologies for biomedical micro- and nano swimmers *Adv. Mater. Technol.* **4** 1800575

Rishabha Malviya, Deepika Yadav, Sonali Sundram, Seifedine Kadry and Gurvinder Singh Virk

Chapter 7

The development of active nanorobots in personalized healthcare

In recent years, significant progress has been seen in the area of nanotechnology, leading to the advancement of novel possibilities for creative applications across several sectors, such as healthcare. The use of active nanorobots, characterized by their unique ability to change matter at the nanoscale, has emerged as a potential sector within the field of personalized healthcare. Starting with the definition of nanorobotics and its application to healthcare, this chapter emphasizes the different benefits that nanorobots provide in terms of targeted medication administration, diagnostics, and treatment. Nanotechnology is a field that is significantly altering the field of medical investigation. Nanorobots have significant potential to be used as valuable instruments in the field of future medicine. 'Nanorobotics' refers to the technological field concerned with the design and fabrication of machines or robots that operate at or near the minuscule size of a nanometer (10^{-9} m). Nanobots can travel through their surroundings by engaging in the consumption of molecules as a means to acquire energy. This chapter presents a comprehensive survey of the progression and prospective uses of active nanorobots within the field of personalized healthcare. The chapter analyzes the methodologies and substances used in the construction of active nanorobots, emphasizing the difficulties encountered and the advancements made in the development and regulation of these tiny devices. These devices are also regarded as valuable tools in medication delivery, a critical component of medical therapy. Nanorobots can execute several functions, such as actuation, sensing, signaling, processing data, and intelligence, at the nanoscale. The chapter mainly focuses on the numerous uses of active nanorobots in personalized medicine, e.g. the potential use of nanoscale agents in achieving targeted medication delivery to specific cells, tissues, or organs. This is intended to reduce the occurrence of systemic adverse effects and improve the

doi:10.1088/978-0-7503-6019-7ch7

overall effectiveness of treatments. Furthermore, the potential of nanorobots in the fields of early illness detection, diagnostics, and monitoring is demonstrated by concrete illustrations of diagnostic platforms that use nanorobot technology. Active nanorobots, which are very tiny devices with the capability to manipulate matter on the nanoscale, have recently gained significant attention as a possible transformative subdomain of the field of personalized healthcare. This chapter describes their development and uses, highlighting their potential to change healthcare. It focuses on the practical use of nanorobots in the fields of medication administration and illness detection, with an emphasis on their significance in the field of precision healthcare.

7.1 Introduction

The term 'nano' has its historical origins in the Greek word 'nanos,' which refers to 'dwarf.' The concept of nanotechnology was first presented by Nobel Prize-winning physicist Richard Feynman in 1959 in a lecture titled 'There's plenty of room at the bottom.' Subsequently, nanotechnology has been used in an extensive variety of applications, including dental diagnostics, materials, and treatments [1]. The word 'nanotechnology' was first introduced by a student studying at a scientific institution in Tokyo in 1974 [2]. Nanotechnology includes the extensive investigation, conceptualization, generation, manipulation, and utilization of substances, apparatuses, and structures at the nanoscale. Nanotechnology is most accurately characterized as a field that involves operations conducted at the atomic or molecular scale, which has practical applications in the macro environment. A nanometer, denoted by nm, is equivalent to one billionth of a meter. To provide a visual comparison, this length corresponds to approximately 1/80 000th of the diameter of a human hair or roughly ten times the dimensions of the hydrogen atom [3–5]. Nanotechnology is a specialized branch of applied science that concentrates on the deliberate manipulation and precise control of matter at the atomic and molecular scales [6]. Significant progress in the field of robotics technology is now reducing the gap between human beings and robots. Robotic systems have shown the capability to assist and interact with those who have disabilities, as well as the elderly. Micromachines show significant promise in several biological fields, such as active drug delivery, biological sensing, micromanipulation, and minimally invasive intervention [7–13]. The use of nanoscale medical robots has become more prevalent in several aspects of everyday life [14–17].

The utilization of surgical robots, such as the widely recognized da Vinci robot system, offers several advantages in the field of minimally invasive procedures. These advantages include improved dexterity, enhanced precision, a reduction in the hand tremors experienced by surgeons, user-friendly ergonomic interfaces, and the capability to remotely access surgical sites using miniature instruments [18, 19]. Robotic devices have been created to help patients with movement impairments to regain function, including upper-limb therapy [20] and lower-limb support [21]. This chapter provides a comprehensive overview of and emphasizes current advancements in the field of self-powered wearable nanorobots for personalized healthcare [22–31].

It enhances the ability of healthcare providers to give personalized healthcare to each patient. The field of personalized medicine discovery has the potential to reveal opportunities that might otherwise remain unexplored. Precision healthcare has seen significant progress, resulting in concrete advantages such as the ability to diagnose diseases at an early stage and the increasing prevalence of personalized therapies in the healthcare sector [32, 33]. Active nanorobots, which are miniature marvels of engineering, have emerged as a beacon of hope for changing individualized healthcare in this era of fast technological innovation. Nanoscale devices provide remarkable capabilities for the precise manipulation of matter, presenting a transformative promise in the fields of disease diagnosis and treatment. Research into active nanorobots has provided knowledge about their evolution, functionalities, and use within the area of personalized healthcare. The field of nanorobotics has the potential to revolutionize healthcare by enabling specialized medicines, improving diagnostics, and facilitating personalized medicine. The potential and prospects of active nanorobots in the field of healthcare provide an enticing vision of a future characterized by highly accurate and completely personalized medicinal treatments. The ability of personalized medicine to personalize healthcare is facilitated by various technologies for data collection and analytics. Nanorobots, as a significant category of miniature medical robotics, have considerable potential to advance biomedicine. Nanorobotics includes the development of robotic mechanisms designed to carry out various functions, such as actuation, monitoring, manipulation, signaling, information processing, and intelligence, specifically at the nanoscale [34].

Small-scale nanorobotic systems are often referred to as nanorobots, or they can be intentionally engineered to engage with materials at the nanoscale, in which case they are generally referred to as nanomanipulators [35]. Nanorobotics has great importance in the field of biomedicine. The concept of personalized medicine [36] raises various critical concerns that require consideration. These include the need for accurate and complete disease diagnosis customized to individual patients, the identification of potential drugs that may provide therapeutic benefits, assistance provided to physicians in formulating specific treatment strategies, etc. To address these concerns, it is essential to understand individual patients' health conditions at the single-molecule level. This is because certain biomolecules present in diseased cells serve as indicators of illness, and there are linkages between these biological molecules and drug molecules that directly affect drug efficacy [37, 38]. Nanorobotics is necessary for the robotic manipulation of biomolecules, since single biomolecules are nanoscale entities [39]. As a result, the emerging field of personalized medicine has significant prospects for the advancement of medical nanorobotics.

7.2 Nanorobots

Nanorobots are nanodevices utilized for preventing humans from being infected by pathogens, or treating such infections. They are small devices with nanoscale dimensions of 1–100 nm that are intended to accurately accomplish a certain activity or function. These devices are expected to operate at the atomic, molecular, and cellular scales to carry out various industrial or medical tasks [6]. Based on the principles of nanorobotic theory, it is hypothesized that nanorobots will possess a small physical scale and hence require a substantial collective presence to effectively execute both microscopic and macroscopic activities [1]. Technological developments in the areas of robotics, medicine, bioinformatics, and nanotechnology may assist with the development of nanorobotic drug delivery systems and the associated computing. Nanorobots may present a wide variety of forms, such as those used for surgery, eating microbes, repairing cells, and breathing. The field of robotics is now seeing advancements that are specifically targeted toward its use in the areas of biological and medical research. Robotic systems can be programmed to execute repetitive surgical operations. Nanobiotechnology is a novel domain in the field of nanorobotics, or nanobots for short, and is the product of advances in robotics. Miniaturized nanobots will be introduced into the body via blood vessels or at the ends of catheters into different veins and other cavities in humans, rather than carrying out treatments from outside the body. Surgeon-programmed surgical nanorobots have the potential to function as independent surgeons inside the human body. Their onboard computers can carry out and coordinate many operations, including searching for diseased tissues, diagnosing conditions, and conducting the necessary procedures for the removal or repair of lesions by nanomanipulation. These concepts, which were once classified as science fiction, have been accepted as potentially achievable. Nanorobots will be able to perform intracellular surgery that is more accurate and exact than the surgery that humans perform using their hands.

Nanorobots designed for use in biomedicine have been the subject of comprehensive investigation and fast advancement over the last decade; as a result, they are now capable of transporting payloads to specific locations inside organisms while operating in a controlled laboratory environment. Nanorobots are not intended to remain in the patient indefinitely; they must also be capable of escaping the host. The construction of nanorobots involves integrating several components, including sensors, actuators, control mechanisms, power sources, communication systems, and interfaces. These components enable the interaction and coordination to take place between nanorobots at different spatial scales, between inorganic and organic matter, and in abiotic as well as biotic systems. A useful approach for accelerating progress in nanorobotics is the manipulation of natural nanomachine systems using engineering techniques. This enables the development of novel and artificial biological devices. In practical applications, a nanorobot may be classified as either an inactive or active structure with the capability to detect, transmit, and process information. The constrained dimensions of these devices dictate restricted functionalities and decreased computational resources [1, 40, 41]. Consequently, it becomes essential to promote collaboration among devices by employing design methodologies such as swarm intelligence. This approach facilitates the realization of intricate systems by enabling interaction and cooperation between elementary agents. The objective is to effectively manage substantial groups of nanorobots that engage in complex interactions inside tumor settings to enhance therapeutic effects. The swarm phenomena that are of particular interest include the ability to amplify, optimize, map, build, move collectively, synchronize, and make decisions [5]. A nanorobot is a specialized mechanism capable of deliberately and reliably altering its immediate environment by operating at the molecular or even atomic level. The future development of medical nanorobots is anticipated to result in their dimensions being comparable to those of bacteria. These nanorobots are expected to consist of several mechanical components at the molecular scale, potentially resembling structures such as gears, bearings, and ratchets. They might be made of a tough, diamond-like substance. To facilitate movement and manipulation, nanorobots require the incorporation of motors for locomotion and manipulators such as arms or prosthetic legs. These autonomous systems will need a power source, sensors for navigation, and an onboard computer for behavior management. Nanorobots, unlike ordinary robots, are smaller than red blood cells and can fit through the body's tiniest capillaries. Nanorobots refer to small, mobile devices operating at nanoscale dimensions, which possess the capability to execute precise activities as required. These duties may be accomplished either automatically or by using external sources of power, after a viable process of design and manufacturing. The field of nanotechnology and small-scale manufacture has seen significant progress, leading to the development of different structures of nanorobots (NRs) that exhibit efficient mobility in varied physiological conditions [1, 40–45]. Furthermore, the presence of functional components gives these devices capabilities such as the ability to carry cargo, react to their microenvironment [46], work collaboratively [47], and exhibit biocompatibility [48].

In the future, nanorobotics may contribute to early cancer diagnosis and personalized therapy. A potential use of nanotechnology involves the development of a nanodevice that can serve both diagnostic and therapeutic purposes. This nanodevice might be surgically implanted as a preventive step in patients who do not show any apparent symptoms of a tumor. Subsequently, the position of the nanodevice could be tracked by independent remote monitoring. The proposed technology would have the ability to freely circulate inside the body and effectively identify cancer at an early stage, thereby facilitating the administration of suitable therapeutic interventions. Before implantation, the safety and biodegradability of such a device would have to be ensured. This would be the maximum level of personalized cancer prevention management. Early detection improves cure rates. This technology has benefits over periodic biomarker detection in bodily fluids, which is less precise than continuous *in vivo* analysis [49]. A variety of nanorobotic devices, such as nanorobots, have been created for various biomedical purposes. These advancements have effectively demonstrated the remarkable abilities of nanorobotics in addressing biomedical challenges with exceptional spatial accuracy. Consequently, they have greatly enhanced the field of medical robotics. Nanorobots, characterized by their nanoscale size, and nanomanipulators, characterized by their macroscale size and end effectors capable of manipulating nanoscale objects, are two distinct categories of nanorobotic devices within the field of nanorobotics and nanomanipulation in the context of their applications in the medical sector. The many classifications of nanorobotic devices [50–56] and their primary applications in the field of healthcare are presented in table 7.1 and shown in figure 7.1.

Table 7.1. Various types of nanorobotic systems [50–56].

Types of nanorobotic systems		Size range	Application
Nanorobots	Molecular machines	1–20 nm	A molecular machine refers to a collection of molecular components that have been purposefully constructed to execute mechanical motions in response to certain external inputs.
	Nanomotors	10 nm–10 μm	DNA nanorobots are fabricated using DNA origami techniques and can encapsulate and deliver therapeutic compounds to specific sites using molecular recognition mechanisms.
	DNA nanorobots	5∼100 nm	A nanomotor is a device at the nanoscale that can autonomously convert energy from many environmental sources, including chemical, optical, magnetic, ultrasonic, and electrical energy, into movement.
Nanomanipulators	Based on optical/magnetic/acoustic/techniques	Macroscale	Nanomanipulators that use tweezers as their end effectors, such as optical, magnetic, or acoustic tweezers, are employed for the manipulation of biological samples at the nanoscale without direct touch.
	Based on atomic force microscopy (AFM)	Macroscale	AFM-based nanomanipulators employ a nanoscale tip as their terminal component to perform mechanical manipulation of biological samples under diverse settings, including both gaseous and liquid environments.
	Based on electron microscopy (EM)	Macroscale	EM-based nanomanipulators carry out robotic procedures on biological samples inside a vacuum or gaseous environment while being directed by EM imaging.

These techniques complement each other by enabling various robotic operations to take place at multiple levels, particularly in the field of personalized healthcare. The most effective characteristics of nanorobots are as follows:

- Nanorobots are required to possess dimensions ranging from 0.5 to 3 μm, and their constituent components should measure between 1 and 100 nm.
- Nanorobots bigger than the dimensions noted above impede capillary flow.

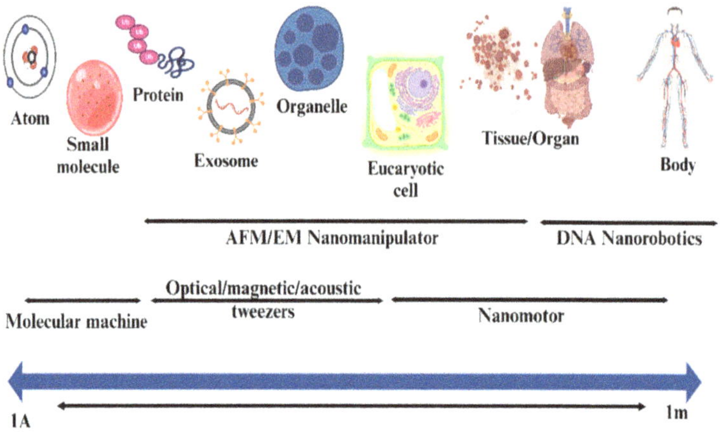

Figure 7.1. The most important biomedical uses of various types of nanorobotic systems. Different nanorobotic systems can be used to study biological materials at different scales from single molecules to the scale of the human body.

- Their passive, diamond exteriors will protect them from being damaged by the immune system.
- The system will establish communication with the physician by sending messages via the transmission of acoustic signals at carrier wave frequencies ranging from 1 to 100 MHz.
- Self-replication, or the production of additional copies for the purpose of replacing worn-out units, could be a potential development [6].

7.3 Nanorobots in healthcare

The development of nanorobots in the field of healthcare signifies a significant connection between nanotechnology and biomedicine, introducing a new era of personalized healthcare. These important nanoscale devices, often measuring just a few nanometers in size, have been appropriately designed and manufactured to traverse the complicated geography of the human body. The process of creating such items involves the use of advanced materials, such as biocompatible chemicals, to minimize any negative consequences of introducing them into the bloodstream or specific regions of concern. This progress has been closely associated with the development of complementary technologies, including magnetic controls and nanostructures [57]. In 2005, the first instances of nanoscale robots were documented, one of which was a nano car mostly made from fullerene molecules [58] During the 2010s, three primary classifications of nanorobots surfaced: helices, referred to as nano swimmers; nanorods, sometimes known as nano swimmers, nanomotors, or, in cases of increased length, nanowires; and DNA nanorobots. Table 7.2 presents a non-exhaustive collection of examples of nanorobots. These three categories typically satisfy the provisional definition of nanorobots. since they possess both nanoscale dimensions and the capability to execute certain functions. Nevertheless, in some cases, the complete realization of the job at hand has not been

Table 7.2. Non-exhaustive examples of nanorobots. Here, NA stands for 'not available.'

	Nanorobot	Materials	Size (nanometer)	Reference
Helices	Helical propeller	Glass, cobalt	200–300 nm wide	[59]
	Repolymerized flagellum-bound nanoparticles	Magnetic material, bacterial flagella	Nanoparticles: 40–400 nm. Flagella: 20 nm	[60]
	Artificial bacterial flagella	Indium, gallium, arsenic, nickel, and gold	200 nm wide	[61]
Nanorods	V-shaped nanorods	Platinum	700 nm wide	[62]
	Match-like nanorods	Silica, silver, silver chloride	<210 nm wide	[63]
	Nanorods with a flagellum tail	Gold, nickel, polymer	300–600 nm wide	[64]
	Light-driven nanorods	Gold, iron oxide	300 nm wide	[65]
	Drug-delivering nanorods	Gold, nickel, polymer	250 nm wide	[66]
	Nanofish	Gold, nickel, silver	200 nm wide	[67]
DNA nanorobots	DNA walker	DNA	NA	[68]
	Tetrahedron DNA	DNA	8×10 nm	[69]
	Nanosheet/tubular Nanorobot	DNA	90 × 50 × 2 nm	[70]
	Molecular spider	Protein, DNA	NA	[71]

achieved by certain nanorobot designs. However, there is often a strong aspiration to successfully carry out medication administration or other related tasks, such as biological imaging. Overall, it seems that nanorods and DNA nanorobots have made significant progress in the field of medication delivery and related activities. The development of these nanorobots requires an accurate and comprehensive approach, emphasizing the development of complicated structures that can effectively respond to distinct biological signals, adapt to changing surroundings, and perform a wide array of functions, including medication administration and cellular-level analysis. In addition, the advancement of nanorobots has required significant advancements in control and communication systems. Nanoscale agents often possess advanced onboard sensors and actuators, enabling them to effectively detect and react to their immediate environment. Furthermore, the ability to interface with other devices allows for real-time monitoring and remote-control capabilities. The degree of accuracy and flexibility shown in healthcare is unparalleled, presenting the opportunity for personalized therapies that are carefully adjusted to an individual's distinct physiology and genetic composition. Nanorobots are small, with a maximum size of 3 μm, allowing for easy penetration into the body without hindering capillary flow. The cost of mass production can be reduced by batch processing, even if the initial development costs are high. Because the use of nanorobots is minimally invasive, it necessitates a lower amount of post-treatment care [43]. Nanorobots' path from concept to reality has been marked by constant innovation and collaboration across numerous scientific fields, such as materials science, robotics, and biotechnology. Investigators have overcome numerous technical obstacles, including ensuring the biocompatibility, stability, and controlled locomotion of nanorobots within the body. As these obstacles are overcome, nanorobots will play crucial roles in personalized healthcare, revolutionizing the way in which clinicians diagnose diseases, administer treatments, and track patient responses. Their vast range of potential applications, from targeted drug delivery to early disease detection, makes them a beacon of hope for more effective, minimally invasive, and patient-centered healthcare solutions.

7.3.1 Helices

Several examples have been reported of robots that move using helical or screw-shaped tails. These robots frequently resemble bacterial flagella or other biological structures. The majority of them, including the MagnetoSperm and the MOFBOTS, are more accurately described as microrobots. However, there are examples of robots with helix-like structures that are gradually advancing towards the nanometer scale [59], measuring 200–300 nm wide and 1–2 μm long. The propeller is designed to replicate the swimming behavior of a bacterial flagellum. The propeller is capable of being manipulated and directed within magnetic fields, in both the forward and backward directions, due to the presence of a magnetic cobalt layer. This enables the propeller to achieve speeds of approximately 40 μm s^{-1}. Controlled navigation in an aqueous solution has been demonstrated through the utilization of the propeller's trajectory to trace out micrometer-scale letters and symbols, such as 'R,' '@,' and 'H.'

Multiple propellers can be simultaneously controlled using this method. An additional helical configuration that can be classified as a nanorobot is the fabricated bacterial flagellum proposed by Zhang *et al* [60]. The dimensions of this particular design are 200 nm in thickness, 2.5 μm in width, and 2.5 μm in length. The structure comprises a head composed of magnetic chromium–nickel–gold connected to a tail made of indium gallium arsenide–gallium arsenide–chromium. The structure in question bears a resemblance to a bacterial flagellum in terms of both its size and shape, with a notably smaller tail portion. In addition, the head of this structure possesses the capability to facilitate magnetic propulsion and control. The artificial bacterial flagellum is capable of moving at an average velocity of 1.2 μm s^{-1} when exposed to a magnetic field, due to the presence of its magnetic head. The artificial bacterial flagellum, like the helical glass propellers, has the ability to navigate through water-based environments by modifying the shape of its helix and responding to the magnetic field's orientation. This enables the flagellum to move in multiple directions, including forward, backward, and turning movements.

It has been demonstrated that bacterial flagella can manipulate polystyrene microparticles by exerting both pushing and rotating forces. In addition, several helix-like nanorobots have been established, most of which are microscale and some of which fall within the nano- to microscale range [72]. Bacterial flagella can be used through the depolymerization of the flagellin proteins, followed by their repolymerization and subsequent attachment to magnetic particles ranging in size from 40 to 400 nm [61]. Several flagella can be bonded to the same nanoparticle, but during the depolymerization process, a functional group is capable of attaching to the nanoparticles. The depolymerized flagella exhibit outer diameters of approximately 20 nm and lengths ranging from 5 to 10 μm and are capable of assuming various shapes (such as normal, curly, and coiled), depending on the presence of either ethylene glycol or dimethyl sulfoxide. This concept suggests that altering its geometric structure could potentially offer advantages in moving through diverse biological surroundings, such as the human body, in contrast to motion in a homogeneous medium such as water. The nanoparticle–flagella clusters are capable of achieving velocities of up to 2.5 μm s^{-1} using magnetic fields. One notable benefit of the helical nanorobot design is its ability to interchange specific nanoparticles for diverse applications while preserving the repolymerized flagella for locomotion. However, the nanoparticles must be magnetic to support both propulsion and navigation.

7.3.2 Nanorods

Nanorods are generally cylindrical rods composed of various metal segments, although alternative shapes are also employed for similar objectives. A significant example from a medical perspective was a rod measuring 250 nm in width and 1800 nm in length, consisting of gold–nickel–gold segments [66]. The movement of these nanorods was attributed to the application of ultrasound waves. In serum, their velocity reached approximately 50 μm s^{-1}, while in saliva, their speed was slightly lower at around 10 μm s^{-1}. The utilization of nickel's magnetic properties enabled the controlled manipulation of nanorods along predetermined pathways.

As an example, the developers programmed the system to generate trajectories that accurately depicted the letters 'U,' 'C,' 'S,' and 'D.' The nanorods were able to undergo functionalization, thereby enabling them to serve as carriers for drug cargos. One significant prospective utilization of the gold–nickel–gold nanorod was demonstrated through its functionalization with a polypyrrole–polystyrene sulfonate segment. The organic segment was able to form a binding interaction with the antiseptic drug brilliant green. Subsequently, it facilitated the targeted delivery of this drug to specific locations. The drug was subsequently released as a result of alterations in pH. Kiristi *et al* [73] demonstrated an additional potential medical application of nanorods. They employed ultrasound-assisted porous gold nanorods with a width of less than 300 nm and modified them with lysozyme, a bactericidal agent capable of eliminating both Gram-negative and Gram-positive bacteria. The investigators demonstrated that gold nanorods functionalized with lysozyme exhibited the ability to eliminate approximately 80% of Gram-positive bacteria *Micrococcus lysodeikticus* in a short period.

The mortality rate of the bacteria was found to be dependent on the quantity of nanorods; approximately 5000 nanorods were necessary to achieve a mortality rate of 80%. The glycosidic bonds present in bacterial cell walls serve as biological receptors for lysozyme. Despite the absence of navigation control for the nanorobot, its movement significantly enhanced the interactions between lysozyme and the bacteria, consequently increasing the bactericidal efficacy compared to the use of pure lysozyme alone. Numerous nanorod configurations have been developed to detect and treat cancer. MicroRNAs (miRNAs) are a class of short RNA molecules, some of which have been implicated in the pathogenesis of medical conditions such as diabetes and tumors. A study conducted by Uygun *et al* employed gold nanowires 200 nm wide, which were coated with graphene oxide. These nanowires were utilized for miRNA detection. The utilization of ultrasound-driven nanowires enabled cancer cells to be infiltrated, facilitating the detachment of DNA strands from the surface of graphene oxide and their subsequent binding to miRNA. The interaction between graphene oxide and gold nanowires resulted in the emission of a fluorescent signal, enabling the identification of a particular miRNA and potentially indicating the presence of a cancerous cell. Gold–nickel–gold–polymer nanowires were used as a very efficacious agent for combating cancer, taking the field of cancer research beyond detection and into treatment [74]. The nanowires were propelled by ultrasound at a normal velocity of [73] $\mu m\ s^{-1}$ in a solution of human serum. In addition, the nanowires were guided by magnetic forces facilitated by the presence of nickel.

In addition, the researchers incorporated asparaginase enzymes into the polymer segment, which effectively removed the important amino acid asparagine from the cancer cells, consequently preventing their proliferation. Lymphoma cancer cells were inhibited by 92% when asparagine was bound to nanowires, compared to only 17% when asparagine was free. Various mechanisms, such as chemical reactions (hydrogen decomposition), magnetic forces, acoustic waves (ultrasound), and biological interactions (the attachment of bacterial flagella), have traditionally served as the primary means for propelling and navigating nanorods. However, a recent study has also demonstrated the utilization of light as a propulsion mechanism for nanorods [75]. An example involves gold–iron oxide nanorods with a width of 300 nm. These nanorods may be triggered by visible light in a solution of dilute hydrogen peroxide. As a consequence of the breakdown of hydrogen peroxide at the iron oxide end, these nanorods are capable of achieving speeds in the range of micrometers per second [65, 73]. The utilization of superparamagnetic iron enables magnets to steer rods along predetermined paths. Similarly, silicon nanowires coated with platinum nanoparticles in a quinone solution can be propelled by visible or near-infrared light. The light power intensity determines their speed, which lies in an achievable range of 5–35 $\mu m\ s^{-1}$. The manipulation of the nanowire's surface structure has the potential to generate a wide range of propulsion patterns, including both linear and circular movements. Light-propelled nanorods include a specific kind of nanorod, namely a silver–silica nanorod with a silver chloride tail, which has a width of less than 210 nm [63]. Nanorods can travel at a speed of 4–14 $m\ s^{-1}$, depending on their length. However, there have been advancements in the development of nanorobots that possess shapes different from purely cylindrical structures, yet possess similarities with nanorods. An example is a V-shaped platinum nanorod with a width of 700 nm and a length ranging from 4000 to 4500 nm [62]. The movement of the object took place within a medium of hydrogen peroxide, facilitated by the decomposition of hydrogen peroxide:

$$H_2O_2 \rightarrow H_2 + O_2.$$

The nanorobot's directional movement was due to its V shape, as the hydrogen peroxide decomposition primarily took place at one end of the robot. However, the nanorobot's rotational movement was limited to circles with a diameter of micrometers, and there was no implementation of navigational control. Another study used a nanorod with multiple cylinder segments, namely a gold head, two nickel body segments, a gold caudal fin segment, and three flexible porous silver hinges [67]. This nanofish was capable of magnetic propulsion as a result of its nickel segments, and it moved by undulating its tail like a real fish. The position of the nickel segments within the fish body was a continuous process that varied depending on the introduction of a magnetic field. As a result, the gold segment located in the tail fin displayed undulatory motion, which allowed the nanofish to achieve a velocity of approximately 31 $\mu m\ s^{-1}$. Another example of a nanorobot that differed from the strictly cylindrical nanorod category was a two-armed nanoswimmer that could be manipulated using magnetic forces. This nanoswimmer was composed of nickel–gold–nickel segments, each measuring 200 nm in width, with silver hinges connecting them [76].

7.3.3 DNA nanorobots

DNA nanorobots are composed of deoxyribonucleic acid (DNA) molecules and make use of DNA as the building material for nanoscale devices [77, 78]. Sometimes, DNA origami serves as the foundation for these structures, wherein DNA fragments are manipulated and folded to generate intricate patterns and forms [48]. An example of a nanorobot that exemplified this concept was the DNA walker created by Gu *et al* [68]. This nanorobot was composed of a triangular configuration of double helices. The 'feet' of the nanorobot functioned as ligands. The DNA attachments possessed the ability to attach themselves to a larger DNA origami structure, referred to as a 'landscape.' The DNA walker was able to traverse this landscape by rotating at an angle of 120° and subsequently attaching to a fresh bioreceptor at each step. The transportation of cargo across the DNA sheet to a specified location was facilitated by the DNA walker, as demonstrated in a study in which multiple 5 nm gold nanoparticles were successfully delivered. Another type of structure that is capable of traversing a DNA origami structure is known as a molecular spider. These spiders are composed of protein bodies that possess three DNA legs and an additional capture leg, which is synthesized by DNA enzymes [71].

DNA nanorobots have been deployed *in vivo* situations with live things. An example is a DNA nanorobot referred to as the I-switch, which comprised a triad of DNA strands [79]. The I-switch was able to alter its configuration in response to changes in pH. This property enabled the nanorobot to remain in two different shapes. Furthermore, when the nanorobot was labeled with a fluorescent molecule, each of these shapes emitted light of a unique wavelength. Fluorescence-labeled I-switches were transported to specific nematode cells and internalized via receptor-mediated endocytosis, allowing for the temporal and spatial mapping of pH alterations within these cells. These DNA nanorobot may have various potential applications in mapping due to their sensitivity to changes in pH within the range that influences cellular phenomena such as neurodegeneration and spermatogenesis. Therapeutics were also successfully delivered *in vivo* via tetrahedral DNA nanoparticles [69]. The tetrahedral structure consisted of six self-assembling DNA strands and six strands of siRNA, which has the potential to effectively suppress the expression of specific genes within tumors. The application involved injecting tetrahedral-bound siRNA into the tail vein of nude mice to target tumors. The cage-like icosahedral DNA nanocapsule is another type of DNA nanorobot that works in the same way. It can be used to enclose biomacromolecules [80]. The development of DNA origami technology has introduced a novel approach to the investigation of nanorobot construction. DNA is a material that can be programmed, and by combining sequence-complementary domains, DNA molecules can be put together into pre-planned shapes [81]. Nanorobots made using DNA techniques are classified as nanomotors [82].

DNA origami, a technology developed in 2006 [83], involves the use of programmed combinations of many short complementary 'staple' oligonucleotides to manipulate a single strand of 'scaffold' DNA, resulting in the formation of precise two-dimensional (2D) and three-dimensional (3D) structures. The stability of these structures is maintained by the presence of several base pairs [84]. The DNA origami technique allows for the controlled construction of discrete items through a bottom-up approach. These objects exhibit very accurate characteristics at the subnanometer scale and have dimensions ranging from nanometers to micrometers. In addition, they may have molecular weights that extend up to the gigadalton scale [85]. The use of DNA origami has facilitated the fabrication of diverse functional static nanostructures and dynamic nanodevices [86]. These advancements have provided the basis for the advancement of DNA nanorobotics at the level of individual molecules. The authors of a further study [71] described the locomotive actions of DNA walkers in a two-dimensional DNA origami environment. These DNA walkers were composed of a streptavidin molecule as the body and three deoxy ribozymes as the legs. The study demonstrated the potential of DNA technology in achieving programmed robotic behaviors. In 2018, Kopperger *et al* [87] designed a nanoscale robotic arm that self-assembled using DNA origami and electric fields. The actuator unit of the system comprised a DNA origami plate with dimensions of 55 nm×55 nm, which included a 25 nm long arm. This design enabled the electrical manipulation and movement of nanoparticles over distances of several nanometers. The speed of the robotic motions produced in trials was equivalent to those of adenosine triphosphatase-driven biohybrids and greater than those of DNA motor systems described in the past. DNA nanorobots may also insert themselves onto 2D DNA crystalline substrates at particular places [88] as well as sorting (picking up, transporting, and dropping off) cargo [89, 90]. Significant advancements have been made in the field of DNA nanorobotics for healthcare purposes, particularly in the domain of drug delivery, over the last ten years. DNA nanorobotic structures can be fabricated with a cavity that can accommodate molecular payloads, such as antibody fragments that can bind to specific antigens. These structures possess the capability to undergo conformational changes, transitioning between open and closed states. As a result, they may either expose or hide their cargos, depending on the presence of certain chemical triggers [91]. Empirical data has substantiated the preliminary therapeutic potential of DNA nanorobotic systems in the precise administration of pharmaceutical agents to neoplastic masses, while concurrently mitigating harm to unaffected biological tissues [92, 93].

7.4 Applications of nanorobots in personalized healthcare

Nanorobots possess a wide variety of applications within the field of personalized healthcare, providing the potential to revolutionize the methods by which investigators ascertain, address, and manage personalized healthcare. Nanorobots have the potential to initiate a major change in the field of medicine, presenting a wide range of innovative potential that possess the potential to significantly alter the provision of healthcare to patients. Nanorobots possess abilities, particularly in the field of targeted drug delivery, which represent a significant departure from the non-specific impacts associated with conventional drug administration methods. These tiny machines can deliver therapeutic agents directly to tumors, infected tissues, and damaged organs by nanoscale navigation through the human body. This improves therapeutic efficacy and reduces the detrimental side effects of conventional treatments. Furthermore, the use of nanorobots in the treatment of cancer is highly promising. These microscopic agents can be individualized to target and destroy cancer cells while preserving surrounding healthy tissue, allowing for surgical precision without the need for invasive procedures. These microscopic marvels can deliver drugs to specific cells or tissues, thereby reducing off-target effects and improving treatment efficacy. By detecting biomarkers in real-time and providing

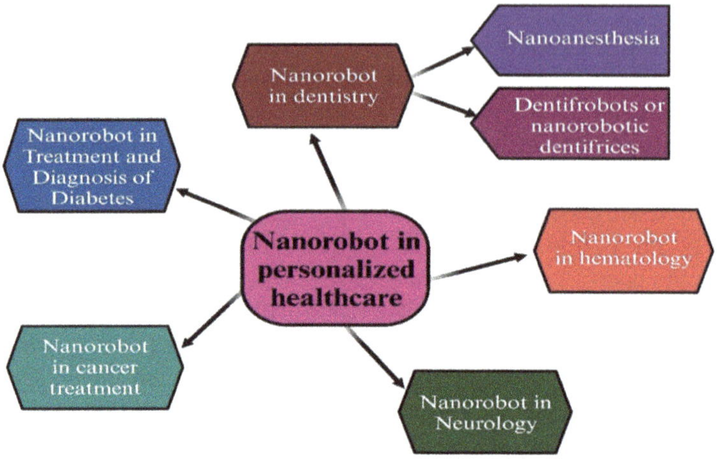

Figure 7.2. Various applications of nanorobots in personalized healthcare.

timely interventions, they excel at early disease detection. Nanorobots possess the capability to facilitate customized therapeutic interventions, effectively addressing the unique requirements of individual patients and dynamically adjusting to evolving circumstances. Their ability to perform minimally invasive surgeries and precise tissue repairs improves patient-centric care. However, ethical, safety, and regulatory concerns must be addressed as the full potential of nanorobots in personalized healthcare is realized, ushering in an era of more effective, individualized, and minimally invasive medical solutions (figure 7.2).

Nanorobots with diagnostic and imaging capabilities can revolutionize disease detection and monitoring beyond drug delivery. These nanobots can travel through the circulatory system and report the presence or absence of certain biomarkers or disease indicators as they are detected. This enables quick medical interventions and decisions, potentially saving lives through early disease detection. Nanorobots provide unparalleled precision in microsurgery. They can be programmed to repair damaged tissues, remove blood clots, and unblock arteries at the cellular or molecular level. When conventional surgical techniques are either too invasive or inaccurate, these tools can be invaluable. Nanorobots can be programmed to react to particular biological cues or signals within the body, making them more than passive agents and enabling truly personalized therapies. As the field of nanorobotics develops and overcomes technical challenges, it has the potential to reshape medical conditions by providing patients with more effective, less invasive, and highly personalized healthcare solutions. The utilization of nanorobots represents an important development in the field of healthcare, providing the potential for enhanced precision and effectiveness in the treatment of diseases, thus paving the way for a promising future in healthcare. Nanorobots are predicted to facilitate novel therapeutic interventions for individuals afflicted with various medical conditions, thereby leading to an important step in the progression of medical science. The utilization of nanorobots has the potential to enhance biomedical interventions by enabling minimally invasive surgical procedures and facilitating the continuous monitoring of physiological processes for patients. In addition, nanorobots may contribute to improving treatment efficacy by enabling the early detection of potentially severe diseases (figure 7.2). For example, nanorobots can attach to inflammatory or white blood cells, accelerating tissue healing. Several applications of nanorobots are described below.

7.4.1 The use of nanorobots in dentistry

7.4.1.1 Dentifrobots or nanorobotic dentifrices

When administered through the use of mouthwash or toothpaste, these substances can cover all subgingival surfaces, leading to the conversion of trapped organic matter into vapors that are both odorless and harmless. Dentifrobots that are appropriately configured can detect and eliminate pathogenic bacteria present in both plaque and other areas. These dentifrobots are purely mechanically powered devices that, once swallowed, safely deactivate themselves. They are so small that they are almost invisible [1]. Nanorobotic dentifrices are an innovative methodology for maintaining oral hygiene. When introduced via oral washes or toothpaste, these tiny mechanical devices possess the ability to access and efficiently address all subgingival surfaces within the oral cavity. Their exceptional metabolism converts trapped organic matter into harmless, odorless vapors. Dentifrobots have also been developed to detect and eliminate pathogenic bacteria that are found in plaque and various regions of the oral cavity, thereby enhancing oral health. Significantly, these virtually invisible nanorobots have been engineered with safety in mind, and they deactivate themselves if they are ingested. This advanced technology could revolutionize oral care by providing a fast, painless way to clean teeth and prevent dental issues. Nanorobots are becoming more popular as a means of treating dentine hypersensitivity. The quantity of dentinal tubules in teeth that have hypersensitivity is greater than that of teeth that are considered normal. Nanorobots exhibit the capability of selectively eliminating dentinal tubules upon penetration, thereby preventing the transmission of stimuli that would normally produce a pain response. Nanorobots have been found to contribute to dental care through their integration into mouthwash and toothpaste. The regular use of these products allows for direct manipulation of the periodontal tissues, thereby assisting in the process of tooth repositioning [94].

7.4.1.2 Nanoanesthesia

Oral anesthesia is a prevalent procedure in dental practice. Nanoanesthesia is an innovative and significant development in the field of dentistry, providing a transformative method for pain control during oral interventions. In this novel approach, dental practitioners apply a colloidal suspension consisting of a large number of active analgesic dental nanorobot 'particles' at the micron scale directly onto the patient's gingiva. This migration occurs without causing any pain as the nanorobots effortlessly traverse the lamina propria, which is a thin layer of loose tissue measuring approximately 1–3 μ in thickness, located at the cement–dentinal junction. Upon reaching the dentin layer, the nanorobots penetrate the dentinal tubules, which are cylindrical channels with diameters ranging from 1 to 4 μ. Subsequently, they advance towards the pulp region, following a path determined by a combination of chemical gradients, temperature variations, and positional navigation. These movements are orchestrated by an embedded nanocomputer, which operates according to the instructions provided by the dentist. The microscopic nanorobots possess the necessary precision to specifically target pain receptors and administer anesthesia with remarkable accuracy.

Nanoanesthesia reduces pain and suffering compared to conventional methods by providing targeted and potent pain relief without the need for injections. The utilization of this technique not only improves the overall patient experience but also optimizes the efficiency of dental procedures by ensuring the rapid and precise administration of anesthesia. Nanoanesthesia has the potential to revolutionize the field of oral anesthesia by enhancing the comfort and efficiency of dental treatments. This advancement can ultimately enhance patient outcomes and satisfaction in the field of dental care. The diameter of the tubules exhibits an increase in proximity to the pulp, potentially enhancing the potential for nanorobot movement. After they are implanted within the dental pulp and achieve regulation of nerve impulse transmission, the analgesic dental nanorobots can be instructed by the dentist to deactivate all sensory perception in a specific tooth that requires dental intervention. Subsequently, as shown the handheld controller's display, the designated tooth promptly experiences a state of anesthesia. Once the oral procedures have been concluded, the dentist instructs the nanorobots to reinstate all sensory perception, relinquish their regulation of nerve activity, and become fully engaged, subsequently followed by aspiration. Nanorobotic analgesics enhance patient comfort and reduce anxiety, eliminating the need for needles. They also offer improved selectivity and controllability of the analgesic effect, along with rapid and fully reversible switchable action. In addition, these analgesics help to minimize the occurrence of side effects and complications [95].

7.4.2 The use of nanorobots in cancer treatment

The prognosis for cancer treatment is generally more favorable when the disease is detected at an earlier stage. Nanosensors, specifically nanorobots equipped with chemical biosensors, have been employed for the early detection of tumor cells during the initial stages of cancer progression. These nanosensors can detect the existence of cancerous cells within the human body. The narrow therapeutic index of the majority of anticancer drugs often leads to toxicity in normal stem cells as well as adverse effects on hematological and gastrointestinal systems, among others. Conventional chemotherapeutic agents function by targeting and eliminating neoplastic cells, primarily due to their characteristic of rapid cell division. Doxorubicin, a commonly employed anticancer medication, finds application in various cancer types, including Hodgkin's disease (HD). In the treatment of HD, doxorubicin is typically administered alongside other antineoplastic agents to mitigate their toxic effects. Nanorobots offer an innovative approach to cancer treatment due to their extraordinary drug delivery, targeted therapy, and real-time monitoring capabilities. These tiny devices, with dimensions on the order of nanometers, possess the capacity to significantly transform the field of cancer treatment by effectively addressing multiple crucial obstacles. These entities possess the ability to traverse the circulatory system, actively locating areas of tumor growth with exceptional precision and administering chemotherapy medications directly to malignant cells. This targeted approach yields a substantial reduction in adverse effects on the body as a whole, while simultaneously enhancing the efficacy of therapeutic interventions. Nanorobots possess the capability to undergo surface modifications, thereby facilitating their ability to selectively identify and target cancer cells while minimizing any potential harm to healthy tissue.

Certain nanorobots are equipped with sensors that enable the continuous monitoring of a tumor's response to treatment, thereby presenting the potential for personalized adaptive therapies based on the specific requirements of each patient. Moreover, these nanoscale agents possess the capability to perform photothermal therapy, wherein they convert external energy sources, such as light, into localized heat with high precision and selectivity, thereby effectively eliminating cancer cells. Nanorobots can also deliver immunostimulants directly to tumors, thereby improving immunotherapy. Furthermore, these technologies possess potential applications in the early detection of cancer due to their ability to facilitate the identification of distinct biomarkers or molecules associated with cancer within the circulatory system. Although several challenges must be overcome, such as ensuring safety, obtaining regulatory approval, and achieving scalability, the potential of nanorobots to significantly transform cancer treatment by enhancing effectiveness and reducing adverse effects renders them a highly promising and pivotal area of ongoing research and development in the struggle against cancer. Because nanorobots can move around as blood-borne devices, they can help with some of the most important aspects of treating cancer.

Nanorobots possessing integrated chemical biosensors have the potential to facilitate the early-stage identification of tumor cells within the anatomical confines of the patient's body. Researchers have employed genetic modification techniques to alter salmonella bacteria, rendering them attracted to tumors through the release of chemicals emitted by cancerous cells. The bacteria transport nanoscale robots measuring approximately 3 μm, which autonomously release drug-filled capsules upon reaching the tumor. The nanorobots, which the research team dubbed bacteriobots, reduce the patient's exposure to chemotherapy's negative effects by targeting only the tumor and not healthy cells [6, 41].

7.4.3 The application of nanorobots in the treatment and diagnosis of diabetes

Nanorobots have developed as a promising field within the healthcare industry, providing potential advancements in medical instrumentation, diagnostic procedures, and the management of diabetes. Individuals diagnosed with diabetes are required to regularly obtain small blood samples throughout the day to effectively manage and regulate their glucose levels. These types of procedures are painful and very inconvenient. Medical nanorobotics allow for continuous glucose monitoring, which can help to prevent such difficulties. To reduce such issues, the monitoring of blood sugar levels can be achieved through the implementation of medical nanorobotics for continuous glucose monitoring. A prototype model of a simulated nanorobot incorporated nanobioelectronics based on complementary metal–oxide–semiconductor technology. It was 2 μm in size, which allowed it to operate freely within the body. The nanorobot used an embedded chemosensor mechanism that entailed the modulation of glucosensor activity in the hSGLT3 protein. By utilizing its integrated chemical sensor, the nanorobot was capable of accurately determining whether the patient needed the administration of insulin or any additional measures, such as the consumption of clinically prescribed medication. Glucose levels were detected by these entities as they circulated alongside red blood cells within the bloodstream. The nanorobots aimed to maintain blood glucose levels within a target range of approximately 130 mg dl^{-1}, which is considered a typical glucose concentration. The medical nanorobot architecture automatically transferred important data to the patient's mobile phone via RF signals. The nanorobot alerted the user via their mobile phone if the glucose levels became critical.

Nanorobots have the potential to significantly advance the diagnosis and management of diabetes through the use of novel approaches. These nanoscale devices have the capability to continually assess blood glucose levels with high precision, offering real-time data that facilitates proactive management and decreases diabetics' dependency on invasive blood tests. Nanorobots possess the capability to directly deliver insulin or other therapeutic substances to the specific cells involved in glucose regulation, thereby facilitating treatment that is personalized and precisely targeted. Their ability to navigate the complex networks of blood vessels and deliver therapies at the cellular level has the potential to revolutionize diabetes care, providing greater control over blood sugar levels, reducing complications, and ultimately improving the quality of life for diabetics. However, it is imperative to continue conducting research and development to successfully address the safety, regulatory, and scalability challenges that must be overcome before nanorobotic solutions can be widely integrated into diabetes management protocols [1].

7.4.4 The application of nanorobots in neurology

The utilization of nanorobots in the field of neurology is growing as a significant and flexible area of practical investigation and advancement. The utilization of nanotechnology and the integration of nanorobots have the potential to offer significant advantages in the field of neurosurgery. These advancements can contribute to a range of applications, including enhanced detection of pathological conditions, intracranial monitoring with fewer invasive procedures, and enhanced drug administration among many more. One of the primary challenges encountered involves the re-establishment of severed nerves and the facilitation of axonal regeneration using enhanced scaffolds. The activation of the restoration function is contingent upon the reconnection of the impaired nerves. The physicians' limitation is performing surgery on such a small scale. The ability to manipulate individual axons is facilitated through the utilization of nanoscale devices. A surgical instrument with a diameter of 40 nm, commonly referred to as a nano knife, has demonstrated efficacy in performing surgical procedures on axons. Dielectrophoresis is a process utilized in the surgical field to control the motion of axons by manipulating polarizable objects within an electric field. Subsequently, the connection between the two ends of the nerves is established through a process of electrofusion or laser-induced cell fusion [94]. A brain aneurysm is the occurrence of a thrombus within the cerebral blood vessels responsible for delivering oxygen to the brain. This potentially fatal intracranial hemorrhagic condition arises from the leakage or rupture of an aneurysm, primarily located in the region between the cranial base and the lower part of the brain. Nanotechnology has played a significant role in the advancement of nanoscale robots to diagnose brain aneurysms.

The construction of nanorobots includes three fundamental concepts: the prototype of the equipment, the production technique, and the intracorporeal connection. The manufacturing methodology centers on the development of a robot that incorporates a biochip, utilizing biomaterials, photonics, and nanobioelectronics. 'Intracorporeal contact' refers to how well the nanorobots fit together and work with the body's parts and chemical processes. The morphology of the nanorobots is influenced by cellular morphology, proteomics, and microbiology. Nanorobots created specifically to diagnose brain aneurysms should be able to effectively detect endothelial injury by following the blood vessel pathways before the onset of subarachnoid hemorrhage. The use of chemical nanobiosensors facilitates the detection process for nanorobots, as the reliable detection of small biomolecules poses a significant challenge. The detection of intracranial aneurysm can be facilitated by assessing the level of nitric oxide synthase (NOS) in the brain. Protein expression levels are used to calibrate the detection thresholds so that a 50 nA signal is sent if the NOS level is found to be in the low microgram range. When the level of nitric oxide synthase exceeds a certain threshold, such as that of proteomic signal transduction, it provides compelling evidence for the presence of an intracranial aneurysm. Subsequently, the nanorobots transmit data about the vessel's coordinates and the dimensions of the bulb [96].

7.4.5 The application of nanorobots in hematology

Nanorobotics have applications in the field of hematology, but these applications are still in the investigative phase. The utilization of nanorobots in the field of hematology includes a wide spectrum of applications, including the administration of non-blood oxygen carriers during transfusions and the restoration of primary hemostasis. A nanorobot being developed for use in blood transfusions is called a respirocyte. The robot is expected to measure 1000 nm, and its constituent parts are expected to be fabricated at the nanoscale. The system will include an onboard computer 58 nm in diameter. The primary purposes of a nanorobot known as a respirocyte, during its passage through the bloodstream, include the retrieval of oxygen from the respiratory system and the utilization of circulating glucose to generate energy for its operations. Compared to red blood cells, this robot can carry

236 times as much oxygen per unit of volume. Nanorobotics studies focus on the application of hemostasis. Different promoters and inhibitors are needed at different stages of hemostasis to maintain a healthy equilibrium between thrombosis and fibrinolysis.

Hemostasis stops bleeding and improves blood vessel repair when it works properly. The typical bleeding period in physiologic hemostasis is a significant difficulty, lasting for around five minutes. The utilization of nanorobotics has the potential to address this issue. During the process of platelet transfusion, patients may potentially deal with infections from pathogens, which can subsequently trigger an immune response. To replicate this function, a mechanical artificial platelet and clottocyte nanorobot has been proposed. The dimensions of the proposed robot are 2 μ, accompanied by a mesh size of 0.8 nm. In addition, it is equipped with a hemostasis-promoting protein that will be utilized for binding vessel injuries during the process of hemostasis.

Another potential use of nanorobots in the field of hematology is as phagocytic agents. The proposed nanorobots have been designated as microbivores. The microbivore, developed by Robert A. Freitas, is an artificial mechanical phagocyte that has been specifically designed to effectively eliminate blood-borne pathogens safely. It is a nanomedical device in the shape of an oblate spheroidal ball that is composed of 610 billion precisely arranged structural atoms as well as 150 billion gas molecules. The external surface of the nanorobot is equipped with a wide range of customizable binding sites that can effectively interact with antigens and pathogens. It is widely believed that this treatment has the potential to effectively cure septicemia within a few hours of being administered, exhibiting a significantly higher efficacy rate of nearly 80 times that of innate phagocytic performance. The implementation of nanorobotics applications has the potential to be advantageous in the management of infections [96].

7.5 Future perspectives

The rapid advancements in the field of nanorobotics have greatly expanded the potential applications for healthcare robotics at the nanoscale. Nanoscale robots are highly suitable for *in vivo* use as transporters of therapeutic substances [97]. On the other hand, nanomanipulators are primarily well-suited to recognizing the structures and characteristics of biological samples. Nanorobots provide a novel therapeutic strategy for diseases, including tumors. Many studies have been conducted on the utilization of nanoparticles to deliver drug molecules to tumors. However, it has been observed that these nanoparticles have not yet demonstrated the ability to overcome all the necessary biological barriers to successfully achieve this objective [98]. Thus, the clinical application of nanoparticles has been considerably restricted [99]. The field of DNA nanorobotics enables the fabrication of nanorobots that possess adjustable three-dimensional architectures, thereby facilitating the execution of intricate robotic functions aimed at selectively and exclusively transporting drug molecules to cancer locations [92]. Nanorobots have great potential for use in medicine, with applications ranging from disease elimination to anti-aging therapies.

They will offer personalized treatments with enhanced efficacy and diminished side effects that are not currently available. They will offer synergistic benefits, such as diagnostic tests provided with pharmaceuticals, imaging agents that double as therapeutics, and real-time guidance for diagnosis during surgical procedures. Nanorobotics has the potential to revolutionize healthcare and the way in which diseases are treated in the future, even though it currently sounds like science fiction. The future of the field of medicine will display a shift from a focus on medical science to medical engineering, in which the anticipated emergence of nanorobotic technology will act as a revolutionary force. The field of nanorobotics includes a wide range of scientific activities. The typical progress made in the field of nanorobotics proves that nanorobotics can be used in health applications, which will have a big effect on the next step of personalized precision healthcare [100–106] and provide further information on a variety of related topics related to nanorobotics, including imaging techniques for nanorobots [100], the use of medical nanorobotics in the healthcare sector, including toxicology [102], nanorobots that can detect cancer at an early stage [104], and nanorobots that can be controlled selectively. To be effective in medical applications, nanorobots must be able to bypass the immune systems of organisms. Although tetrahedral DNA nanoparticles [69] and nanosheet/tubular DNA nanorobots did not provoke an immunogenic response in mice, this can be challenging for DNA nanorobots due to the immunogenicity of foreign DNA [70, 107]. To enable future nanorobot use, convenient, large-scale fabrication methods are necessary. Until nanorobot production and use increase, the associated risks will remain low. In the early stages of development, known as the embryonic phase, all technologies are rarely used [108]. Therefore, initial low levels of production and consumption are not indicative of future low levels of production and consumption.

7.6 Conclusions

Nanorobots have emerged as a transformative technology within the healthcare industry, facilitating advancements in disease diagnosis and treatment and personalized healthcare. Nanorobots exhibit site specificity, noninvasiveness, and computer-controlled delivery, thereby reducing the adverse effects associated with conventional treatments. This improves early disease diagnosis and offers the prospect of low-cost treatment. Nanorobots may soon be used for conventional diagnosis and treatment. In conclusion, the development of active nanorobots in the field of personalized healthcare is placed at the center of a transformative revolution in the healthcare industry. These tiny but effective devices are revolutionizing medical science, establishing new diagnostic, drug delivery, and treatment options. The ability of nanorobots to target specific cells or tissues, navigate the complex pathways of the human body with high precision, and ultimately improve patient wellbeing is the key to lowering the risk of unwanted side effects, increasing the treatment's overall effectiveness, and ultimately making patients healthier. However, there are many challenges in the way, such as safety evaluations, regulations, and ethical considerations. Yet, the potential impact of nanorobots in revolutionizing healthcare by enabling personalized treatments for each patient is incontrovertible. In conclusion, the use of active nanorobots in personalized healthcare has the potential to completely change the field of medicine. These tiny marvels can deliver targeted drugs, diagnoses, and adaptive therapies, marking a precision medicine revolution. Despite the presence of ongoing ethical and legal challenges, the advancement of nanorobot research holds great potential for revolutionizing healthcare. It offers the possibility of personalized healthcare treatments that respond to the differing attributes of individuals, resulting in enhanced efficacy, reduced invasiveness, and a patient-centered approach. Consequently, these developments can substantially enhance patient outcomes and overall quality of life.

References

[1] Kumar S S, Nasim B P and Abraham E 2018 Nanorobots a future device for diagnosis and treatment *J. Pharm. Pharm.* **5** 44–9

[2] Kshirsagar N, Patil S, Kshirsagar R, Wagh A and Bade A 2014 Review on application of nanorobots in health care *World J. Pharm. Pharm. Sci.* **3** 472–80

[3] Sivasankar M and Durairaj R 2012 Brief review on nanorobots in biomedical applications *Adv. Robot. Autom.* **1** 2

[4] Ummat A, Sharma G, Mavroidis C and Dubey A 2016 Bio-nano-robotics: state of the art and future challenges *Tissue Engineering and Artificial Organs* (Boca Raton, FL: CRC Press)

[5] Hussan Reza K, Asiwarya G, Radhika G and Bardalai D 2011 Nanorobots: the future trend of drug delivery and therapeutics *Int. J.Pharm. Sci. Rev. Res.* **10** 60–8

[6] Kharwade M, Nijhawan M and Modani S 2013 *Res. J. Pharm., Biol. Chem. Sci.* **4** 1299–1307

[7] Zhang H, Li Z, Gao C, Fan X, Pang Y, Li T, Wu Z, Xie H and He Q 2021 Dual-responsive biohybrid neutrobots for active target delivery *Sci. Robot.* **6** eaaz9519

[8] Mhanna R, Qiu F, Zhang L, Ding Y, Sugihara K, Zenobi-Wong M and Nelson B J 2014 Artificial bacterial flagella for remote-controlled targeted single-cell drug delivery *Small* **10** 1953–7

[9] Xie M *et al* 2020 Bioinspired soft microrobots with precise magneto-collective control for microvascular thrombolysis *Adv. Mater.* **32** 2000366

[10] Zhang Y, Yuan K and Zhang L 2019 Micro/nanomachines: from functionalization to sensing and removal *Adv. Mater. Technol.* **4** 1800636

[11] Wang Q, Yang L and Zhang L 2021 Micromanipulation using reconfigurable self-assembled magnetic droplets with needle guidance *IEEE Trans. Autom. Sci. Eng.* **19** 759–71

[12] Nelson B J, Kaliakatsos I K and Abbott J J 2010 Microrobots for minimally invasive medicine *Annu. Rev. Biomed. Eng.* **12** 55–85

[13] Wang B, Chan K F, Yuan K, Wang Q, Xia X, Yang L, Ko H, Wang Y X J, Sung J J Y and Chiu P W Y 2021 *Sci. Robot.* **6** eabd2813

[14] Martel S 2017 Beyond imaging: macro-and microscale medical robots actuated by clinical MRI scanners *Sci. Robot.* **2** eaam8119

[15] Sitti M, Ceylan H, Hu W, Giltinan J, Turan M, Yim S and Diller E 2015 Biomedical applications of untethered mobile milli/microrobots *Proc. IEEE* **103** 205–24

[16] Taylor R H, Menciassi A, Fichtinger G, Fiorini P and Dario P 2016 Medical robotics and computer-integrated surgery *Springer Handbook of Robotics* (Cham: Springer) 2nd edn 1657–84
[17] Taylor R H 2006 A perspective on medical robotics *Proc. IEEE* **94** 1652–64
[18] Troccaz J, Dagnino G and Yang G Z 2019 Frontiers of medical robotics: from concept to systems to clinical translation *Annu. Rev. Biomed. Eng.* **21** 193–218
[19] Burgner-Kahrs J, Rucker D C and Choset H 2015 Continuum robots for medical applications: a survey *IEEE Trans. Rob.* **31** 1261–80
[20] Maciejasz P, Eschweiler J, Gerlach-Hahn K, Jansen-Troy A and Leonhardt S 2014 A survey on robotic devices for upper limb rehabilitation *J. Neuroeng. Rehab.* **11** 29
[21] Huo W, Mohammed S, Moreno J C and Amirat Y 2014 Lower limb wearable robots for assistance and rehabilitation: a state of the art *IEEE Syst. J.* **10** 1068–81
[22] Yang G Z *et al* 2017 Medical robotics—regulatory, ethical, and legal considerations for increasing levels of autonomy *Sci. Robot.* **2** eaam8638
[23] Yang G Z *et al* 2018 The grand challenges of science robotics *Sci. Robot.* **3** eaar7650
[24] Bergeles C and Yang G Z 2013 From passive tool holders to microsurgeons: safer, smaller, smarter surgical robots *IEEE Trans. Biomed. Eng.* **61** 1565–76
[25] Li J, Esteban-Fernández de Ávila B, Gao W, Zhang L and Wang J 2017 Micro/nanorobots for biomedicine: delivery, surgery, sensing, and detoxification *Sci. Robot.* **2** eaam6431
[26] Huang H W, Sakar M S, Petruska A J, Pané S and Nelson B J 2016 Soft micromachines with programmable motility and morphology *Nat. Commun.* **7** 12263
[27] Hu W, Lum G Z, Mastrangeli M and Sitti M 2018 Small-scale soft-bodied robot with multimodal locomotion *Nature* **554** 81–5
[28] Ren Z, Hu W, Dong X and Sitti M 2019 Multi-functional soft-bodied jellyfish-like swimming *Nat. Commun.* **10** 2703
[29] Diller E and Sitti M 2013 Micro-scale mobile robotics *Found. Trends Robot.* **2** 143–259
[30] Feinberg A W 2015 Biological soft robotics *Annu. Rev. Biomed. Eng.* **17** 243–65
[31] Ceylan H, Giltinan J, Kozielski K and Sitti M 2017 Mobile microrobots for bioengineering applications *Lab Chip* **17** 1705–24
[32] van der Schee M, Pinheiro H and Gaude E 2018 Breath biopsy for early detection and precision medicine in cancer *Ecancermedicalscience* **12** ed84
[33] Hartmaier R J *et al* 2017 High-throughput genomic profiling of adult solid tumors reveals novel insights into cancer pathogenesis *Cancer Res.* **77** 2464–75
[34] Mavroidis C and Ferreira A 2012 Nanorobotics: past, present, and future *Nanorobotics: Current Approaches and Techniques* (New York, NY: Springer) 3–27
[35] Oldham K, Sun D and Sun Y 2018 Focused issue on micro-/nano-robotics *Int. J. Intell. Robot. Appl.* **2** 381–2
[36] Collins F S and Varmus H 2015 A new initiative on precision medicine *New Engl. J. Med.* **372** 793–5
[37] Copeland R A 2016 The drug–target residence time model: a 10-year retrospective *Nat. Rev. Drug Discov.* **15** 87–95
[38] Leemans C R, Snijders P J and Brakenhoff R H 2018 The molecular landscape of head and neck cancer *Nat. Rev. Cancer* **18** 269–82
[39] Fernandez-Leiro R and Scheres S H 2016 Unravelling biological macromolecules with cryo-electron microscopy *Nature* **537** 339–46

[40] Chiranjib D B, Chandira R M and Jayakar B 2009 Role of nanotechnology in novel drug delivery system *J. Pharm. Sci. Technol.* **1** 20–35
[41] Singh C, Kumar L, Dewangan B, Sen P and Bohidar S 2014 A study on vehicle differential system *Int. J. Sci. Res. Manag.* **2** 1680–3
[42] GléciaVirgolino da Silva L, KleberVânio G B, Fábio Vladimir Calixto de A, Gabriela Barbosa da S, Pedro Augusto Ferreira da Silva, Roxana Claudia I C, Lourdes and M B 2016 Nanorobotics in drug delivery systems for treatment of cancer: a review *J. Mater. Sci. Eng.* A **6** 167–80
[43] Mishra J, Dash A K and Kumar R 2012 Nanotechnology challenges; nanomedicine: nanorobots *Int. Res. J. Pharm.* **2** 112–9
[44] Abhilash M 2010 Nanorobots *Int. J. Pharm. Bio Sci.* **1** 1–10
[45] Sharma K R 2013 Nanorobot drug delivery system for curcumin for enhanced bioavailability during treatment of Alzheimer's disease *J. Encapsul. Adsorpt. Sci.* **3** 24–34
[46] Erkoc P, Yasa I C, Ceylan H, Yasa O, Alapan Y and Sitti M 2019 Mobile microrobots for active therapeutic delivery *Adv. Therap.* **2** 1800064
[47] Yu J, Wang B, Du X, Wang Q and Zhang L 2018 Ultra-extensible ribbon-like magnetic microswarm *Nat. Commun.* **9** 3260
[48] Soto F, Karshalev E, Zhang F, Esteban Fernandez de Avila B, Nourhani A and Wang J 2021 Smart materials for microrobots *Chem. Rev.* **122** 5365–403
[49] Jain K K 2005 Role of nanobiotechnology in developing personalized medicine for cancer *Technol. Cancer Res. Treat.* **4** 645–50
[50] Pezzato C, Cheng C, Stoddart J F and Astumian R D 2017 Mastering the non-equilibrium assembly and operation of molecular machines *Chem. Soc. Rev.* **46** 5491–507
[51] Ellis E, Moorthy S, Chio W I K and Lee T C 2018 Artificial molecular and nanostructures for advanced nanomachinery *Chem. Commun.* **54** 4075–90
[52] Zhang L, Marcos V and Leigh D A 2018 Molecular machines with bio-inspired mechanisms *Proc. Natl Acad. Sci.* **115** 9397–404
[53] Xu T, Gao W, Xu L P, Zhang X and Wang S 2017 Fuel-free synthetic micro-/nano-machines *Adv. Mater.* **29** 1603250
[54] Toebes B J, Cao F and Wilson D A 2019 Spatial control over catalyst positioning on biodegradable polymeric nanomotors *Nat. Commun.* **10** 5308
[55] Li S, Jiang Q, Ding B and Nie G 2019 Anticancer activities of tumor-killing nanorobots *Trends Biotechnol.* **37** 573–7
[56] Sitti M 2007 Microscale and nanoscale robotics systems [grand challenges of robotics] *IEEE Robot. Autom. Mag.* **14** 53–60
[57] Martel S 2016 Swimming microorganisms acting as nanorobots versus artificial nanorobotic agents: a perspective view from a historical retrospective on the future of medical nanorobotics in the largest known three-dimensional microfluidic networks *Biomicrofluidics* **10** 021301
[58] Shirai Y, Osgood A J, Zhao Y, Kelly K F and Tour J M 2005 Directional control in thermally driven single-molecule nanocars *Nano Lett.* **5** 2330–4
[59] Ghosh A and Fischer P 2009 Controlled propulsion of artificial magnetic nanostructured propellers *Nano Lett.* **9** 2243–5
[60] Zhang L, Abbott J J, Dong L, Kratochvil B E, Bell D and Nelson B J 2009 Artificial bacterial flagella: fabrication and magnetic control *Appl. Phys. Lett.* **94** 064107

[61] Ali J, Cheang U K, Martindale J D, Jabbarzadeh M, Fu H C and Jun Kim M 2017 Bacteria-inspired nanorobots with flagellar polymorphic transformations and bundling *Sci. Rep.* **7** 14098
[62] Bao J, Yang Z, Nakajima M, Shen Y, Takeuchi M, Huang Q and Fukuda T 2013 Self-actuating asymmetric platinum catalytic mobile nanorobot *IEEE Trans. Robot.* **30** 33–9
[63] Wang Y *et al* 2018 photocatalytically powered matchlike nanomotor for light-guided active SERS sensing *Angew. Chem.* **130** 13294–7
[64] Ahmed D, Baasch T, Jang B, Pane S, Dual J and Nelson B J 2016 Artificial swimmers propelled by acoustically activated flagella *Nano Lett.* **16** 4968–74
[65] Zhou D, Ren L, Li Y C, Xu P, Gao Y, Zhang G, Wang W, Mallouk T E and Li L 2017 Visible light-driven, magnetically steerable gold/iron oxide nanomotors *Chem. Commun.* **53** 11465–8
[66] Garcia-Gradilla V, Orozco J, Sattayasamitsathit S, Soto F, Kuralay F, Pourazary A, Katzenberg A, Gao W, Shen Y and Wang J 2013 Functionalized ultrasound-propelled magnetically guided nanomotors: toward practical biomedical applications *ACS Nano* **7** 9232–40
[67] Li T *et al* 2016 Magnetically propelled fish-like nanoswimmers *Small* **12** 6098–105
[68] Gu H, Chao J, Xiao S J and Seeman N C 2010 A proximity-based programmable DNA nanoscale assembly line *Nature* **465** 202–5
[69] Lee H *et al* 2012 Molecularly self-assembled nucleic acid nanoparticles for targeted *in vivo* siRNA delivery *Nat. Nanotechnol.* **7** 389–93
[70] Li S *et al* 2018 A DNA nanorobot functions as a cancer therapeutic in response to a molecular trigger *in vivo Nat. Biotechnol.* **36** 258–64
[71] Lund K *et al* 2010 Molecular robots guided by prescriptive landscapes *Nature* **465** 206–10
[72] Chen X Z, Hoop M, Mushtaq F, Siringil E, Hu C, Nelson B J and Pané S 2017 Recent developments in magnetically driven micro-and nanorobots *Appl. Mater. Today* **9** 37–48
[73] Kiristi M, Singh V V, Esteban-Fernández de Ávila B, Uygun M, Soto F, Aktaş Uygun D and Wang J 2015 Lysozyme-based antibacterial nanomotors *ACS Nano* **9** 9252–9
[74] Uygun M, Jurado-Sanchez B, Uygun D A, Singh V V, Zhang L and Wang J 2017 Ultrasound-propelled nanowire motors enhance asparaginase enzymatic activity against cancer cells *Nanoscale* **9** 18423–9
[75] Zhan Z, Wei F, Zheng J, Yang W, Luo J and Yao L 2018 Recent advances of light-driven micro/nanomotors: toward powerful thrust and precise control *Nanotechnol. Rev.* **7** 555–81
[76] Li T, Li J, Morozov K I, Wu Z, Xu T, Rozen I, Leshansky A M, Li L and Wang J 2017 Highly efficient freestyle magnetic nanoswimmer *Nano Lett.* **17** 5092–8
[77] Smith L M 2010 Molecular robots on the move *Nature* **465** 167–8
[78] Krishnan Y 2008 DNA's new avatar as nanoscale construction material *Resonance* **13** 195–7
[79] Surana S, Bhat J M, Koushika S P and Krishnan Y 2011 An autonomous DNA nanomachine maps spatiotemporal pH changes in a multicellular living organism *Nat. Commun.* **2** 340
[80] Bhatia D, Surana S, Chakraborty S, Koushika S P and Krishnan Y 2011 A synthetic icosahedral DNA-based host–cargo complex for functional *in vivo* imaging *Nat. Commun.* **2** 339
[81] Linko V, Ora A and Kostiainen M A 2015 DNA nanostructures as smart drug-delivery vehicles and molecular devices *Trends Biotechnol.* **33** 586–94
[82] Guix M, Mayorga-Martinez C C and Merkoçi A 2014 Nano/micromotors in (bio) chemical science applications *Chem. Rev.* **114** 6285–322

[83] Rothemund P W 2006 Folding DNA to create nanoscale shapes and patterns *Nature* **440** 297–302
[84] Kearney C J, Lucas C R, O'Brien F J and Castro C E 2016 DNA origami: folded DNA-nanodevices that can direct and interpret cell behavior *Adv. Mater.* **28** 5509–24
[85] Schneider F, Möritz N and Dietz H 2019 The sequence of events during folding of a DNA origami *Sci. Adv.* **5** eaaw1412
[86] Zhang F, Nangreave J, Liu Y and Yan H 2014 Structural DNA nanotechnology: state of the art and future perspective *J. Am. Chem. Soc.* **136** 11198–211
[87] Kopperger E, List J, Madhira S, Rothfischer F, Lamb D C and Simmel F C 2018 A self-assembled nanoscale robotic arm controlled by electric fields *Science* **359** 296–301
[88] Ding B and Seeman N C 2006 Operation of a DNA robot arm inserted into a 2D DNA crystalline substrate *Science* **314** 1583–5
[89] Thubagere A J *et al* 2017 A cargo-sorting DNA robot *Science* **357** eaan6558
[90] Blanchard A T and Salaita K 2019 Emerging uses of DNA mechanical devices *Science* **365** 1080–1
[91] Singh H R, Kopperger E and Simmel F C 2018 A DNA nanorobot uprises against cancer *Trends Mol. Med.* **24** 591–3
[92] Tasciotti E 2018 Smart cancer therapy with DNA origami *Nat. Biotechnol.* **36** 234–5
[93] Bradley C A 2018 DNA nanorobots—seek and destroy *Nat. Rev. Drug Discov.* **17** 242 242
[94] Saadeh Y and Vyas D 2014 Nanorobotic applications in medicine: current proposals and designs *Am. J. Robot. Surg.* **1** 4–11
[95] Moezizadeh M 2013 Future of dentistry, nanodentistry, ozone therapy and tissue engineering *J. Dev. Bio. Tissue Eng.* **5** 1–6
[96] Zafar M S, Khurshid Z, Najeeb S, Zohaib S and Rehman I U 2017 Therapeutic applications of nanotechnology in dentistry *Nanostructures for Oral Medicine* (Amsterdam: Elsevier) 833–62
[97] Peng F, Tu Y and Wilson D A 2017 Micro/nanomotors towards *in vivo* application: cell, tissue and biofluid. *Chem. Soc. Rev.* **46** 5289–310
[98] Petros R A and DeSimone J M 2010 Strategies in the design of nanoparticles for therapeutic applications *Nat. Rev. Drug Discov.* **9** 615–27
[99] Wilhelm S, Tavares A J, Dai Q, Ohta S, Audet J, Dvorak H F and Chan W C 2016 Analysis of nanoparticle delivery to tumours *Nat. Rev. Mater.* **1** 1–12
[100] Pané S, Puigmartí-Luis J, Bergeles C, Chen X Z, Pellicer E, Sort J, Počepcová V, Ferreira A and Nelson B J 2019 Imaging technologies for biomedical micro-and nanoswimmers *Adv. Mater. Technol.* **4** 1800575
[101] Martel S 2016 Swimming microorganisms acting as nanorobots versus artificial nano-robotic agents: a perspective view from an historical retrospective on the future of medical nanorobotics in the largest known three-dimensional biomicrofluidic networks *Biomicrofluidics* **10** 2
[102] Soto F and Chrostowski R 2018 Frontiers of medical micro/nanorobotics: *in vivo* applications and commercialization perspectives toward clinical uses *Front. Bioeng. Biotechnol.* **6** 170
[103] Dahmen C, Wortmann T and Fatikow S 2012 Techniques for MRI-based nanorobotics *Nanorobotics: Current Approaches and Techniques* (New York: Springer) 301–22

[104] Cerofolini G F and Amato P 2012 Sensing strategies for early diagnosis of cancer by swarm of nanorobots: an evidential paradigm *Nanorobotics: Current Approaches and Techniques* (New York: Springer) 331–52
[105] Li J *et al* 2016 Enteric micromotor can selectively position and spontaneously propel in the gastrointestinal tract *ACS Nano* **10** 9536–42
[106] Gao W, Dong R, Thamphiwatana S, Li J, Gao W, Zhang L and Wang J 2015 Artificial micromotors in the mouse's stomach: a step toward *in vivo* use of synthetic motors *ACS Nano* **9** 117–23
[107] Surana S, Shenoy A R and Krishnan Y 2015 Designing DNA nanodevices for compatibility with the immune system of higher organisms *Nat. Nanotechnol.* **10** 741–7
[108] Grübler A 2003 *Technology and Global Change* (Cambridge: Cambridge University Press)

IOP Publishing

Rishabha Malviya, Deepika Yadav, Sonali Sundram, Seifedine Kadry and Gurvinder Singh Virk

Chapter 8

Nanozyme-based nanorobots for cancer treatment applications

Complex tasks at the nanoscale can be carried out by a new class of artificial robots called nanorobots. Typically, a nanorobot's system consists of four subsystems: logic control, drive, sensing, and functioning. The production of nanorobots necessitates nanomaterials that are designable, programmable, and multifunctional because of their nuanced structure and complicated activity. As such, we argue that nanozymes, with their adaptable architecture, tunable enzyme-like activities, and nanoscale physicochemical features, are suitable choices for the manufacture of nanorobots. An array of nanorobot systems, or 'systems,' may be combined with the help of nanozymes. In this chapter, we discuss the developments in nanozyme-based systems for making nanorobots, as well as the potential future applications of nanozymes in the field. We anticipate that the special characteristics of nanozymes will inspire new approaches to the development of nanorobotics.

8.1 Introduction

The capacity to examine and comprehend the world around us on ever-smaller scales has been a hallmark of scientific and medical advancement. New treatment options and theoretical frameworks have emerged with each order of magnitude of access to smaller dimensions. The germ hypothesis and microbiology were two of these advancements.

The next step in the relentless pursuit of miniaturization is the advent of nanotechnology, which allows scientists to operate on the nanometer scale for the first time. The National Nanotechnology Initiative (NNI), an American government program to advance nanotechnology, defines nanotechnology as science, research, and technology at the nanoscale [1]. According to the NNI, this scale is between 1 and 100 nm. To provide some perspective on the nanoscale, a cell surface receptor

doi:10.1088/978-0-7503-6019-7ch8

is on the order of 40 nm in size, a DNA strand is on the order of 2 nm in size, and an albumin molecule is on the order of 7 nm in size.

To date, nanotechnology has enabled developments such as better imaging techniques to improve the sensitivity of cancer and disease detection [2], more accurately target drug treatments [3], reduce the adverse effects of chemotherapy, and increase the effectiveness of other antineoplastic therapies such as cryotherapy [4] and ultrasound [5]. Outside the medical sector, developments in agriculture [6], energy [7], electronics [8], and many other areas are also being fueled by nanotechnology.

Dr Richard Feynman, a world-renowned physicist, is credited for originally conceptualizing nanotechnology in a seminar titled 'There's Plenty of Room at the Bottom,' which he gave to the American Physical Society in December 1959. At a fundamental level, Dr Feynman described the scope and size of nanotechnology, as well as the potential benefits it would bring to industries such as biology, IT, manufacturing, electrical engineering, and others.

Nanobiotechnology, a subset of nanotechnology, applies nanotechnology's concepts and methods to the study and treatment of biological and medical problems. Nanobiotechnology is the usage of nanoscale engineering to learn about biological systems and the production of medicines and mechanical devices for use in diagnosing and treating disease. This chapter examines the way in which nanobiotechnology has progressed in the area of device development, particularly with regards to the creation of nanorobots and their use in medicine. We will look at several case studies from various medical disciplines such as microbiology, hematology, oncology, neurosurgery, and dentistry.

8.2 Nanomedicine and nanotheranostics

Due to their unique nanoscale physicochemical properties [8], materials that have nanoscale (1–100 nm) surface engineering have been proposed for use in biological and sensing applications in recent decades. In addition, nanoscale platforms have demonstrated significant potential in various domains for several reasons. First, their small dimensions enable enhanced accumulation and binding at specific sites. Second, their physicochemical properties, such as their structure, form, stability, and surface charge, may be finely tuned. Third, their enhanced surface area allows them to carry large drug payloads and perform controlled delivery. Fourth, these platforms can easily be functionalized with targeted ligands and biomolecules on their surfaces. Finally, they exhibit multiple uses and modalities, further enhancing their versatility. Due to their ability to accommodate a greater payload than small molecules (a traditional platform) while still circulating unimpeded in the bloodstream, nanoscale platforms are often favored in biomedical applications. Furthermore, these nanoparticles are categorized into three primary types, including metallic, non-metallic, and biotic, demonstrating their flexible medicinal qualities for enhanced medical treatment; this field of study is known as nanomedicine [8]. Nanoscale materials, or 'nanomedicines,' are having a substantial effect on the development of low-priced diagnostic and therapeutic tools. Due to their small size, nanomaterials have shown that they are readily absorbed by cells and distributed uniformly across the diverse tumor microenvironment. The drawback of these nanomedicines is that they aggregate easily.

The future representation and application of theranostics is crucial to the perfect idea of next-generation medication. In short, nanoengineered theranostics provides significant benefits for site-specific imaging and therapy in short timescales using low dosages. The nanoengineering of theranostics presents several challenges, not least of which is preserving the diagnostic and therapeutic efficacy of imaging probes and other nanoscale devices. In 2002, John Funkhouser combined a targeting ligand with imaging and therapeutic probes [9]. Cost, the time spent in diagnosis and treatment, unwanted effects, and other negative outcomes may all be mitigated by theranostic drugs. Nanotheranostics, the nanoscale engineering of theranostics, has appeared as a promising field of study in biomedical studies, particularly for multimodal imagery and combination therapies [1, 2]. Targeting, reaction to various stimuli, regulated administration, enhanced contrast and therapeutic effectiveness, better transportation efficacy, and so on are just some of the many benefits demonstrated by these smart nanotheranostics. Such multimodality and 'all-in-one' capabilities thus hold great promise but must be modified for practical use. Therefore, scientists from a wide range of disciplines are working on developing therapeutically relevant theranostics by refining synthetic techniques without compromising the effectiveness of the manufactured platforms.

8.3 Targeted tumor vessel infarction with nanomedicine

Tumoral vascular infarction, caused by the proliferation of blood vessels during tumor angiogenesis, is an effective method of halting tumor development. Amazingly, it only takes one blood clot to block an artery, resulting in the death of a thousand cells. It is possible to stop a tumor from growing by damaging its blood supply using antiangiogenic and tumor-specific vascular disruption agents [10, 11]. This new method of vascular targeting, known as tumoral vessel infarction caused by coagulation factor, has shown promise in clinical trials. When a tumor's vascular system is in direct contact with vascular endothelial cells, the nonspecific biodistribution of traditional chemotherapeutic medicines leads to insufficient therapeutic levels within the cancer cells. In addition, several other anticancer medicines, antiangiogenic agents, and vasculature-disrupting chemicals have been tested for their ability to halt tumor growth and cut off tumors' blood supply. An intravenous infusion of truncated tissue factor (tTF)-NGR, unlike other fusion proteins, causes thrombosis in blood vessels and completely regresses tumor development. tTF-RGD, Cys-Arg-Glu-Lys-Ala, and tumor-homing pentapeptide are three examples of the many conjugated peptide assemblies being used to trigger vascular infarction in cancers of the breast and lungs. However, their usefulness is limited by inadequate targeting and high-dose delivery [12]. On the other hand, nanomedicine-based techniques have shown their ability to cause local infarction of tumoral vasculature in targeted cancer treatment due to their improved therapeutic effectiveness and safety [13]. The use of nanohybrids, and more specifically those with nucleic acid incorporated into them, to target tumoral vasculature is a relatively new field in onconanomedicine [14–19]. Furthermore, hydrogel crosslinked with tetra(aniline) nanoparticles and conductive hydrogel with hydrogen sulfide emission have also been explored for their ability to cause localized infarction in arteries. In addition, it has been suggested that the design of smart nanotherapeutics should be tailored to the unique anatomical and physiological characteristics of tumoral blood vessels. Importantly, the treatment of arterial infarction in solid tumors has been successfully addressed by the use of nanohybrids, which exhibit the ability to selectively restrict blood flow to the tumor, resulting in significant cellular demise. Tissue necrosis and vascular infarction have been seen in experimental studies in which polyethylene glycol (PEGF)-conjugated retargeted tissue factor and thrombin-loaded DNA nanorobots were administered by intratumoral arterial injection [14, 15]. The use of DNA-integrated nanoassembly, often referred to as nanorobotics, has been explored in several uses such as targeted imaging, biosensing, and cargo delivery. Recently, DNA-based nanohybrids have gained a lot of attention due to their potential to selectively occlude tumoral arteries, thereby limiting the supply of nutrients and oxygen to tumor cells and hastening their demise. In this method, platelet aggregation control is used to prevent obstinate thrombosis, which results from platelet activation and the conversion of fibrinogen to fibrin. Therefore, it is essential and crucial to target the delivery of thrombin specifically to tumor locations in a highly regulated way to minimize its effects on healthy tissues. In summary, DNA nanorobotic systems may serve as a source of innovation in the development of cancer therapies via the administration of small interfering ribonucleic acid (siRNA) as well as chemotherapeutic antitumor or peptide medicines. In addition, these DNA nanorobotic systems, when used in conjunction with other treatment techniques, may be effective in the complete elimination of solid tumors [14, 20].

The resulting conjugates are subsequently assessed for their ability to induce localized infarction of tumor vessels. Platelet-supported polymeric nanoparticles, often referred to as nanoplatelets, are considered to be recently developed targeted delivery strategies. The ability of these synthetic hybrids to transport the thrombolytic medication rtPA has been evaluated. These customized nanoplatelets had a lower risk of causing bleeding problems *in vivo* than free rtPA, which is surprising. In addition, the innate aiming molecules on the blood plasma membrane of these platelets aid in maintaining the integrity of the injured endothelium and avoid the major hurdles of active aiming approaches when used with thrombolytic drugs [21]. Therefore, nanoplatelets have become more effective in achieving thrombolysis than the previously available molecularly focused nanotherapeutics. Finally, these hybrid biomimetic nanoplatelets showed promise as a means to improve the effectiveness and decrease the risk of bleeding associated with thrombolytic treatment across a variety of thrombotic disorders. However, there are still challenges with these nanoscale platforms, such as limited targeting capabilities, short half-lives, and unrestrained hemorrhage problems.

8.4 Targeted tumor drug delivery systems

8.4.1 Passively targeted drug delivery systems

In the field of tumor therapy, passively targeted drug delivery systems (PTDDSs) rely heavily on the enhanced permeation and retention (EPR) effect, which in turn is heavily dependent on the specific pathophysiological features of tumors, the properties of nanomaterials, and the parameters of plasma flow (such as circulation time, phagocytosis, etc) [22]. To maximize the therapeutic benefit of the EPR effect, scientists have developed a wide range of passive drug carriers that account for both the physiological and nanomaterial aspects that influence it. There are six basic pathophysiological features shared by most tumors: significantly elevated levels of permeability mediators, aberrant vasculature, misaligned endothelial cells, faulty angiotensin II receptors, reduced lymphatic drainage/recovery, and the absence of a smooth muscle layer. The specific characteristics of each tumor are used to optimize targeted drug delivery systems (TDDSs) [22]. Drug distribution also critically depends on further aspects, such as size, shape, surface charge, and surface wettability.

So far, nanocarriers have been broken down into five distinct categories: the types of nanoparticles often used in research and applications include lipid-based nanoparticles, such as nanoparticles made of polymers, micelles, dendrimers, carbon, and metallic and magnetic materials. Liposomes are lipid-based vesicles that have gained significant attention in the field of drugs. They may be either unilamellar or multilamellar and range in size from 20 to 1000 nm. These are spherical vesicles that assemble themselves and provide the following benefits: (1) they efficiently encapsulate hydrophilic and hydrophobic medicinal substances, (2) shield the encapsulated pharmaceuticals from environmental deterioration, and (3) they can be functionalized for a variety of purposes (e.g. the use of ligand-mediated selective targeting). The synthesis of the appropriate composition and the lengthening of the vesicles' half-life in the circulation are the key factors in this research. Polymeric micelles are structures that undergo self-assembly and spontaneously evolve into monolayers under favorable circumstances. They may elude renal excretion and avoid absorption by the mononuclear phagocyte system owing to their hydrophilic corona and tiny size (100 nm). Dendrimers are polymeric molecules that have well-established host–guest trapping capabilities, definite molecular weights, and a large number of surface functional groups. They radiate outward from a central core and are made up of several flawlessly branching monomers. Carbon nanotubes (CNTs) and other carbon-based nanocarriers may be thought of as tubes spun from sheets of graphene. CNTs have the benefit of being able to quickly enter any kind of cell, including those that are notoriously difficult to transfect. To conjugate antibodies, ligands, and medicines of interest, metallic nanoparticles may be produced and modified using different chemical functional groups. Applications in magnetic separation, targeted drug administration, and analytic imaging have shown their usefulness in the medical field. However, their use *in vivo* is constrained by issues of biocompatibility and toxicity. Targeted medicine delivery, imaging contrast agents, and the remediation of polluted water are all areas where magnetic particles show great promise.

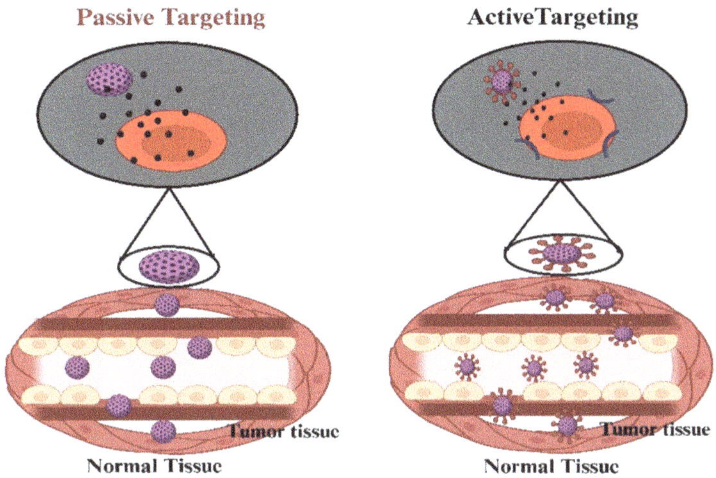

Figure 8.1. Passively and actively targeted medication delivery systems.

Even though PTDDSs (figure 8.1) have advantages over standard chemotherapeutic drugs, such as longer *in vivo* circulation times, decreased uptake by endothelial cells and phagocytes, enhanced drug efficacy, etc. they still have several shortcomings and face several challenges that will require more research to overcome.

8.4.2 Actively targeted medication delivery systems

In actively targeted medication delivery systems (ATDDs), ligands are coupled to carriers and then interact with their relevant receptors to selectively attach to the target cells. In addition to the minor molecules and macromolecules (e.g. peptides) already mentioned, other ligands have also been employed in ATDDSs. In this sense, ATDDSs may also be thought of as nanocarriers that target their payloads through ligands. As well as increasing the bioavailability of chemotherapeutic drugs, ATDDSs may lessen their off-target effects [23]. In addition, certain cutting-edge active drug carriers may transport nanocarriers to their intended areas in response to endogenic (pH, hypoxia, etc.) and exogenous stimuli, allowing for environment-responsive drug administration or regulated drug delivery (in which the method of regulation is, for example, ultrasound, light, heat, or a magnetic field). For these reasons, among others, ATDDSs have been the subject of substantial study and considerable interest.

Nanomaterial-based TDDSs are a novel approach to treating cancer. Nanocarriers' potential for improved tumor tissue penetration and sustained, targeted medication release stems from their many desirable characteristics, including their small sizes, enhanced surface-to-volume ratios, tunable drug release profiles, and specific alterations. However, there are still issues and obstacles with these novel methods of targeted medication administration: (i) when a nanocarrier interacts with a biological fluid (such as blood serum) or a component of the bioenvironment (such as a protein), it may undergo unfavorable changes in its structure, size, surface qualities, and charges, which in turn have a main impact on the delivery of the nanomedicine; (ii) since there are so many factors that may affect the characterization of nanocarriers—including their composition, size, shape, porosity, and hydrophobicity—it can be difficult to perform an accurate assessment of their toxicity; (iii) knowing where they are and where they are distributed in real time is a challenge. There are other obstacles related to biostability, nanocarrier clearance rate, and body tolerance that prevent their clinical translation. Furthermore, the generated PTDDSs and ATDDSs are unable to self-propel and have poor tumor targeting efficacy (0.7%, median) due to their passive diffusion and short-range recognition (0.5 nm) targeting techniques [22].

8.5 Micro- and nanorobots

Micro- and nanorobots (MNRs) are capable of self-propulsion because they transform ambient energy into mechanical motion, setting them free from the limitations of Brownian movement and small Reynolds numbers that normally restrict the motion of micro- and nanoscale objects. Rather than just floating about in the blood, MNRs may actively navigate through the body, overcoming obstacles such as the thick extracellular matrix, the blood–brain barrier, and the blood–tumor barrier with the aid of their propulsive power. MNRs' capacity to transport drugs specifically to tumors increases drug bioavailability and decreases the required medication dosage, both of which have the potential to lessen unwanted side effects. In the next section, we categorize and exemplify MNRs powered by various processes (figure 8.2) [24–26].

8.5.1 Chemically powered micro- and nanorobots

Moving nonhuman robotics, e.g. MNRs that rely on chemical energy conversion to propel themselves are called chemically powered MNRs. After decades of research

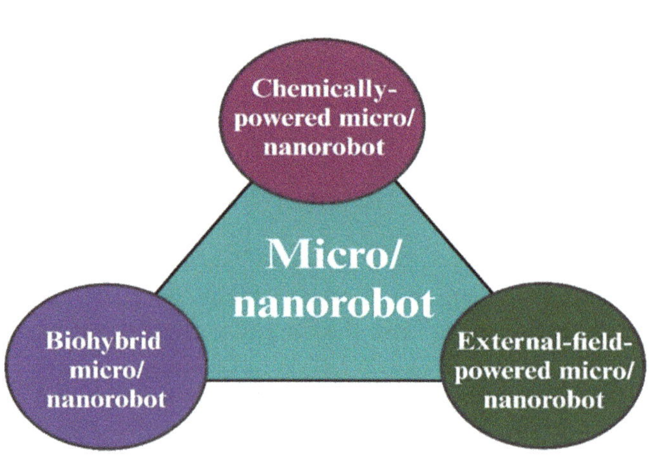

Figure 8.2. Examples of micro- and nanorobots.

and development, we now have access to a wide variety of available MNRs in a wide range of materials, geometries, and surface modifications [27].

The rebound effect of ejected bubbles formed by an interaction between body materials and a biological fuel, which typically comprises peroxide and bioactive liquids, propels the MNRs that use this method of propulsion. Researchers have invested significant time and energy into developing uses for bubble-propelled MNRs in biomedicine because of their remarkable speed. Electrolytic (ionic) diffusiophoresis and non-electrolytic (non-ionic) diffusiophoresis are the two forms of diffusiophoresis [28]. Self-diffusiophoretic MNRs are propelled by a concentration gradient they generate through chemical processes on their surface that use reactants to create products [29]. In contrast to conventional electrophoretic materials, self-electrophoresis-driven MNRs do not generally immediately react to external electric fields. Instead, they move in reaction to electric fields produced by uneven distributions of ions in the environment, which are created by chemical gradients. It is possible to generate a surface tension gradient by constructing the formulation of a solution medium in such a way that an unequal liberation of a preformulated biochemical from the MNRs is achieved. The Marangoni effect describes how a mass flow, triggered by an interfacial energy gradient, may effectively push micro- and nanoscale objects.

The catalytic reaction of H_2O_2 is the foundation of many chemically driven MNRs. However, their potential medicinal use is severely limited due to H_2O_2's harmful effects on living organisms. Consequently, studies have been undertaken to identify potential replacement fuels for MNRs. Among these are the naturally occurring compounds such as glucose, urea, water, and others. Mg-based micromotors that are biocompatible and driven by bubbles were suggested by Mou *et al* [30]. In addition, de Avila *et al* [31] showed that Mg-based MNRs were functional *in vivo*. In a mouse model of gastritis, using stomach acid as fuel, the motor's surface was coated with poly (lactic-co-glycolic acid) (PLGA) and chitosan-carrying clarithromycin (CLR). The H^+ in gastric juices can react with the micromotor's Mg to produce hydrogen bubbles that move the motor forward and raise the juices' pH [32]. Drugs are released into the environment when the Mg core dissolves, causing motor failure. In addition, the positively charged chitosan coating improves local drug release from PLGA and helps the motor to stick to the stomach wall.

Enzymatic MNRs may use biocompatible fuels such as glucose and urea, both of which are readily accessible substances. Sanchez *et al* reported independent locomotion in silica microbots loaded with urease [33], which catalyzed the degradation of urea into ammonia and carbon dioxide, importantly for their potential use in cancer treatment. They were also able to load the microbots with a substantial quantity of antitumor drugs (doxorubicin (DOX)) and rapidly transport them toward tumor cells [34]. Recently, Mou *et al* [35] discovered that ZnO-based micromotors are extremely sensitive to CO_2 dissolved in water, allowing them to be driven by ultralow levels of CO_2 and to exhibit highly effective chemotaxis towards a CO_2 source. Thus, by autonomously following the metabolic CO_2 signals released by certain cells and pathogens, the micromotors were able to 'hunt out' these targets and carry out targeted biomedical procedures [36].

8.5.2 External-field-powered micro- and nanorobots

Fuel-free MNRs that are activated by an outside field, such as light, ultrasound, an electrical field, or a magnetic field, are known as external-field-powered MNRs. The benefits of external-field-powered MNRs over chemically powered MNRs include greater controllability, a longer lifespan, and fewer hazardous unintended effects, resulting in a greater potential for widespread use. Fluctuating magnetic fields (i.e. spinning, oscillating, and on–off magnetic fields) are the primary power source for attractive field-driven MNRs [37]. Typically, there are two directions of motion for MNRs that are pushed or pulled by a magnetic field. The first is that when subjected to magnetic fields that rotate or oscillate, MNRs may move in fluids with a low Reynolds number by undergoing nonreciprocal body deformation. For instance, helical microrobots may counter-rotate in a magnetic field's direction to produce a corkscrew-like motion of translation [38]. Because MNRs encounter increased hydrodynamic resistance close to a wall surface compared to that farther away, magnetic fields may accelerate them by forming an asymmetric force field in the region of a wall.

Many people are interested in ultrasound because it is a potent, biocompatible energy source that may be used in clinical and research settings with little or no special equipment. Typically, surface standing waves may be generated by an interdigital transducer, whereas ultrasonic standing waves can be generated using a bulk acoustic wave device. The acoustic radiation forces that MNRs experience in an ultrasound field are the primary radiation force (PRF), which is the strongest force in the field of acoustic waves responsible for MNR migration, and the secondary radiation force (SRF), a weaker force than the axial PRF. The SRF is responsible for MNR repulsion and attraction [14]. Three different ways of using ultrasound as a propellant have been suggested. A proposal for a self-acoustophoretic process for metallic nanowires suggests that the nanorods' compositional or geometrical asymmetry might lead to nonuniform motion in response to an ultrasonic field [18]. To illustrate the second mechanism, a hollow conical microcannon was filled with nanobullets composed of silica or fluorescent nanospheres. A perfluorocarbon emulsion on the microcannon's inner surface underwent immediate evaporation when subjected to ultrasonic energy [39]. This caused the nanobullets to be rapidly expelled, boosting the microcannon's maximum speed. Such a characteristic may be employed for tissue penetration. The final category includes MNRs that contain trapped air bubbles. Sonic currents may be generated and propelled by an external ultrasonic field. Ultrasonic fields have been utilized to do more than just push MNRs; they have also been used to direct the movement of MNRs (such as bubble-propelled microtubes) and to create swarming behaviors [40, 41].

Light's utility as a renewable energy source has been shown by its ability to activate MNRs, regulate movement, orchestrate group behavior, etc. Both intentionally creating an asymmetric structure and applying a nonuniform light field result in nonuniform gradient fields. For example, by taking advantage of the asymmetric photocatalytic processes and chemical gradients between their lighted and shaded sides, isotropic TiO_2 micromotors may be driven by UV irradiation. The motion of these motors is caused by the interaction between the photoresponsive material and light, which has little to no dependence on environmental factors such as the ionic strength of the surrounding medium, and is inspired by microorganisms found in nature [42]. Due to their programmable geometric forms and the use of different lighting configurations, these biomimetic morphing microswimmers are capable of swimming in a variety of ways. For instance, a simple cylindrical microrobot may cause traveling-wave body deformation and move in the opposite direction to that of the wave when exposed to periodic moving monochromatic light with a certain geometry [43].

There are four common ways to harness the energy of electric fields for MNRs. The first is to use an alternating current (AC) electric field to induce opposing polarizations in the metal and dielectric halves of a Janus microparticle, which in turn causes the microparticle to be propelled away from the metal side using asymmetric electroosmotic fluxes. A second strategy makes use of a diode's rectification of an AC electric field into a direct current (DC) electric field, which produces electrokinetic fluxes and accomplishes self-actuation. The third strategy involves inducing chemical reactions using an electromagnetic field. The final technique uses the Quincke effect. To propel themselves through a low-conductivity liquid medium to the intended destination, dielectric micromotors may be rotated by an AC electric field, which induces an electrokinetic effect [44]. Although electric-field-propelled MNRs can be handled with great accuracy and flexibility using electric tweezers, the restricted locomotion range of electric tweezers and their incompatibility with highly ionic biomedia may limit their bioapplications.

8.5.3 Biohybrid micro- and nanorobots

Biohybrid MNRs are created when nonliving devices are combined with living components at the molecular, cellular, organismal, and tissue levels. This makes it possible to achieve desired functions that combine the advantages of both nonliving systems (such as high accuracy, high strength, and controllability) and living biological materials [45]. The construction of biohybrid MNRs that can exhibit biomimetic behavior and carry out on-demand activities requires appropriate structural design, functional modification (e.g. ligands, antibodies), and the use of controlling actuators (e.g. living cells, critters) [46]. For instance, near-infrared (NIR) laser irradiation was used to create a cellular engine called a 'muscular fin.' Sun and his colleagues conducted another fascinating investigation. Cardiomyocyte-driven soft robots were reported that had features such as snakeskin-like claws, a layer of CNT-assisted myocardial tissue, and a structural color indication layer [47]. The parallel aligned CNT layer induced orientation and had electrical properties that improved the beating ability. The asymmetric claws aided the soft robots to perform directional movement by serving as supporting points [48]. Biohybrid MNRs may be used with a microfluidic system for drug screening assessment in addition to the advantages already described. More recent and significant research into biohybrid MNRs has been conducted [49].

Synthetic MNRs have made great strides, but there are still several obstacles that prevent them from being used in medicine. In future medical applications, organic hybrid drug delivery systems may work as possible perfect drug delivery mechanisms. Biologically designed motile organisms or cells have shown outstanding abilities to safeguard overloaded medications and prevent them from having adverse effects on regular cells or tissues by encapsulating pharmaceuticals within them, because of their great physiological flexibility and functional immunosuppression [50, 51]. Their superior biocompatibility and cell affinity also aid in boosting lesions' medication absorption. In addition, they may release their cargo selectively in response to both external cues, such as food, and endogenous cues, such as light, ultrasound, magnetic fields, and electric fields [51].

Living things have honed their actuation systems into a wide variety of efficient variants that allow them to power themselves and adapt to their surroundings within a narrow range. Bacteria, for instance, may use environmental nutrients by metabolizing them into energy. Bacteria, within a given range, may make the correct modifications in response to environmental change, improving their ability to adapt and survive. They may be guided to their intended targets with pinpoint accuracy using a mix of chemotaxis and exterior field direction, where they can then release their cargo of therapeutic agents. Scientists have fused one or more bacterial strains with magnetic microparticles or nanoparticles. These magnetic particles, when exposed to a magnetic field, move in the direction of the field. The germs then follow the magnetic field's direction of travel. With the help of DOX and a coating of magnetic nanoparticles, researchers were able to attach *Escherichia coli* bacteria to microparticles [52]. This study found that by placing cancer cells in a Petri dish, researchers were able to remotely regulate the program of drug-carrying bacterial robots using magnets. When compared to just adding drug microparticles to tumor cells, this technique may enhance drug targeting [53].

In biohybrid MNRs derived from sperm, high-quality biological properties are essential for clinical use. To propel themselves through thick biofluids, MNRs may make use of the powerful driving forces provided by sperm, which can also be used to carry therapeutic medications or imaging chemicals [54]. Second, immunosuppression may prevent the clearance of loaded medications due to numerous molecules on the membrane. Since the drug absorption of target cells is aided by the sperm's unique acrosome structure, drug-loaded sperm were attached to a magnetic tetrapod-like microtube. With the aid of a magnetic field, it was guided to the designated targets. This microrobot delivered drugs directly into tumor cells by squeezing the sperm into the cancer cell and fusing it with the cell membrane. The use of this sperm-biohybrid MNR medium shows promise for use in medication delivery to treat cancer and other reproductive system illnesses. Biohybrid MNRs have emerged as a hot topic in recent years due to their impressive *in vitro* and *in vivo* experimental outcomes. However, there are still a lot of obstacles to be addressed [51, 55]. Understanding how to keep biohybrid MNRs alive and well in a hostile bioenvironment is crucial for their medicinal use.

8.6 Difficulties with cancer nanomedicines

When a nanosystem is introduced into an organism, it is affected by a complex set of variables. Problems in aiming, dynamic *in vivo* modifications of resources, and numerous biological obstacles are especially relevant in limiting the efficacy of antitumor nanostructures. Multifunctionality is essential for overcoming such intricately linked challenges, which need layered approaches to mitigation.

Numerous pathogenic events [56], many of which are non-tumor-specific but include typical physiological processes altered by the illness, contribute to the cumulative effect of cancer's growth. Pathological variations exist across cancer types, between patients, and within tumors because cancer cells are very diverse and have high mutation rates. Combinatorial or multiple-target treatments based on nanostructures are being investigated to address this diversity. By combining approaches that specifically target tumor cells with those that work to alter the tumor microenvironment (TME), it is possible to customize treatment for individual tumors. The release of growth features and pro-inflammatory cytokines may be suppressed and nanostructure-delivered therapies can be distributed into the dense stroma [57–59] in highly fibrotic tumors by targeting both cancer cells and cancer-associated fibroblasts (CAFs). The co-delivery of doxorubicin, a chemotherapeutic agent that aids in the eradication of tumor sites that are less inhabited by blood vessels, may further reduce the reoccurrence of tumors following vascular obstruction by the targeted administration of thrombin [60].

Improving the pharmacokinetics and biodistribution of a less precise medicine may significantly boost its effectiveness, even though developing a tumor-specific treatment is highly challenging. Indeed, tumor-targeted delivery has been regarded as a fundamental benefit of nanomedicines in cancer treatment [2], whether they function through active targeting or drug release in response to stimuli, or passive targeting based on the EPR effect. However, multifunctional nanostructures' *in vivo* behavior and fate are more complex than those of conventional medication formulations, which might make them particularly susceptible to discrepancies between persons and between preclinical models and clinical applications [61].

When nanostructures enter a living organism, their characteristics are immediately modified by connections at the nano–bio boundary. The delivery efficiency and biosafety of nanostructures [62] may be drastically impacted by instabilities caused by these interactions, such as the accumulation of particles, deterioration, loss of functioning components, or release of hazardous species. The protein corona that forms on a nanostructure's surface once it comes into touch with a bodily fluid might conceal surface properties (such as targeting ligands) and obstruct drug release [63]. Poly (ethylene glycol) (PEG) coating is a popular antifouling modification used to reduce protein interactions between nanoparticles. Alternatives based on biomolecules, in particular proteins and peptides, have also been reported [64, 65]. For example, pre-adsorbed antibodies on polymeric nanoparticles preserve their targeting capability better than chemically attached molecules, probably as a result of more robust surface coverage; however, this relies on the functionalization approach used. The composition of the protein corona may be altered and exploited by nanosurface changes to enhance circulation, lessen toxicity, or fine-tune targeting [63–67]. For instance, the liver-targeting protein apolipoprotein E may be recruited onto the surface of cholesterol-containing lipid nanoparticles *in vivo* [68] using Onpattro, a commercially offered siRNA formulation. To increase transport across the blood–brain barrier, scientists have experimented with the use of short peptides to change the ways in which serum apolipoproteins attach to the surface of nanoparticles [69]. Although nonspecific adsorption interference has been precisely described [70], it was hypothesized that method allowed coronal proteins to be modulated with more precision, allowing for their possible use in a wider variety of applications.

The reticuloendothelial system (RES) [71] clears the blood of protein corona-coated nanostructures because phagocytes easily attach to them through specialized receptors. Therefore, antifouling coatings such as PEG are routinely utilized to increase nanostructures' duration in the circulation. However, the use of PEG only partially decreases immunogenicity, and the induction of PEG-binding antibodies has prompted safety concerns [72, 73]. Motifs based on CD47 [74, 75], a self-marker protein that inhibits phagocytosis or removes blood cell membranes (displaying CD47 on their surface) [73, 76] may be used as active antifouling techniques to aid nanomaterials in avoiding clearance by phagocytes. These strategies have displayed better stealth qualities than PEGylation [73, 74, 77] in mouse models. Indeed, macrophage- or RES-targeted organ delivery may likewise benefit from corona-mediated clearance. Cationic liposomes, for instance, may be used to selectively distribute genes to the liver and spleen by switching their charge.

It has long been believed that the leaky tumoral blood vasculature allows nanosystems to extravasate from the circulation and reach tumor tissue [26]. However, the therapeutic importance of the EPR effect is debatable [27, 78, 79] due to the wide variation it exhibits from tumor to tumor and even within a single tumor. By generating local hypertension, relaxing blood vessels, or causing further damage to tumor blood vessels, multifunctional nanoparticles may actively promote intratumoral extravasation. It is possible to partially resolve the issue of EPR heterogeneity via such methods [78–80], but patient classification and imaging-guided customized therapy will be necessary to fine-tune nanomaterial-based treatment techniques.

It has been shown that the properties of nanomaterials affect their ability to extravasate; for instance, spherical nanoparticles in flowing blood tend to remain around the center of the stream, but rod- or plate-shaped objects have the propensity to drift towards the vessel walls and, because of their greater contact area, demonstrate robust interactions with endothelial cells. [26, 80]. The softness of the surface of extracellular vesicles has a major effect on their capability to be taken up by cells *in vivo* [81]. Covering nanoparticles with cell membranes produced from leukocytes [49] increases endothelial adherence and, in turn, extravasation. Paracellular leakage is the most widely accepted method for extravasation; nevertheless, active transport by endothelial cells [79, 82] similarly plays a role and is gaining interest in the field of nanosystem design and targeting [83, 84].

To combat cancer, nanoformulations are often administered intravenously. For instance, the issue of intravenously injected nanomaterial accretion in the liver has not yet been addressed by multifunctional strategies; this might enhance general tolerance and lessen the medication toxicity experienced by other tissues [12], but remains a problem for effective drug delivery to the tumor. The biodistribution pattern of medications is largely determined by the mode of delivery; hence, for some malignancies, researchers are investigating alternatives to intravenous injection along with targeted tactics. Some forms of administration, such as intradermal and subcutaneous injection, may be more effective than others for tumor immunization through the lymphatic system [85], whereas colon cancer [86] may be targeted by the oral administration of nanoparticles.

The tumor and the TME also act as a roadblock for drugs delivered via nanostructures. Nanostructures are hindered in their ability to penetrate tissues due to the increased interstitial liquid pressure and desmoplastic stroma [26]. In addition, there are fewer blood arteries in the deeper tumor locations. Moreover, tumor-associated macrophages (TAMs) rather than cancer cells may engulf nanoparticles after extravasation [85]. These tumor-intrinsic problems have prompted the creation of TME-targeting techniques (see box 1), which take advantage of prospective targets that are more easily reached than cancer cells. Several targets in the TME have previously been used for nanoparticle administration, including the fibroblast activation protein on CAFs [58], the fibrin–fibronectin composite in tumor blood vessels [60], and TAMs [87–89]. Gene and antigen delivery treatments, as well as other intracellular therapies, rely on cellular uptake and endosomal escape. Nanoparticles, on the other hand, do not passively diffuse across the plasma membrane like hydrophobic tiny medicines. To increase cellular uptake [90], ligands that specifically target membrane proteins or fusogenic materials are used.

8.7 Future perspectives

Nanostructures based on biomolecules combine the material and functional benefits of these naturally occurring building blocks to create drug carriers with potential applications. However, the clinical translation of such nanostructures becomes increasingly difficult as the complexity of their materials increases. In addition, the potential of biomolecule-based anticancer nanostructures will only be achieved through a complete comprehension of nanomaterial–tumor interactions [65]. *In vivo*, biomolecule-derived nanomaterials may interact with and disrupt biological processes and exhibit a wide range of molecular and supramolecular structural variations. As a result, the performance of nanostructures based on biomolecules might be highly dependent on the molecular composition of their constituent parts, making system optimization difficult. Tripeptides that form hydrogels have been discovered using molecular dynamics simulations [91], which is just one instance of the way in which computer simulation and statistical models aid in the logical design of nanostructures based on biomolecules. Using these methods, it is possible to mimic drug release, cell uptake, protein adsorption, and extravasation. Structure–activity correlations can also be developed for safety analyses [92]. However, in contrast to inorganic or polymeric nanostructures, the *in vivo* behaviors of biomolecule-based systems are notoriously difficult to forecast due to their complexity and the absence of rigorous experimental *in vivo* data. Systems with very complex spatial structures and response mechanisms have been used [93, 94] to investigate the multifunctional benefits of nanoparticles. However, there is still a lack of reliable and repeatable production techniques for complicated structures. Unlike proteins, the supramolecular behaviors (and thus the structural creation) of nucleic acids and peptides may reliably be planned. The creation and analysis of nanomaterials may now be automated and monitored with the use of microfluidic and high-throughput techniques.

However, if therapeutic benefits are only triggered by a multistep process, current methods (such as chromatography-based small-molecule drug quantification) may not be able to distinguish between the many drug forms associated with nanostructures. Further, it is sometimes difficult to figure out how to include active components in biomolecule-based nanostructures. Liposomes and polymeric micelles are two common types of drug-encapsulating nanoformulations used in clinical trials because their simple structures allow for uniformity of *in vivo* evaluation and contrast with unrestricted medication compositions. Therefore, researchers need to create theoretical and statistical models that are specific to these systems to preclinically study the action and behavior of biomolecule-based nanostructures *in vivo*.

Furthermore, the use of studies of the high-resolution, *in vivo* imaging of nanostructures may aid in accurate delivery evaluation. Ideal versions of these probes would be able to tell the difference between various nanostructure types. Since the effect of living barriers on the transportation of nanostructures varies from person to person, nanomedicines may be combined with imaging agents (nanotheranostics) to allow actual delivery evaluation [35]. Nanomedicine screening and medication response prediction may be possible through animal-free assessments of nanomaterial delivery. However, at this time, these models cannot reliably predict the effectiveness of intratumor administration for specific patients. Using machine learning techniques, researchers may be able to analyze diverse datasets and discover novel imaging indicators [36]. AI has potential in two areas: patient categorization and the creation of personalized nanostructure delivery techniques. Tumor cell metastasis is still the leading cause of mortality from cancer. It is not always the case that metastatic cancer cells have similar hereditary or functional features to those of the initial tumor cells [37], which can be exploited in the treatment process. In particular, nanoparticle-based techniques have a hard time targeting early metastases because they lack targetable TME properties such as fully established vasculatures. Primary metastases, pre-metastatic tissues, and circulating cancer cells are being targeted for therapy using nanomedical treatments. For instance, platelet and neutrophil-34-derived biological membrane-coated nanoparticles have been studied for anti-metastatic medication delivery. Since it is still challenging to locate metastatic regions for surgical removal or targeted therapies, it makes sense that using nanostructures that can precisely attach to and target metastatic tumor cells might be beneficial. The incorporation of imaging modalities into multifunctional nanostructures is crucial for the growth of nanomedicines with anti-metastatic properties.

8.8 Conclusions

This chapter has emphasized the great potential of prototype nanozyme-based nanorobots for cancer therapy applications. These nanorobots, equipped with nanozymes, allow precision cancer cell targeting, controlled drug release inside the tumor microenvironment, and the manipulation of tumor conditions, promising to boost therapy effectiveness while reducing systemic adverse effects. The absence of methods to predict and assess *in vivo* performance is a significant barrier to the creation of nanomedicines that specifically target tumors. Nanostructures' mechanisms of action, such as multimeric and aggregation-induced effects, cannot always be described using traditional pharmacokinetic parameters alone. However, researchers need to confront obstacles related to biocompatibility and scalability in their pursuit of the clinical implementation of this innovative technology. This technology has the potential to significantly transform cancer treatment and enhance patient outcomes.

References

[1] Shi J, Kantoff P W, Wooster R and Farokhzad O C 2016 Cancer nanomedicine: progress, challenges and opportunities *Nat. Rev. Cancer* **17** 20

[2] Chen H, Zhang W, Zhu G, Xie J and Chen X 2017 Rethinking cancer nanotheranostics *Nat. Rev. Mater.* **2** 17024

[3] Douglas S M, Bachelet I and Church G M A 2012 Logic-gated nanorobot for targeted transport of molecular payloads *Science* **335** 831–4

[4] Zhao Z, Ukidve A, Kim J and Mitragotri S 2020 Targeting strategies for tissue-specific drug delivery *Cell* **181** 151–67

[5] Cheng Z, Al Zaki A, Hui J Z, Muzykantov V R and Tsourkas A 2012 Multifunctional nanoparticles: cost versus benefit of adding targeting and imaging capabilities *Science* **338** 903

[6] Datta L P, Manchineella S and Govindaraju T 2020 Biomolecules-derived biomaterials *Biomaterials* **230** 119633

[7] Liu K, Jiang X and Hunziker P 2016 Carbohydrate-based amphiphilic nano delivery systems for cancer therapy *Nanoscale* **8** 16091–156

[8] Habibi N, Kamaly N, Memic A and Shafiee H 2016 Self-assembled peptide-based nanostructures: smart nanomaterials toward targeted drug delivery *Nano Today* **11** 41–60

[9] Prasad R, Jain N K, Conde J and Srivastava R 2020 Localized nanotheranostics: recent developments in cancer nanomedicine *Mater. Today Adv.* **8** 100087

[10] Seeman N C and Sleiman H F 2018 DNA nanotechnology *Nat. Rev. Mater.* **3** 17068

[11] Lammers T, Kiessling F, Ashford M, Hennink W, Crommelin D and Storm G 2016 Erratum: Cancer nanomedicine: is targeting our target? *Nat. Rev. Mater.* **1** 16076

[12] Seidi K, Neubauer H A, Moriggl R, Jahanban-Esfahlan R and Javaheri T 2018 Tumor target amplification: implications for nano drug delivery systems *J. Control. Release* **275** 142–61

[13] Zhang Y and He J 2021 Tumor vasculature-targeting nanomedicines *Acta Biomater.* **134** 1–2

[14] Li T, Wan M and Mao C 2020 Research progress of micro/nanomotors for cancer treatment *Chempluschem.* **85** 2586–98
[15] Li Z, Seo Y, Aydin O, Elhebeary M, Kamm R D and Kong H 2019 Biohybrid valveless pump-bot powered by engineered skeletal muscle *Proc. Natl Acad. Sci. USA* **116** 1543–8
[16] Liang X, Mou F, Huang Z, Zhang J, You M and Xu L 2020 Hierarchical microswarms with leader–follower-like structures: electrohydrodynamic self-organization and multimode collective photoresponses *Adv. Funct. Mater.* **30** 1908602
[17] Liao M J, Din M O, Tsinring L and Hasty J 2019 Rock-paper-scissors: engineered population dynamics increase genetic stability *Science* **365** 1045–9
[18] Lin R, Yu W, Chen X and Gao H 2021 Self-propelled micro/nanomotors for tumor targeting delivery and therapy *Adv. Healthc. Mat.* **10** 2001212
[19] Liu X, Chen W, Zhao D, Liu X, Wang Y and Chen Y 2022 Enzyme-powered hollow nanorobots for active microsampling enabled by thermoresponsive polymer gating *ACS Nano* **16** 10354–63
[20] Kong X, Gao P, Wang J, Fang Y and Hwang K C 2023 Advances of medical nanorobots for future cancer treatments *J. Hematol. Oncol.* **16** 74
[21] Zenych A, Fournier L and Chauvierre C 2020 Nanomedicine progress in thrombolytic therapy *Biomaterials* **258** 120297
[22] Zhang D, Liu S, Guan J and Mou F 2022 Motile-targeting' drug delivery platforms based on micro/nanorobots for tumor therapy *Front. Bioeng. Biotechnol.* **10** 1002171
[23] Lima A C, Ferreira H, Reis R L and Neves N M 2019 Biodegradable polymers: an update on drug delivery in bone and cartilage diseases *Exp. Opinion Drug Deliv.* **16** 795–813
[24] An M, Feng Y, Liu Y and Yang H 2023 External power-driven micro/nanorobots: design, fabrication, and functionalization for tumor diagnosis and therapy *Prog. Mater. Sci.* **9** 101204
[25] Feng Y, An M, Liu Y, Sarwar M T and Yang H 2023 Advances in chemically powered micro/nanorobots for biological applications: a review *Adv. Funct. Mater.* **33** 2209883
[26] Agrahari V, Agrahari V, Chou M L, Chew C H, Noll J and Burnouf T 2020 Intelligent micro-/nanorobots as drug and cell carrier devices for biomedical therapeutic advancement: promising development opportunities and translational challenges *Biomaterials* **260** 120163
[27] Akolpoglu M B, Alapan Y, Dogan N O, Baltaci S F, Yasa O and Tural G A 2022 Magnetically steerable bacterial microrobots moving in 3D biological matrices for stimuli-responsive cargo delivery *Sci. Adv.* **8** eabo6163
[28] Velegol D, Garg A, Guha R, Kar A and Kumar M 2016 Origins of concentration gradients for diffusiophoresis *Soft Matter* **12** 4686–703
[29] Yang F, Rallabandi B and Stone H A 2019 Autophoresis of two adsorbing/desorbing particles in an electrolyte solution *J. Fluid Mech.* **865** 440–59
[30] Mou F, Chen C, Ma H, Yin Y, Wu Q and Guan J 2013 Self-propelled micromotors driven by the magnesium–water reaction and their hemolytic properties *Angew. Chem. Int. Ed.* **52** 7208–12
[31] Esteban-Fernandez de Avila B, Angsantikul P, Li J, Lopez-Ramirez M A, Ramirez-Herrera D E and Thamphiwatana S 2017 Micromotor-enabled active drug delivery for *in vivo* treatment of stomach infection *Nat. Commun.* **8** 272
[32] Hansen-Bruhn M, de Avila B E F, Beltran-Gastelum M, Zhao J, Ramirez-Herrera D E and Angsantikul P 2018 Active intracellular delivery of a cas9/sgRNA complex using ultrasound-propelled nanomotors *Angew. Chem. Int. Ed.* **57** 2657–61

[33] Medina-Sanchez M, Xu H and Schmidt O G 2018 Micro- and nano-motors: the new generation of drug carriers *Ther. Deliv. 9* 303–16
[34] Hortelao A C, Patino T, Perez-Jimenez A, Blanco A and Sanchez S 2018 Enzyme-powered nanobots enhance anticancer drug delivery *Adv. Funct. Mat.* **28** 1705086
[35] Mou F, Chen C, Zhong Q, Yin Y, Ma H and Guan J 2014 Autonomous motion and temperature-controlled drug delivery of Mg/Pt-poly (N-isopropyl acrylamide) Janus micromotors driven by simulated body fluid and blood plasma *ACS Appl. Mat. Interfaces* **6** 9897–903
[36] Mou F, Xie Q, Liu J, Che S, Bahmane L and You M 2021 ZnO-based micromotors fueled by CO2: the first example of self-reorientation-induced biomimetic chemotaxis *Natl Sci. Rev.* **8** nwab066
[37] Mou F, Zhang J, Wu Z, Du S, Zhang Z and Xu L 2019 Phototactic flocking of photochemical micromotors *Iscience* **19** 415–24
[38] Jin D and Zhang L 2021 Collective behaviors of magnetic active matter: recent progress toward reconfigurable, adaptive, and multifunctional swarming micro/nanorobots *ACC. Chem. Res.* **55** 98–109
[39] Zhao S, Sun D, Zhang J, Lu H, Wang Y, Xiong R and Grattan K T 2022 Actuation and biomedical development of micro-/nanorobots–a review *Mater. Today Nano* **18** 100223
[40] Li J, Mayorga-Martinez C C, Ohl C D and Pumera M 2022 Ultrasonically propelled micro- and nanorobots *Adv. Funct. Mater.* **32** 2102265
[41] Zhang Z, Wang L, Chan T K, Chen Z, Ip M, Chan P K, Sung J J and Zhang L 2022 Micro-/nanorobots in antimicrobial applications: recent progress, challenges, and opportunities *Adv. Healthcare Mater.* **11** 2101991
[42] Alapan Y, Yasa O, Schauer O, Giltinan J, Tabak A F and Sourjik V 2018 Soft erythrocyte-based bacterial microswimmers for cargo delivery *Sci. Robot.* **3** eaar4423
[43] Dreyfus R, Baudry J, Roper M L, Fermigier M, Stone H A and Bibette J 2005 Microscopic artificial swimmers *Nature* **437** 862–5
[44] Moo J G, Mayorga-Martinez C C, Wang H, Khezri B, Teo W Z and Pumera M 2017 Nano/microrobots meet electrochemistry *Adv. Funct. Mater.* **27** 1604759
[45] Wang J, Dong Y, Ma P, Wang Y, Zhang F, Cai B, Chen P and Liu B F 2022 Intelligent Micro-/Nanorobots for Cancer Theragnostic *Adv. Mater.* **34** 2201051
[46] Banerjee H, Suhail M and Ren H 2018 Hydrogel actuators and sensors for biomedical soft robots: a brief overview with impending challenges *Biomimetics* **3** 15
[47] Shang Y, Chen Z, Fu F, Sun L, Shao C, Jin W, Liu H and Zhao Y 2018 Cardiomyocyte-driven structural color actuation in anisotropic inverse opals *ACS Nano* **13** 796–802
[48] Sun L, Chen Z, Bian F and Zhao Y 2020 Bioinspired soft robotic caterpillar with cardiomyocyte drivers *Adv. Funct. Mater.* **30** 1907820
[49] Aydin O, Zhang X, Nuethong S, Pagan-Diaz G J, Bashir R and Gazzola M 2019 Neuromuscular actuation of biohybrid motile bots *Proc. Natl Acad. Sci. USA* **116** 19841–7
[50] Gao L, Akhtar M U, Yang F, Ahmad S, He J and Lian Q 2021 Recent progress in engineering functional biohybrid robots actuated by living cells *Acta Biomater.* **121** 29–40
[51] Hasebe A, Suematsu Y, Takeoka S, Mazzocchi T, Vannozzi L and Ricotti L 2019 Biohybrid actuators based on skeletal muscle-powered micro-grooved ultrathin films consisting of poly (styrene-block-butadiene-block-styrene) *ACS Biomater. Sci. Eng.* **5** 5734–43
[52] Alapan Y, Bozuyuk U, Erkoc P, Karacakol A C and Sitti M 2020 Multifunctional surface micro rollers for targeted cargo delivery in physiological blood flow *Sci. Robot.* **5** eaba5726

[53] Luo M, Feng Y, Wang T and Guan J 2018 Micro-/nanorobots at work in active drug delivery *Adv. Funct. Mater.* **7** 1706100
[54] Li Z, Seo Y, Aydin O, Elhebeary M, Kamm R D and Kong H 2019 Biohybrid valveless pump-bot powered by engineered skeletal muscle *Proc. Natl Acad. Sci. USA* **116** 1543–8
[55] Prinz V Y and Fritzler K B 2023 3D printed biohybrid microsystems *Adv. Mater. Technol.* **8** 2101633
[56] Valkenburg K C, de Groot A E and Pienta K J 2018 Targeting the tumor stroma to improve cancer therapy *Nat. Rev. Clin. Oncol.* **15** 366–81
[57] Ji T *et al* 2016 Transformable peptide nanocarriers for expeditious drug release and effective cancer therapy via cancer-associated fibroblast activation *Angew. Chem. Int. Ed.* **55** 1050–5
[58] Han X *et al* 2018 Reversal of pancreatic desmoplasia by re-educating stellate cells with a tumor microenvironment-activated nanosystem *Nat. Commun.* **9** 3390
[59] Li S *et al* 2020 Combination of tumor-infarction therapy and chemotherapy via the co-delivery of doxorubicin and thrombin encapsulated in tumor-targeted nanoparticles *Nat. Biomed. Eng.* **4** 732–42
[60] Metselaar J M and Lammers T 2020 Challenges in nanomedicine clinical translation *Drug Deliv. Transl. Res.* **10** 721–5
[61] Nel A E, Mädler L, Velegol D, Xia T, Hoek E M, Somasundaran P, Klaessig F, Castranova V and Thompson M 2009 Understanding physicochemical interactions at the nano–bio interface *Nat. Mater.* **8** 543–57
[62] Cai R and Chen C 2019 The crown and the scepter: roles of the protein corona in nanomedicine *Adv. Mater.* **31** 1805740
[63] Banerjee I, Pangule R C and Kane R S 2011 Antifouling coatings: recent developments in the design of surfaces that prevent fouling by proteins, bacteria, and marine organisms *Adv. Mater.* **23** 690–718
[64] Chelmowski R, Köster S D, Kerstan A, Prekelt A, Grunwald C, Winkler T, Metzler-Nolte N, Terfort A and Woll C 2008 Peptide-based SAMs that resist the adsorption of proteins *J. Am. Chem. Soc.* **130** 14952–3
[65] Tonigold M *et al* 2018 Pre-adsorption of antibodies enables targeting of nanocarriers despite a biomolecular corona *Nat. Nanotechnol.* **13** 862
[66] Hamad-Schifferli K 2015 Exploiting the novel properties of protein coronas: emerging applications in nanomedicine *Nanomedicine* **10** 1663–74
[67] Setten R L, Rossi J J and Han S P 2019 The current state and future directions of RNAi-based therapeutics *Nat. Rev. Drug Discov.* **18** 421–46
[68] Zhang Z *et al* 2019 Brain-targeted drug delivery by manipulating protein corona functions *Nat. Commun.* **10** 3561
[69] Mirshafiee V, Kim R, Park S, Mahmoudi M and Kraft M L 2016 Impact of protein pre-coating on the protein corona composition and nanoparticle cellular uptake *Biomaterials* **75** 295–304
[70] Owens D E and Peppas N A 2006 Opsonization biodistribution, and pharmacokinetics of polymeric nanoparticles *Int. J. Pharm.* **307** 93–102
[71] Zhang P, Sun F, Liu S and Jiang S 2016 Anti-PEG antibodies in the clinic: current issues and beyond PEGylation *J. Control. Release* **244** 184–93
[72] Hu C M, Zhang L, Aryal S, Cheung C, Fang R H and Zhang L 2011 Erythrocyte membrane-camouflaged polymeric nanoparticles as a biomimetic delivery platform *Proc. Natl Acad. Sci.* **108** 10980–5

[73] Rodriguez P L, Harada T, Christian D A, Pantano D A, Tsai R K and Discher D E 2013 Minimal 'self' peptides that inhibit phagocytic clearance and enhance delivery of nanoparticles *Science* **339** 971–5

[74] Kim J, Sinha S, Solomon M, Perez-Herrero E, Hsu J, Tsinas Z and Muro S 2017 Co-coating of receptor-targeted drug nanocarriers with anti-phagocytic moieties enhances specific tissue uptake versus non-specific phagocytic clearance *Biomaterials* **147** 14–25

[75] Kang T *et al* 2017 Nanoparticles coated with neutrophil membranes can effectively treat cancer metastasis *ACS Nano* **11** 1397–411

[76] Cheng Q, Wei T, Farbiak L, Johnson L T, Dilliard S A and Siegwart D J 2020 Selective organ targeting (SORT) nanoparticles for tissue-specific mRNA delivery and CRISPR–Cas gene editing *Nat. Nanotechnol.* **15** 313–20

[77] Abbott J J, Nagy Z, Beyeler F and Nelson B J 2007 Robotics in the small, part I: microbotics *IEEE Robot. Autom. Mag.* **14** 92–103

[78] Alapan Y, Bozuyuk U, Erkoc P, Karacakol A C and Sitti M 2020 Multifunctional surface micro rollers for targeted cargo delivery in physiological blood flow *Sci. Robot.* **5** eaba5726

[79] Alapan Y, Yasa O, Schauer O, Giltinan J, Tabak A F and Sourjik V 2018 Soft erythrocyte-based bacterial microswimmers for cargo delivery *Sci. Robot.* **3** eaar4423

[80] Ash C, Dubec M, Donne K and Bashford T 2017 Effect of wavelength and beam width on penetration in light-tissue interaction using computational methods *Lasers Med. Sci.* **32** 1909–18

[81] Aubry M, Wang W A, Guyodo Y, Delacou E, Guigner J M and Espeli O 2020 Engineering *E. coli* for magnetic control and the spatial localization of functions *ACS Synth. Biol.* **9** 3030–41

[82] Aziz A, Pane S, Iacovacci V, Koukourakis N, Czarske J and Menciassi A 2020 Medical imaging of microrobots: toward *in vivo* applications *Acs Nano* **14** 10865–93

[83] Bae Y H and Park K 2011 Targeted drug delivery to tumors: myths, reality and possibility *J. Control. Release* **153** 198–205

[84] Bourdeau R W, Lee-Gosselin A, Lakshmanan A, Farhadi A, Kumar S R and Nety S P 2018 Acoustic reporter genes for noninvasive imaging of microorganisms in mammalian hosts *Nature* **553** 86–90

[85] Andhari S S, Wavhale R D, Dhobale K D, Tawade B V, Chate G P and Patil Y N 2020 Self-propelling targeted magneto-nanobots for deep tumor penetration and pH-responsive intracellular drug delivery *Sci. Rep.* **10** 4703

[86] Calvo-Marzal P, Sattayasamitsathit S, Balasubramanian S, Windmiller J R, Dao C and Wang J 2010 Propulsion of nanowire diodes *Chem. Commun.* **46** 1623–4

[87] Camp E R, Wang C, Little E C, Watson P M, Pirollo K F and Rait A L 2013 Transferrin receptor targeting nanomedicine delivering wild-type p53 gene sensitizes pancreatic cancer to gemcitabine therapy *Cancer Gene Ther.* **20** 222–8

[88] Canale F P, Basso C, Antonini G, Perotti M, Li N and Sokolovska A 2021 Metabolic modulation of tumors with engineered bacteria for immunotherapy *Nature* **598** 662–6

[89] Ceylan H, Dogan N O, Yasa I C, Musaoglu M N, Kulali Z U and Sitti M 2021 3D printed personalized magnetic micromachines from patient blood-derived biomaterials *Sci. Adv.* **7** eabh0273

[90] Che S, Zhang J, Mou F, Guo X, Kauffman J E and Sen A 2022 Light-programmable assemblies of isotropic micromotors *Research* **2022** 1–12

[91] Katyal P, Mahmoudinobar F and Montclair J K 2020 Recent trends in peptide and protein-based hydrogels *Curr. Opin. Struct. Biol.* **63** 97–105
[92] Sethi B, Kumar V, Mahato K, Coulter D W and Mahato R I 2022 Recent advances in drug delivery and targeting to the brain *J. Control. Release* **350** 668–87
[93] Llopis-Lorente A, Garcia-Fernandez A, Lucena-Sanchez E, Diez P, Sancenon F and Villalonga R 2019 Stimulus-responsive nanomotors based on gated enzyme-powered Janus Au-mesoporous silica nanoparticles for enhanced cargo delivery *Chem. Commun.* **55** 13164–7
[94] Llopis-Lorente A, Garcia-Fernandez A, Murillo-Cremaes N, Hortelao A C, Patino T and Villalonga R 2019 Enzyme-powered gated mesoporous silica nanomotors for on-command intracellular payload delivery *ACS Nano* **13** 12171–83

IOP Publishing

Integrating Nanorobotics with Biophysics for Cancer Treatment

Rishabha Malviya, Deepika Yadav, Sonali Sundram, Seifedine Kadry and Gurvinder Singh Virk

Chapter 9

Progress in the bioelectrochemical and biophysical diagnostic profiling of malignant cancer cells

The examination of cancer biomarkers has significant potential to expand our knowledge of molecular pathology and facilitate more accurate and prompt disease detection and subsequent monitoring. The liquid biopsy method serves as a nonintrusive replacement for the traditional tissue biopsy approach, enabling the detection of many circulating biomarkers without causing any harm to healthy tissue. These biomarkers include microRNA (miRNA), exosomes, circulating tumor DNA (ctDNA), circulating tumor cells (CTCs), and proteins. This chapter examines the use of surface plasmon resonance (SPR) and localized SPR (LSPR) technologies in the identification of various cancer biomarkers in liquid biopsy samples, evaluating the significance and practicality of these technologies in this context. It begins by critically analyzing current problems and challenges with the collection and interpretation of biomarkers. In addition, we identify the prevailing concerns that need to be resolved before SPR biosensors can be used in clinical environments. Ultimately, the focus is directed toward the latest advancements (within the last five years) in SPR-based systems used in the analysis of patient samples. These systems aim to identify and measure biomarkers, serving as a less invasive liquid biopsy technique for individuals diagnosed with cancer. In conclusion, an analysis of many example assays using SPR biosensor technology is presented, highlighting the numerous advantages it offers in terms of enhanced sensitivity, specificity, precision, and a more efficient workflow.

9.1 Introduction

There are two distinct hypotheses for the cause of carcinogenesis, often known as oncogenesis or tumorigenesis. The somatic mutation theory (SMT) has dominated cancer studies for almost sixty years; it claims that cancer arises from the accretion

doi:10.1088/978-0-7503-6019-7ch9

of many DNA mutations in a single somatic cell. Hence, tumor formation is a multistep process in which accumulating mutations create favorable physiologic compatibility [1]. Several aspects of cancer, including familial malignancies and the effectiveness of gene-targeting tumor medicines, may be explained by the SMT [1]. Nevertheless, the lack of mutations in certain cancers and the use of non-genotoxic agents that generate cancer without any DNA alterations disprove this notion [2, 3]. In response to this perspective, the tissue organization field theory was introduced in 1999, positing the notion that cancer arises from issues in tissue organization, as opposed to beginning only at the cellular level. Carcinogenic substances can alter the microenvironments in which parenchymal cells may undergo proliferation and migration. This is achieved by interfering with the intercellular connections that are responsible for maintaining tissue architecture, healing processes, and overall homeostasis [4].

According to the tissue organization field hypothesis of carcinogenesis, cells communicate primarily via bioelectric control that, when disrupted, may lead to changes in tissue organization. The importance of bioelectricity in the activity and functioning of non-neural cells has just lately become known, in contrast to the substantial research done on cells originating in the brain. Figure 9.1 summarizes the most significant advances and breakthroughs in our understanding of cancer propagation. Improvements in identifying the function of bioelectric signaling in carcinogenesis have resulted from an increased knowledge of the bioelectric processes underlying cancer and the advancement of molecular techniques for monitoring and manipulating the electric fields associated with it. The process of

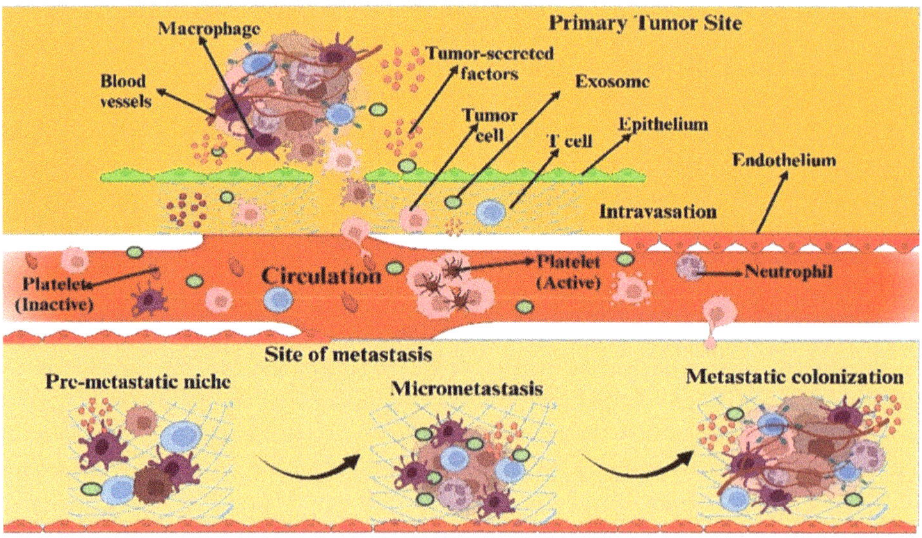

Figure 9.1. The tumor metastasis process. Cancerous cells first break the basement membrane and travel across the stroma. Following intravasation into arteries, cancer cells migrate through the circulation to reach the secondary metastatic location. After extravasation via the endothelial barrier, cancer cells colonize the metastatic target organ and establish a secondary cancer. Adapted from [6]. CC BY 4.0.

synthesizing and transmitting intercellular communication between cells of various tissue types relies on the release of extracellular vesicles (EVs) and contributes to the preservation of tissue homeostasis. Tumor microenvironment (TME) EVs produced by malignant tumors mediate connections between malignant and nonmalignant cells and play a role in all stages of carcinogenesis [5]. One further mechanism by which cancer disrupts cellular bioelectrical signaling pathways is the abnormal synthesis of EVs.

Recent research has examined the bioelectric control of cancer processes, including migration and metastasis [6–9]. In this chapter, we take a broader look at the role of bioelectric control in the progression of malignancy and its spread. We also examine the current technology and methods used to assess and control the bioelectric characteristics of cells *in vivo*, and key ion channels connected to cancer are discussed. Each cell has a distinctive electrical property called the membrane potential (V_{mem}). Plasma-membrane-localized molecular machines such as pumps, carriers, and ion channels create the electric characteristics of the membrane's electrical potential, which in turn generates endogenous electrical fields (EFs) [10]. Transmembrane voltage gradients have been shown to regulate several cellular processes, including cell growth; they cause both excitable and unexcitable cells to move, differentiate, and position themselves; and they also influence brain communication via gap junctions [11, 12].

Whether a cell is excitable or unexcitable depends on the presence or absence of a plasma membrane electric potential gradient. A cell is said to be depolarized when its internal environment, i.e. the cytoplasm, acquires a higher electrical potential than the surrounding area. When the plasma membrane has a lower charge than the extracellular region, the cell is highly polarized and possesses a negative V_{mem}. V_{mem} is not only an important feature of cells themselves but also of their surrounding microenvironment, where it exerts both spatial and temporal influences on cell activity [9]. This is accomplished by allowing cells to take actions depending on the conditions in nearby cells [13]. V_{mem} is physiologically relevant between −90 and −10 mV, albeit this value varies widely across cell types and physiological states [12, 14]. In addition, V_{mem} is mostly generated by ion channels that are controlled post-translationally; two cells can have similar genomic and transcriptional states but very distinct bioelectric states [15]. Finally, cytotoxic T-cells produce granzyme B, which stimulates perforin, a membrane-bound channel, to initiate the third pathway. Finally, as seen in figure 9.2, during the execution of this process, all three approaches converge when caspase 3 is triggered, resulting in programmed cell death.

9.2 The use of biosensors in clinical assessment

Histopathology, cytology, enzyme-linked immunosorbant assay (ELISA), next-generation sequencing (NGS), and polymerase chain reaction (PCR) are commonly employed in laboratory diagnostics [16]. These techniques are favored due to their ability to yield test results that are both highly sensitive and precise. Moreover, they possess the advantage of being universally applicable to diverse classes of biomolecules and have been optimized to efficiently process large quantities of samples.

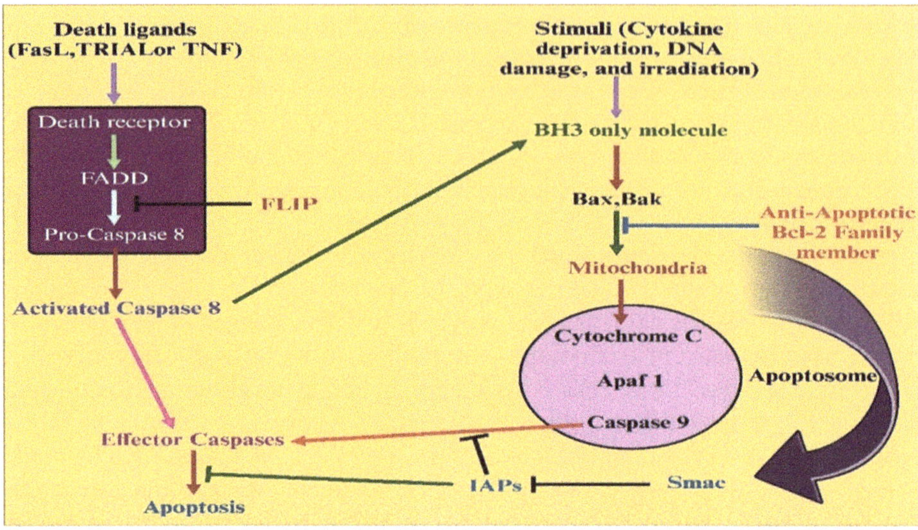

Figure 9.2. A summary of apoptotic signaling pathways, the properties of pro-survival signals, and the microenvironment of tumors. It includes Fas Ligand (FasL), tumor necrosis factor (TNF), and TNF-related apoptosis. Adapted from [6]. CC BY 4.0.

The sample techniques described in this chapter are characterized by their complexity, requiring meticulous attention to detail. The analytic timeframes for DNA sequencing and PCR-related methods are somewhat long, spanning several days and hours, respectively. Moreover, the input volumes for these procedures are rather substantial, often about 1 ml of biofluids. It is essential to acknowledge that these variables may introduce possible sources of bias, such as sample contamination and mistakes in the PCR process. These problems, coupled with the relatively high cost per analysis, are just some of the drawbacks of traditional methods. Even if these technologies were more widely available, their long analysis times and high price tags would limit their use to only the most advanced research facilities [17].

Identifying and quantifying a large number of biomolecules all at once has become much easier thanks to microarray technology. A microarray substrate is a solid support with a pattern of DNA sequences or proteins that have the potential to attach to complementary nucleotide sequences. This binding ability allows them to identify mutations or biomarkers in a given sample. To facilitate their detection, these DNA sequences or proteins may carry a fluorescent tag. Nanomaterials and nanofabrication techniques, which originated in the 1980s, have undergone significant advancements in recent times. These advancements have enhanced the multiplication capability and detection sensitivity of nanotechnology. Consequently, this technology now offers precise, fast, and highly efficient screening methods. These methods have already been employed in the examination and characterization of the underlying factors responsible for various human diseases, as well as in the development of novel therapeutic drugs [18].

Biosensor devices are expected to emerge as very promising possibilities for the identification and surveillance of significant illnesses, such as allergies, diabetes, neurological illnesses, and cancer, because they can provide quick and accurate biomedical testing with small sample amounts and short preparation times [18]. Biosensors are very effective analytical instruments for both accurate clinical assessment and a comprehensive understanding of the molecular mechanisms underlying disease. Such an understanding is crucial because it provides innovative biomarkers that may be used to assess the effectiveness of potential drug therapies. *De novo* mutations that confer resistance may be identified, as well as mutations that are not amenable to clinical therapy but may be to other targeted treatments, thanks to molecular research. Also, such molecular testing addresses the fact that cancerous cell clones are resistant to treatment and patient monitoring during targeted cancer therapy [19]. From this perspective, the use of biosensor platforms for genetic biomarker assessment has the potential to significantly enhance prognostic capabilities and increase survival rates. This advancement has the potential to alleviate the burden of disease and contribute to socioeconomic advancement, ultimately facilitating greater accessibility to healthcare services on a global level. Plasmonic sensor platforms can analyze various categories of biomolecules that have clinical significance. The development of the SPR technique, in particular, has solidified its position in clinical diagnosis. This is primarily due to its capacity to monitor interactions without the need for labeling as well as its ability to qualitatively identify biological molecules in real time at maximum throughput. This retrospective analysis examines the advancements made in the last five years of SPR and LSPR technologies for the recognition and characterization of multiple cancer-related biomarkers in liquid biopsy specimens [16]. Initially, researchers addressed outstanding problems in biomarker capture and analysis by elucidating the existing difficulties inherent in the use of SPR biosensors in clinical settings. In particular, the specificity, sensitivity, and accuracy of the analytical methods used to select the proposals for possible use in clinical diagnostics were assessed using biological fluids, rather than just a buffer.

9.3 Electrochemical biosensors

9.3.1 Various electrochemical measurement methods

In biochemistry, a constant applied voltage is used to oxidize or reduce an electroactive species, depending on the goal, and the currents generated by these reactions are measured using amperometry. This approach has found extensive use in research into cancer biomarkers and the identification of cancerous cells. For instance, Kim *et al* [20] used amperometric immunosensing techniques for analysis and achieved a limit of detection (LOD) of 280 ± 8.0 pg ml^{-1}. Annexin II and MUC5AC are two of the most important biomarkers for the diagnosis of lung cancer. It has been reported that biological sensing prototypes based on a graphite nanocomposite with functioning gold nanoparticles (AuNPs) may detect human cancer of the cervical cavity. CTCs have also been detected through the use of amperometric techniques. For instance, fast CTC detection was achieved through the use of gold array electrodes to identify circulating prostate cancer cells. A linear range (LR) of 50 to 105 cells ml^{-1} and an LOD of 23 ± 2 cells ml^{-1} were achieved by an amperometric biosensor developed to detect cancer cells using an impermeable glycoprotein nanoprobe [21].

Chronoamperometry is another kind of amperometry, in which a square-wave potential is used at the functional electrode to determine the current's time-dependent value under steady-state conditions. A chronoamperometric immunosensor was developed for the recognition of tumor necrosis factor (TNF). The findings of this research showcased remarkable efficacy within the therapeutically significant concentration range. The precision of the immunosensor was determined to be 8%, while the LOD was established to be 0.3 pg ml^{-1}. The chronoamperometric approach was shown to be a viable option for quickly determining the vitality of breast cancer cells [21–24].

When the cell current is off, the electrical potential difference between electrodes may be measured using a potentiometric instrument. The progress of cancerous cells and the occurrence of biomarkers have both been tracked using potentiometric methods.

In early cancer, biomarker concentrations are minimal, making a low LOD (108–1011 M) beneficial for early detection [25]. A light-addressable potentiometric sensor (LAPS) was used to identify the liver cancer biomarker hPRL-3. This investigation detected hPRL-3 and MDA-MB-231 breast cancer cells at LR values of 2.5–250 ng ml^{-1} and 0–105 cells ml^{-1}, respectively, demonstrating their sensitivity and specificity [26]. Another investigation proposed a potentiometric biosensor based on the use of surface molecules to detect carcinoembryonic antigen (CEA) in LoVo human colon cancer cells [27]. The label-free potentiometric detection of HAPLN1, a proteinaceous biomarker that is overexpressed in malignant pleural mesotheliomas (MPM), has been successfully implemented, resulting in a LOD in the pM range and a rapid reaction time of 2–5 min in the sample [28]. A potentiometric microarray based on hybridization has been created to identify exosomal miRNA [29]. In addition, potentiometric methods have been used to analyze microenvironmental electrochemistry while focusing on cancer cells as a target, since they often generate lactate, which causes the pH of their medium to fluctuate. Using this principle, Shaibani and colleagues achieved a LOD of 103 cells ml^{-1} while targeting cancer cells (MDA-MB-231). This investigation also verified alterations in the pH flux in the area around the neoplasm comprised of cancer cells, suggesting a link to the changed cellular metabolism [30]. Using a similar approach to that of LAPS, a potentiometric biosensor based on graphene oxide functionalized with anti-EpCAM was developed for the specific identification of prostate cancer CTCs [31].

Chronopotentiometry is a method for measuring potential changes in response to a constant or square-wave current over time. The prostate-specific antigen (PSA) was studied by Belicky *et al* using chronopotentiometry stripping (CPS) in conjunction with lectins that could recognize PSA glycans in both healthy persons and patients with carcinoma of the prostate [32]. As an electroanalytical technique, voltammetry involves changing an applied potential and then measuring the resultant current to learn more about an analyte. Several voltammetric techniques have been developed because of the wide variety of potential changes that may be made, including square-wave voltammetry (SWV) and stripping voltammetry (SV). In the field of voltammetry, the two most popular techniques are SWV and differential pulse voltammetry (DPV) because of their great sensitivity. Furthermore, they have seen extensive application in the screening of a wide range of media for cancer biomarkers. Several markers (IL-10, HER2, HT-29, PSA, CA-153, HCT, etc.) are only a few of the cancer biomarkers that have been detected using voltammetric methods [33, 34].

As a result of their high sensitivity, short response time, and low excitation voltage, impedimetric methods have also been shown to be a potential tool for detecting cancer biomarkers. They have the added benefit that they can be employed for long-term on-site detection [35]. In terms of frequency of application, electrochemical impedance spectroscopy (EIS) is a popular technique. The excitation voltage for EIS only has to be 5 mV or 10 mV, but the excitation voltage for voltammetric techniques often ranges from 200 to 600 mV [36]. This technology's low excitation voltage makes it a more durable detection method. Electrode heating is an issue in long-term monitoring systems for bioelectrochemical analysis because the electrodes may be harmed and the microenvironment of the body could be altered. Since EIS's low excitation voltage does not generate much heat, it is more appropriate for long-term detection in real time. In addition, EIS offers a wealth of surface biosensor characteristics. Changes in electron transfer resistance (Ret) are measured using a redox pair, commonly a ferricyanide–ferrocyanide combination.

Most electron transfer rates (Ret) are inversely linked to Ret. Double-layer capacitance (CPE) and resistance explain the electrode–electrolyte interface's dielectric and isolation characteristics [37, 38]. EIS may detect cellular, protein, and nucleic acid cancer biomarkers. Volatile organic compounds (VOCs) are unique biomarkers; hence EIS electrochemical detection is not suitable for their detection. A comprehensive slope study of impedance curves at different development phases shows that MDA-MB-231 can multiply despite dietary and space constraints due to its rapid proliferation rate and intrinsic cell death resistance.

9.4 Conventional apoptotic and metastatic cell detection methods

As previously discussed, metastasis is the challenging method by which primary tumor cells spread to develop new tumors in a region of the body that may be either close to or distant from the original spot. The early detection of metastatic illness and aggressive therapy drugs that target these found metastases are still critical for the efficient treatment of individuals with advanced malignancies. Due to their reliance on the circulatory and lymphatic systems for long-distance dissemination, CTCs are often regarded as the most accurate indicators of metastasis. However, cell-enrichment preprocessing is laborious and necessary for the identification of a small number of CTCs [39, 40].

Several potential biomarkers for early cancer diagnosis are secreted or produced by various biological processes. Metastatic cell surface epitopes such as epithelial cell adhesion molecule (EpCAM), mesenchymal cell vimentin, embryonic stem cell/ ectopic mesenchymal transition (Oct4), nanog, and twitch are used to identify CTCs [41]. Apoptosis, like necrosis, is characterized by unique biomarkers, such as the intrinsic pathways involved (caspases, cytochrome- C, Bcl-2, and p53) [42, 43]. Yet, metastatic and apoptotic cells have a distinct appearance from healthy cells that can be monitored, differentiated, and considered during real-time identification. Metastatic cell morphology varies depending on the origin of the metastasis, which may be investigated to pinpoint the initial tumor location. Apoptosis may be identified morphologically using observed characteristics such as chromatin condensation, nuclei that are evenly packed, extensive plasma membrane blebbing, karyorrhexis, and the formation of apoptotic bodies by the detachment of cell fragments.

Understanding metastasis and apoptosis is crucial to the administration of efficient cancer therapy; thus, many conventional methodologies have been devised, refined, and successfully implemented to this end. The underlying technique, such as morphology, biochemistry, immunology, or arrays is most commonly used to categorize this wide range of methods. The response evaluation criteria in solid tumors (RECIST) was formerly regarded as a standard approach to the study of treatment responses in solid tumors. Therapeutic effectiveness may be determined by imaging changes in tumor size and cancer cell morphology using the RECIST [44].

Biosensors, bioelectrochemical techniques (such as cyclic voltammetry), and electron microscopy methodologies are extensively used as contemporary alternatives to the traditional techniques mentioned above. These advanced methods offer additional information for identification, characterization, and quantitative analysis [45]. The induction of apoptosis in cancer cells is primarily studied for its relevance to therapeutic efficacy. The spread of metastases is the single most deadly aspect of cancer. A key barrier to improving clinical outcomes for cancer patients is metastasis, despite tremendous advances in cancer detection and therapy over the last century or more. Despite this, significant advancements in understanding the mechanisms of cancer spread and developing new tools to study it have been completed in the last 200 years. Several novel technologies have been developed as a result of scientific and technological progress, especially since the turn of the millennium [46].

Metastasis is a biological process that has been slowly revealed with the help of innovative technologies. The revelations include the epithelial–mesenchymal transition (EMT) of cancerous cells, the role of CTCs and CTC clusters in seeding metastatic colonies, and the complex relations between cancerous cells. Effective metastasis-targeting drugs are expected to become available shortly, since the 'black box' of metastasis is slowly being uncovered. An intricate multistep process, cancer metastasis begins with primary site invasion and continues with the process of intravasation, which refers to the entry of cancer cells into the bloodstream, followed by their survival inside the circulation. Subsequently, extravasation occurs, which denotes the cancer cells' exit from the bloodstream. Finally, the cancer cells adhere to and colonize the metastatic location, facilitating the establishment of secondary tumors. CTCs are cancer cells that have detached from the primary tumor and been carried away by the body's bloodstream or lymphatic system. To date, most studies of CTCs have looked at CTCs in the blood. Ashworth first identified CTCs in 1869, when he saw 'some cells' in the blood of a metastatic tumor patient that looked like tumor cells from the source tumors [47].

The hypothesis that CTCs serve as the metastatic process's substrate has gained traction. Despite their origin in primary cancer, the EMT properties of CTCs allow them to escape the primary tumor and enter the bloodstream via intravasation, form clusters that increase their metastatic potential, and exhibit stemness features that increase metastasis. Yet the vast majority of CTCs die off in the bloodstream, and only a tiny fraction of them can penetrate distant organs. Among the many factors thought to contribute to CTCs' ability to metastasize is their interaction with the blood environment. This includes the way in which CTCs might evade immune monitoring in the blood. Due to the unique technological obstacles involved in isolating these relatively uncommon CTCs from the enormous pool of circulating blood cells, it took scientists almost a century to uncover the important function of CTCs in the spread of malignancy. Nevertheless, in the last two decades, innovative technology for isolating CTCs has made it possible to study CTC biology and to use CTCs in clinical settings for cancer screening, therapeutic response tracking, and prognosis assessment [48].

9.5 Bioelectricity in cancer processes

Some crucial behaviors that are relevant to cancer are known to be controlled by the bioelectric characteristics of the cellular composition and the electrochemical status of cells inside the microenvironment [49–51]. Researchers have discussed the most prominent ion channels that are linked to cancer.

9.5.1 Cancer and ion channels

Ion channels are types of transmembrane proteins that regulate the movement of ions across cellular membranes, resulting in the establishment of concentration gradients for certain cations and anions. The fundamental function of ion channels is to modulate the movement of ions into and out of cells. However, they also serve as important regulators of other molecular signaling pathways. Calcium ions (Ca^{2+}), sodium ions (Na^+), potassium ions (K^+), and chloride ions (Cl^-) are the principal ions that are widely used in establishing the resting membrane potential (V_{mem}) of a cell. The Goldman equation establishes a connection between the concentrations and permeability values of certain ion species and the overall transmembrane potential. The resting potential V_{mem} is influenced by several factors, including the concentrations of K^+, Na^+, and Cl^- ions, as well as the temperature of the environment and the permeability of each ion species. Modifications in ion channel expression and activity are associated with tumor growth, progression, and metastasis of cancer. For example, several ion channels have been associated with a metastatic phenotype which is characterized by aberrant expression patterns in cancer cells. A plethora of recent literature studies have been published, focusing substantially on the examination of ion channels that have been associated with the development and progression of cancer [27, 28]. The deregulation of ion channel expression disrupts essential signaling pathways in cancer [28–31]. The mitogen-activated protein kinase (MAPK), extracellular signal-regulated kinase (ERK), and c-Jun N-terminal kinase (JNK) signaling pathways, the Wnt/β-catenin system, the phosphoinositide 3-kinase (PI3K)/Akt route, the Notch signaling network, and the Rac and Rho pathways are all illustrative instances of such signaling pathways.

9.5.2 Calcium channels

Ca2+ ion diffusion is tightly regulated by two primary classes of ion channels: calcium channels that are voltage-gated (VGCCs) and transient receptors potential (TRP) ion channels. Epithelial cells from a healthy human breast (HMECs) do not contain VGCCs, while cancerous breast cells do. The impact of calcium ions on cell growth was investigated by Berzingi *et al* [23] After 5 days in culture, MCF7 breast cancer cells grew virtually no larger in a media devoid of Ca2+ ions than they did in a medium containing 2 mM Ca2+ ions, reaching almost 100% confluence in the latter. Furthermore, Verapamil's ability to prevent the entry of Ca2+ ions from the outside world via voltage-gated calcium channels resulted in a significant reduction in cell proliferation in MDA-MB-231 breast cancer cells [23]. Cell cytoskeletal dynamics, protease activity, cellular volume, and pH are all controlled by intracellular calcium concentration, making it an important factor in cancer cell metastasis [52–54]. Epithelial–mesenchymal transition (EMT) pathways and matrix metalloproteinase activity are both influenced by calcium, making the extracellular matrix (ECM) more degradable and facilitating cell invasion. In addition, different types of cancer have diverse regulatory patterns for several TRP channels. Certain breast and ovarian malignancies, as well as cancers of the liver, stomach, and brain (TRPC6), show high levels of TRPC3 expression [55]. The TRPC1-mediated Ca2+ entry and related signaling were shown to imitate proliferation through activation of the Pl3K/Akt and MAPK downstream pathways in non-small-cell lung malignancy cells [56]. Ca2+ activity is increased to mimic apoptosis through many TRP channels, including TRPC1 [57], TRPC3 [58], TRPC6 [59], TRPM2 [60–62], and TRPM8 [63]. An increase in TRPC6-mediated calcium influx has been seen in human glioblastoma multiforme (GBM) and GBM-derived cell lines were also observed to disrupt the Notch pathway, resulting in tumorigenesis [64]. Cancer cell adhesion and migration are both regulated by the Rho signaling system, of which TRPV4 is an essential regulator [65, 66].

9.5.3 Sodium channels

When used properly, Na^+ flow may have an indirect effect on cancer cell metastasis and the metastatic phenotype. For example, fluctuations in Na+ flow may cause localized zones of depolarization, which in turn may induce the migration of Ca^{2+} and H^+ ions. Researchers have demonstrated that the functioning of Na^+/Ca^{2+} exchangers located in the plasma membrane of cells is also associated with increased ECM breakdown and cell invasion using MDA-MB-231 breast cancer cells that promote a voltage-gated sodium channel (VGSC) [67]. Additional transcriptional mechanisms by which NaV1.7 expression promotes cellular invasion include signaling via epithelial growth factor (EGF) and EGF receptor kinases (ERK1/2) [68]. The activation of the MAPK and the extracellular signal-regulated ERK1/2 pathway is associated with depolarization generated by NaV1.5 activity and results in the production of genes involved in invasion in colon cancer cells [69, 70]. A genetic network that controls the invasion of colon cancer has been discovered to be controlled by the sodium channel SCN5A [70]. It has been shown that the activation of certain sodium channels in prostate and breast cancer cell lines may mimic the production of other sodium channels. Cells may dramatically boost ion flow by forming a helpful response loop in which channel activation stimulates channel expression [71]. Last but not least, shifts in cellular pH may be caused by variations in intracellular Na^+ concentration. Cell adhesion is regulated by integrin-mediated focal adhesion contacts, and it is well established that a change in the pH of the tumor microenvironment affects these contacts [72–74].

9.5.4 Intracellular potassium channels

Keeping a cell at its resting potential requires K^+ ions to mostly migrate from the inside of the cell to the outside. Since K^+ promotes Ca^{2+} entrance into the cell, it has an indirect effect on the V_{mem}. K^+ flow is regulated by voltage-gated potassium channels [75–79], which are also critical for tumor cell growth. KV10.1 [80], KV11.1 (HERG) [81], or both channels are expressed by a wide range of tumor cells. One hundred percent of cervical cancer biopsies tested positive for the expression of the K^+ channel EAG, and it has been shown that human cells overexpressing EAG stimulate cell growth *in vitro* [82]. Cell migration mediated by cadherin-11 and MAPK signaling has also been shown to be driven by K^+ channel overexpression in breast cancer cells. KCa3.1, a calcium-dependent K^+ channel, was shown to facilitate cell division by direct interaction with the extracellular signaling kinases ERK1/2 and JNK. Finally, KCa1.1 and other Ca^{2+}-sensitive K^+ channels were shown to be involved in migration in part because Ca^{2+} flow via TRPM8 controls their activation [83, 84]. By initiating the AKT glycogen synthase kinase-3 β (GSK-3β) signaling pathway, TRPM8 overexpression in breast cancer cells boosted their metastatic capacity [85].

9.5.5 Chloride channels

It is common for chloride to travel with more positively charged cations such as calcium, sodium, and potassium. Because chloride channels are responsible for maintaining cell volume, they play a significant role in cancer cell migration [86]. Cell line investigations of gliomas have shown a function for Cl^- channels in glioblastomas [87, 88]. Chloride channels have been demonstrated to regulate cell size and proliferation in human prostate cancer cell lines [89]. Through controlling cell volume, the chloride ion channel-4 Cl^-/H^+ exchanger has been reported to promote glioma and colon cancer cell motility, invasion, and metastasis. Reducing

ClC-3 by genetic knockdown has been shown to significantly slow glioma cell motility [90].

9.5.6 Piezoelectric channels

Various mechanical stimuli, including compression, stretching, membrane tension, and suction, have the potential to imitate the gating mechanism of piezo channels. These channels, known for their nonselective permeability to calcium ions (Ca^{2+}), may be influenced by the aforementioned mechanical forces acting on the plasma membrane. [91–93]. Piezo channels, as shown in recent research, share a high degree of voltage sensitivity with other voltage-gated ion channels [94]. Piezo1 and Piezo2 are two key piezo channels found to be expressed predominantly in particular tissues. Certain malignancies, such as breast, stomach, and bladder tumors, have been linked to an increase in piezo channel expression, whereas others have been linked to a decrease. Numerous *in vitro* and *in vivo* investigations have shown that Piezo channel activation may generate a Ca^{2+} influx, thus influencing important mechanisms associated with the migration, proliferation, and angiogenesis of cancer cells are reliant on the presence of Ca^{2+} [95]. Researchers have shown that Piezo1 overexpression promotes prostate cancer growth by activating the Akt/mTOR pathway [96]. Piezo2's mechanism of action also involves an increase in Wnt11 expression that is mediated by Ca^{2+} or through β-catenin-dependent signaling [97].

9.6 The detection of bioelectric characteristics

In measuring the electrophysiological characteristics of a single cell, microelectrodes are by far the most powerful instrument currently available. In subcutaneous tumors grown in a study, glass microelectrodes were used to measure intratumor potentials in a murine cancer cell line known as 4T1, which is characterized by its triple-negative phenotype [98]. Nevertheless, because of their tiny size, such electrodes are limited in their ability to assess multicellular area and volume. In addition, the material being studied must be maintained completely still [99, 100]. Recent advances in the form of fluorescent bioelectricity reporters have made it possible to assess electrophysiological qualities without resorting to the use of microelectrodes in situations where this would otherwise be impossible. Subcellular resolution, multiplexed *in vivo* cell measurements, and long-term bioelectric gradient tracking are all possible with the help of these dyes, which are stable and unaffected by cell migration or division. Using voltage-sensitive fluorescent dyes, Chernet and Levin were able to noninvasively identify regions of depolarization in *Xenopus* tumor formations generated by oncogenes [25]. Ion-selective extracellular electrode probes with high sensitivity [101, 102] have been developed to detect the flux of ions at the cell membrane. In addition, reporter proteins [103–106] and techniques capable of reporting the contents of specific ion species, such as protons [107] and sodium [108], are employed as tools for characterizing bioelectrical events [109]. The detection of electromagnetic fields, ionic concentrations, and biological indicators is possible through the use of bioelectronic sensors, commonly known as biosensors [110–114]. Recordings of single cells or populations of cells may be taken either intracellularly or extracellularly, depending on the kind of sensor used. The organic electromechanical transistor (OECT) is widely used as a transistor biosensor device in extracellular recordings because of its high sensitivity to ion species and exterior electric fields. Polystyrene sulfonate (PEDOT: PSS) is commonly acknowledged to be a typical material used in OECTs. Its effectiveness in capturing electrochemical gradients has been shown in several cell types, including both nonexcitable cells (such as Caco-2) and excitable cells [115]. Silicon nanowires are often utilized for intracellular readings because they can traverse the cell membrane without being damaged. The electrical characteristics of these nanowires may be produced and manipulated. Thus, by manipulating the doping levels, a nanoscale field effect transistor (NFET) may be built on a single nanowire. Single cells or even 3D cellular networks may be sensed and recorded in a confined manner using NFETs because of their tunability. Because of their three-dimensional probe presentation, NFETs can circumvent a significant shortcoming of conventional nanoelectronic devices, which are typically designed on a flat, two-dimensional plane. Tian *et al* employed 3D NFETs as targeted probes to take measurements inside cardiomyocytes [116]. Although these techniques are useful for gauging the electrical characteristics of cells, manipulating such qualities is necessary for investigating how state changes affect them.

9.7 Bioelectrical modifications

Bioactuators are devices used for the manipulation of cellular activity that is achieved through the targeted delivery of biophysical signals. Researchers have successfully created biocompatible piezoelectric substances and nanoparticles that can directly interact with cells to alter their resting potential [117–119]. According to a study conducted by Warren and Payne [119], the presence of nanoparticles with amine-modified surfaces resulted in significant depolarization in Chinese hamster ovary (CHO) cells and human cervical cancer (HeLa) cells. Conductive polymers provide an additional classification of materials that can induce cellular or tissue growth through the application of electrical impulses [120–122]. These techniques yield conductive nanofibers, conductive hydrogels, and conductive composite scaffolds [123]. To enhance the positive membrane potential of *Escherichia coli* cells, Jayaram *et al* employed conductive polymer microwires made of PEDOT:PSS [117]. In addition, Thorson and Payne showed that PEDOT:PSS microwires may be used to regulate cardiomyocyte action potentials [124]. Hence, conductive polymer microwires provide a noninvasive platform for the precise spatial manipulation of electrical characteristics inside cells. In-depth evaluations of conductive polymers have already been published [123, 125].

As previously indicated, ivermectin therapy is another technique used to manipulate endogenous chloride channels and hence change the transmembrane potential of a subset of cells. To access their chloride channels, ivermectin seeks cells expressing GlyR. GlyR-expressing cells' transmembrane potential may be adjusted by altering the external chloride levels, allowing for the induction or suppression of chloride ion entry and departure. In the event of insufficient chloride concentration in the extracellular environment, chloride ions exit the cell and migrate toward the surrounding medium, increasing the negative charge of the cell's membrane. To examine the impact of this methodology on metastasis and tumors in an *in vivo* setting, frog models were used to manipulate the membrane potential of a specific group of cells that expressed GlyCl channels. The manipulation of cellular bioelectric properties may be achieved by controlling mechanosensitive Ca^{2+}-permeable Piezo channels. These channels play a crucial role in converting mechanical stress into Ca^{2+}-dependent signals. Various mechanical stimuli, such as stiffness, compression, tension, and shear stress, have the potential to induce the activation of Piezo channels. These channels are expressed in the plasma membrane and are regulated by these specific mechanical forces. Upon activation, these channels facilitate the influx of calcium ions (Ca^{2+}) into the cytoplasm, hence contributing to the regulation of cellular polarity. The pharmacological activation of Piezo1 may be achieved using agonists such as Jedi1, Jedi2, and Yoda1 [126]. Pancreatic cancer cells exhibit an increased depolarized state when subjected to mechanical stimulation at a magnitude of 1 μm using a heat-polished glass probe controlled by a piezoelectric device or by the administration of the agonist Yoda1 [127].

9.8 Electrification and extracellular vesicles

MicroRNA and mRNA are two types of nucleic acids that may be transported via EVs and used in intercellular communication [128]. The establishment of planar cell polarity and tissue development relies heavily on EV-mediated communication [129]. As discussed above, EVs are used in the initiation, advancement, and spread of tumors and are especially abundant in the tumor microenvironment [130, 131]. Recent research by Fukuta *et al* showed that extracellular stimuli, such as low-intensity electric field therapy, may trigger intracellular signaling and thereby boost exosome production. EVs from cultivated cells of murine melanoma B16F1 and murine fibroblast 3T3 S have been shown to be secreted at higher rates and to be of higher quality [128]. When taken as a whole, these findings suggest that the increased production of EVs in the cancer tumor microenvironment may be attributable to the bioelectric dysregulation or depolarization of cells that occurs in cancer. At the same time, a feedback loop is formed between the increased generation of EVs and the disruption of bioelectric homeostasis. Cancer's bioelectric dysregulation may be traced back to several different pathways, including alterations in cell state and the creation of EVs, as well as the dependency between these two processes.

9.9 Biosensors for *in vitro* cancer cell assessment

When it comes to improving healthcare, the field of translational medicine is always pushing forward. Biosensors will enable better tumor staging, earlier cancer diagnosis, and the evaluation of a tumor's response to treatment. Thus, it is crucial that such tools achieve widespread clinical implementation. Biosensors are essential in cancer biology [132, 133] for assessing the effectiveness of antiproliferative and cytotoxic medicines and discovering novel aspects of metastatic disease. When an electrochemical biosensor detects a target biological analyte (such as a cell, protein, nucleotide, or metabolite), a transducer converts the detected signal into a proportionate electrical signal that may be analyzed further [134]. Although a vast variety of transducers are available on the market, this chapter concentrates on electrochemical biosensors.

An essential part of every biosensor is a recognition element, which is responsible for picking up the presence of a predetermined molecular constituent in the test sample. A transducer (electrochemical, optical calorimetric, or mass change) is then used to pick up signals that indicate the occurrence of a recognition event; these signals are amplified and processed for analysis [135]. Potentiometric biosensors and amperometric biosensors are both types of electrochemical detection devices. Potentiometric biosensors rely on ion-selective electrodes to detect alterations in electrical potential that occur upon molecular identification. However, amperometric transducers measure the current between electrodes when a voltage is applied. Electrochemiluminescence biosensors, impedance-based sensors, genosensors, and microfluidic platforms have been created for this purpose, along with other forms of biosensors [136, 137]. The benefits of electrochemical sensing methods include low sample costs, high throughput, accuracy, speed, high sensitivity, portability, and simplicity [138, 139]. The authors of these papers have discussed recent progress in the quest to create electrochemical-based sensors that can detect indicators of apoptosis and metastasis in cancer.

The apoptotic pathway utilizes a wide variety of molecular effectors and may be activated by either endogenous or extrinsic signals. Caspase-3 (Cas-3) is regarded as an important mediator because it activates downstream caspases that ultimately result in cell death. In light of this, clinicians can detect Cas-3 using OECTs. In this configuration, a gold nanoparticle-coated modified glassy carbon electrode served as a host for Cas-3 recognition via gold–sulfur bonds. The results showed that after superficial modification using a peptide monolayer, the transistor's transfer curve was shifted to an inferior gate voltage. The biosensor's performance was evaluated by detecting Cas-3 in aqueous solutions; the findings demonstrated more sensitivity and a detection limit of 0.1 pM. Furthermore, in HeLa cells, the proposed sensor was able to accurately detect ten apoptotic cells per 10 l [140].

The researchers in a study conducted by Deng and colleagues [141] assessed the activity of Cas-3 in HeLa cervical cancer (HCC) cells. This measurement was performed utilizing an electrochemical sensing platform. In this study, electrodes modified with graphene oxide (GO) were used as bioreceptors and subjected to functionalization using a peptide substrate specific to Cas-3. The electrocatalytic characteristics shown by the ATCUN Cu (II) complex are very advantageous in enhancing and accelerating electrochemical signals. The maximum electrical current was seen when the treatment sequence consisted of 5 M staurosporine, followed by doxorubicin, cisplatin, and vitamin C. It was observed that when the concentration of Cas-3 increased, there was a corresponding increase in the current. This relationship was quantified within a measured concentration range of 0.5 pg ml^{-1} to 2 ng ml^{-1} [142].

An additional element of detection serves as the first phase in the series of intrinsic apoptotic pathways. Shamsipur *et al* used EIS to create aptasensors that were capable of detecting Cyt-c. This was achieved by the conjugation of gold nanoclusters (Au-Cys-ssDNA@AgNCs) [143]. The increased surface density of the aptamer units was attributed to the incorporation of AgNCs, which served as the active biosensing layer. This integration led to an increased surface-to-volume ratio and thus enhanced the sensitivity of the device's recognition moieties. It is noteworthy to mention that EIS does not need additional labeling of redox-active moieties, rendering it one of the most efficient *in situ* electrochemical analytical techniques in terms of time and labor. Furthermore, aptamers, i.e. synthetic oligonucleotide sequences, have shown enhanced stability in bioanalytical investigations compared to other biorecognition entities, such as antibodies and oligopeptides.

Zhou and colleagues used a dual-signal electrochemical immunosensor to test nilotinib's ability to induce apoptosis in chronic myeloid leukemia K562-treated cells [144]. After an acid rinse, the sandwiched electrochemical immunosensor released Ag^+ and Cd^{2+} ions for anodic stripping voltammetry. The antigens bound to the electrodes were measured using a voltammetric signal. The proposed biosensor detected cells at lower concentrations than existing methods [144].

Li and colleagues established an antibody-based microfluidic microchannel system to measure Survivin (Sur) mRNA levels [145]. Target moiety studies have focused on protein products. Microchannel cytosensors with attached cognate monoclonal antibodies may capture prostate cancer cells by recognizing prostate stem cell antigen (PSCA). Later, an anti-survivin oligonucleotide sensor-tagged graphene oxide nanocarrier was used to detect intracellular Sur mRNA. The addition of fluorescein isothiocyanate labeling transformed the nanosensor into a signal nanoprobe sensitive to 106 copies/cell. It was also revealed that CTCs express survivin. As a result, CTC analysis offers an alternative to invasive biopsy for detecting cancer's spread and recurrence [145].

The physical features of CTCs, as opposed to any kind of biological affinity, were used to create yet another label-free microdevice. The size and flexibility of CTCs are thought to be greater than those of red blood cells. Lung, breast, and colon cancer patients may have their surviving cancer cells extracted from their blood using this method [146]. Nagrath and colleagues' novel approach included creating a 'CTC chip' that used anti-EpCAM-coated microspots to accomplish affinity-based separation of live CTCs in a laminar flow environment. It was stated that the device's selectivity and sensitivity were on par with those of immunomagnetic beads [147]. It is important to note that CTC-derived *ex-vivo* cultures are crucial for determining the function of CTCs in metastasis and for learning the biology of CTCs; both of these are required to develop a method for individualized cancer treatment testing and disease monitoring [148].

Xu and colleagues developed an impedimetric immunosensor to detect EpCAM, a metastasis-related transmembrane protein [79]. Gold electrodes functionalized with poly(amidoamine) dendrimer (G6-PAMAM) and EpCAM biosensing antibodies served as the assembly layer. Voltammetry and EIS allowed for precise quantification of the electrochemical signal produced upon specific antibody binding to EpCAM antigen. The limit of detection was determined to be 2.1 103 cells ml^{-1} in a biological application utilizing Hep-G2 hepatic cancer cells [79].

Further biosensing research presented by Valverde and colleagues [80] described the electrochemical diagnosis of colon cancer metastases using a new immunosensor to amperometrically monitor secreted IL-13R2. The immunosensor's components included antibody-modified magnetic microbeads (MBs) and biotinylated detecting antibodies, which were used for the selective capture of IL-13R2 (BDAb). Amperometric tests relied on an (H_2O_2)/hydroquinone (HQ) system that was magnetically ladened onto disposable screen-printed carbon electrodes (SPCEs) to detect the affinity response. The expression of IL-13R2 was measured in real time using the developed immunosensor in both lysed and intact colon cancer cells. The developed immunosensor was shown to be very sensitive, being quicker than ELISA, and conserving more material than Western blot. The authors of this paper concluded that this biosensor type may be used to evaluate a cell's ability to metastasize [80].

Electrochemical biosensors have been used to monitor and study both apoptosis and metastasis. For instance, Majidi and colleagues [17] demonstrated that an aptasensor could be built to identify L-tryptophan (Trp) using a current–potentiometric stripping investigation. An increase in Trp metabolism is associated with the presence of cancer cells that have already begun to metastasize, which serves to depress the immune system and further facilitates the spread of the disease. The L-tryptophan aptamer was connected to multiwalled carbon nanotubes (MWCNTs) that had been glued to a gold electrode. The aptasensor's LOD of 6.41 011 M demonstrated its sensitivity. In addition, the rate of Trp consumption was used to effectively differentiate between cancer cell lines with different metastatic potentials [17].

In contrast, biosensing the expression of trypsin in cell lysate, which varies in instances of pancreatic cancer, was used to monitor the spread of pancreatic tumor cells electrochemically [81]. Trypsin has an important role in controlling the invasion and metastasis of pancreatic cancer. Hence, NeutrAvidin-MBS was biotin-linked to a synthetic peptide chain to create the biosensor. Fluorescein isothiocyanate (FITC) was added at the end of this peptide chain. The procedures used to develop the biosensor were employed in the reported instance [81]. When a high concentration of trypsin was present, as found in malignant pancreatic cells, the attached FITC was cleaved off, resulting in a reduced amperometric response. Another study [37] devised alternative electrochemical biosensing. This biosensor worked by capturing target proteins on carboxylic MBs modified with antibodies and then labeling them enzymatically using antibodies tagged with horseradish peroxidase (HRP) [37].

Nano- or microsensor chips located on cell culture flasks can provide electrochemical cell activity measurement during cultivation and growth [19]. Electrochemical chip-based cancer biosensing devices may be useful for tracking cancer growth and therapy efficacy. In addition, cellular respiration under varied incubation conditions has been screened using amperometric oxygen sensors. Moreover, potentiometric pH sensors based on electrodeposited iridium oxide sheets have been used to measure cellular acidification. Electrochemical monitoring systems for 3D cell culture may be built on top of this technology [82]. Biocompatible, performant, flexible chips that are new useful polymeric platforms for cell binding and growth and nanostructured biomaterials that can be used for nano- and microfabrication processes will be the focus of future approaches for cancer electrochemical sensors' designs. Nevertheless, sensing devices integrated into 2D cultures and 3D scaffolds may be used to improve our microscale knowledge of the cell culture microenvironment and to enable future advanced organ-on-a-chip research [18].

9.10 Conclusions

Research into bioelectric signaling is expanding, bringing us closer to an understanding of the whole spectrum of cancer as a disease. According to the somatic mutation hypothesis, much of the biology of cancer has been elucidated.

The importance of EVs in aiding the signaling pathways involved in all stages of carcinogenesis is well recognized. In this chapter, we surveyed what is known to date regarding the bioelectric dysregulation that underpins several cancer processes. Nonetheless, the extent to which these two systems are dependent on one another is poorly understood. Finally, exosomes in particular have been shown to have a function in cancer therapeutics. Normal eukaryotic development relies on apoptosis because it aids in cell and tissue regeneration, aids in the phagocytosis-mediated elimination of unwanted cells, and protects against inappropriate immunological responses. Several investigations (functional, biochemical, and morphological examinations) have been carried out to fully comprehend both metastasis and apoptosis. Nonetheless, more progress is still required in characterizing and analyzing the processes of apoptosis and metastasis. In light of this, this chapter reviewed several biophysical and bioelectrochemical techniques (including cyclic voltammetry and electron microscopy approaches) that have been used to study metastasis and apoptosis. It is important to note, however, that no single approach can provide all the answers, since each approach focuses on distinct aspects of the biological process being studied. Hence, a multiparameter observational strategy should be the most helpful, and this may be developed by combining ideas and procedures relevant to cellular biophysics into standard experimental paradigms. Focusing on cancer biology, this interdisciplinary strategy would bring together the study of atomic force microscopy (AFM) and the mechanobiological features of live cells. In addition, the integration of high-resolution imaging methods, such as AFM and scanning electron microscopy (SEM), which can provide lateral nanoscale information, may aid in distinguishing between benign and malignant morphologies. Finally, the advancement of electrochemical analytical procedures will allow for the creation of sensitive biosensors designed for the accurate measurement of targeted cancer biomarkers. Cancer biologists and biophysicists need to work together to solve experimental issues and glean the most physiologically relevant insights possible.

References and further reading

[1] Hanahan D and Weinberg R A 2011 Hallmarks of cancer: the next generation *Cell* **144** 646–74

[2] Mally A and Chipman J 2002 Non-genotoxic liver carcinogens: early effects on gap junctions, cell proliferation and apoptosis in the rat *Toxicology* **178** 45
[3] Versteeg R 2014 Tumours outside the mutation box *Nature* **506** 438–9
[4] Sonnenschein C and Soto A M 2008 Theories of carcinogenesis: an emerging perspective *Semin. Cancer Biol.* **18** 372–7
[5] Wortzel I, Dror S, Kenific C M and Lyden D 2019 Exosome-mediated metastasis: *communication from a distance Dev. Cell* **49** 347–60
[6] Arafa K K, Ibrahim A, Mergawy R, El-Sherbiny I M, Febbraio F and Hassan R Y A 2022 Advances in cancer diagnosis: bio-electrochemical and biophysical characterizations of cancer cells *Micromachines* **13** 1401
[7] Lobikin M, Chernet B, Lobo D and Levin M 2012 Resting potential, oncogene-induced tumorigenesis, and metastasis: the bioelectric basis of cancer *in vivo Phys. Biol.* **9** 065002
[8] Funk R H 2015 Endogenous electric fields as guiding cue for cell migration *Front. Physiol.* **6** 143
[9] Silver B B and Nelson C M 2018 The bioelectric code: reprogramming cancer and aging from the interface of mechanical and chemical microenvironments *Front. Cell Dev. Biol.* **6** 21
[10] Simanov D, Mellaart-Straver I, Sormacheva I and Berezikov E 2012 The flatworm macrostomum lignano is a powerful model organism for ion channel and stem cell research *Stem Cells Int.* **2012** 167265
[11] Sundelacruz S, Levin M and Kaplan D L 2009 Role of membrane potential in the regulation of cell proliferation and differentiation *Stem Cell Rev. Rep.* **5** 231–46
[12] Blackiston D J, McLaughlin K A and Levin M 2009 Bioelectric controls of cell proliferation: ion channels, membrane voltage and the cell cycle *Cell Cycle* **8** 3527–36
[13] Levin M, Selberg J and Rolandi M 2019 Endogenous bioelectrics in development, cancer, and regeneration: *drugs and bioelectronic devices as electroceuticals for regenerative medicine iScience* **22** 519–33
[14] Al Ahmad M, Al Natour Z, Mustafa F and Rizvi T 2018 Electrical characterization of normal and cancer cells *IEEE Access* **1** 25979–86
[15] Levin M 2014 Molecular bioelectricity: how endogenous voltage potentials control cell behavior and instruct pattern regulation *in vivo Mol. Biol. Cell* **25** 3835–50
[16] Bellassai N, D'Agata R, Jungbluth V and Spoto G 2019 Surface plasmon resonance for biomarker detection: advances in non-invasive cancer diagnosis *Front. Chem.* **7** 570
[17] Majidi M R, Karami P, Johari-Ahar M and Omidi Y 2016 Direct detection of tryptophan for rapid diagnosis of cancer cell metastasis competence by an ultra-sensitive and highly selective electrochemical biosensor *Anal. Methods* **8** 7910–9
[18] Zhou H, Du X and Zhang Z 2021 Electrochemical sensors for detection of markers on tumor cells *Int. J. Mol. Sci.* **22** 8184
[19] Kieninger J, Tamari Y, Enderle B, Jobst G, Sandvik J A, Pettersen E O and Urban G A 2018 Sensor access to the cellular microenvironment using the sensing cell culture flask *Biosensors* **8** 44
[20] Kim H, Kim K, Yu S J, Jang E S, Yu J, Cho G, Yoon J H and Kim Y 2013 Development of biomarkers for screening hepatocellular carcinoma using global data mining and multiple reaction monitoring *PLoS One* **8** 63468
[21] Ilie M, Hofman V, Long E, Bordone O, Selva E, Washetine K, Marquette C H and Hofman P 2014 Current challenges for detection of circulating tumor cells and cell-free circulating nucleic acids, and their characterization in non-small cell lung carcinoma patients. What is the best blood substrate for personalized medicine *Ann. Transl. Med.* **2** 11

[22] Taylor J T, Huang L, Pottle J E, Pottle K, Yang Y and Zeng X 2008 Selective blockade of T-type Ca2+ channels suppresses human breast cancer cell proliferation *Cancer Lett.* **267** 116–2.0000004

[23] Berzingi S, Newman M and Yu H G 2016 Altering bioelectricity on inhibition of human breast cancer cells *Cancer Cell Int.* **16** 72

[24] Guéguinou M, Harnois T, Crottes D, Uguen A, Deliot N and Gambade M 2016 SK3/TRPC1/orai1 complex regulates SOCE-dependent colon cancer cell migration: a novel opportunity to modulate Anti-EGFR mAb action by the alkyl-lipid ohmline *Oncotarget* **7** 36168–84

[25] Chernet B and Levin M 2013 Endogenous voltage potentials and the microenvironment: bioelectric signals that reveal, induce and normalize cancer *J. Clin. Exp. Oncol. Suppl.* **1** S1–002

[26] Arcangeli A, Crociani O, Lastraioli E, Masi A, Pillozzi S and Becchetti A 2009 Targeting ion channels in cancer: *a novel frontier in antineoplastic therapy Curr. Med. Chem.* **16** 66–93

[27] Jiang L H, Adinolfi E and Roger S 2021 Editorial: ion channel signalling in cancer: *from molecular mechanisms to therapeutics Front. Pharmacol.* **12** 711593

[28] Lang F and Stournaras C 2014 Ion channels in cancer: future perspectives and clinical potential *Philos. Trans. R Soc. Lond. B Biol. Sci.* **369** 1638

[29] Litan A and Langhans S A 2015 Cancer as a channelopathy: ion channels and pumps in tumor development and progression *Front. Cell Neurosci.* **9** 86

[30] Prevarskaya N, Skryma R and Shuba Y 2018 Ion channels in cancer: are cancer hallmarks oncochannelopathies? *Physiol. Rev.* **98** 559–621

[31] Dhillon A S, Hagan S, Rath O and Kolch W 2007 MAP kinase signalling pathways in cancer *Oncogene* **26** 3279–90

[32] Belicky S, Černocká H, Bertok T, Holazova A, Réblová K, Paleček E, Tkac J and Ostatná V 2017 Label-free chronopotentiometry glycoprofiling of prostate-specific antigen using sialic acid recognizing lectins *Bioelectrochemistry* **117** 89–94

[33] Su Kim D, Choi Y D, Moon M, Kang S, Lim J B, Kim K M, Park K M and Cho N H 2013 Composite three-marker assay for early detection of kidney cancer *Cancer Epidemiol. Biomarkers Prev.* **22** 390–8

[34] Kroeze S G, Bijenhof A M, Bosch J L and Jans J J 2010 Diagnostic and prognostic tissuemarkers in clear cell and papillary renal cell carcinoma *Cancer Biomarkers* **7** 261–8

[35] Wehland M, Bauer J, Magnusson N E, Infanger M and Grimm D 2013 Biomarkers for anti-angiogenic therapy in cancer *Int. J. Mol. Sci.* **14** 9338–64

[36] Javanbakht M, Khoshsafar H, Ganjali M R, Badiei A, Norouzi P and Hasheminasab A 2009 Determination of nanomolar mercury (II) concentration by anodic-stripping voltammetry at a carbon paste electrode modified with functionalized nanoporous silica gel *Curr. Anal. Chem.* **5** 35–41

[37] Muñoz-San Martín C, Gamella M, Pedrero M, Montero-Calle A, Pérez-Ginés V, Camps J, Arenas M, Barderas R, Pingarrón J M and Campuzano S 2022 Anticipating metastasis through electrochemical immunosensing of tumor hypoxia biomarkers *Anal. Bioanal. Chem.* **1** 1–4

[38] Thiery J P 2002 Epithelial–mesenchymal transitions in tumour progression *Nat. Rev. Cancer* **2** 442–54

[39] Prevarskaya N, Skryma R and Shuba Y 2010 Ion channels and the hallmarks of cancer *Trends Mol. Med.* **16** 107–21

[40] Pardo L A, Contreras-Jurado C, Zientkowska M, Alves F and Stühmer W 2005 Role of Voltage-gated potassium channels in cancer *J. Membr. Biol.* **205** 115–24
[41] Kunzelmann K 2005 Ion channels and cancer *J. Membr. Biol.* **205** 159–73
[42] Kari S, Subramanian K, Altomonte I A, Murugesan A, Yli-Harja O and Kandhavelu M 2022 Programmed cell death detection methods: a systematic review and a categorical comparison *Apoptosis* **27** 482–508
[43] Gonzalez D M and Medici D 2014 Signaling mechanisms of the epithelial-mesenchymal transition *Sci. Signal.* **7** re8–8
[44] Wahl R L, Jacene H, Kasamon Y and Lodge M A 2009 From RECIST to PERCIST: evolving considerations for PET response criteria in solid tumors *J. Nucl. Med.* **50** 122S–50S
[45] Xie Q Z, Lin M W, Hsu W E and Lin C T 2020 Advancements of nanoscale structures and materials in impedimetric biosensing technologies *ECS J. Solid State Sci. Technol.* **9** 115027
[46] Lin D *et al* 2021 Circulating tumor cells: *biology and clinical significance Signal Transduct. Targeted Ther.* **6** 404
[47] Vasantharajan S S, Eccles M R, Rodger E J, Pattison S, McCall J L, Gray E S, Calapre L and Chatterjee A 2021 The epigenetic landscape of circulating tumor cells *Biochim. Biophys. Acta (BBA)-Rev. Cancer* **1875** 188514
[48] Radfar P, Es H A, Salomon R, Kulasinghe A, Ramalingam N, Sarafraz-Yazdi E, Thiery J P and Warkiani M E 2022 Single-cell analysis of circulating tumour cells: *enabling technologies and clinical applications Trends Biotechnol.* **40** 1041–60
[49] Levin M 2009 Bioelectric mechanisms in regeneration: unique aspects and future perspectives *Semin. Cell Dev. Biol.* **20** 543–56
[50] Rajnicek A M, Foubister L E and McCaig C D 2006 Growth cone steering by a physiological electric field requires dynamic microtubules, microfilaments and rac-mediated filopodial asymmetry *J. Cell Sci.*. **119** 1736–45
[51] Becchetti A 2011 Ion channels and transporters in cancer. 1. ion channels and cell proliferation in cancer *Am. J. Physiol. Cell Physiol.* **301** C255–265
[52] Postovit L M, Margaryan N V, Seftor E A, Kirschmann D A, Lipavsky A, Wheaton W W, Abbott D E, Seftor R E and Hendrix M J 2008 Human embryonic stem cell microenvironment suppresses the tumorigenic phenotype of aggressive cancer cells *Proc. Natl Acad. Sci.* **105** 4329–34
[53] Giancotti F G 2013 Mechanisms governing metastatic dormancy and reactivation *Cell* **155** 750–64
[54] Chou J, Lin J H, Brenot A, Kim J W, Provot S and Werb Z 2013 GATA3 suppresses metastasis and modulates the tumour microenvironment by regulating microRNA-29b expression *Nat. Cell Biol.* **15** 201–13
[55] Byers L A *et al* 2013 An epithelial–mesenchymal transition gene signature predicts resistance to EGFR and PI3K inhibitors and identifies Axl as a therapeutic target for overcoming EGFR inhibitor resistance *Clin. Cancer Res.* **19** 279–90
[56] Zhang Z *et al* 2012 Activation of the AXL kinase causes resistance to EGFR-targeted therapy in lung cancer *Nat. Genet.* **44** 852–60
[57] Radisky D C and LaBarge M A 2008 Epithelial-mesenchymal transition and the stem cell phenotype *Cell Stem Cell* **2** 511–2
[58] Ambasta R K, Sharma A and Kumar P 2011 Nanoparticle mediated targeting of VEGFR and cancer stem cells for cancer therapy *Vasc. Cell* **3** 3–9

[59] Marjanovic N D, Weinberg R A and Chaffer C L 2013 Cell plasticity and heterogeneity in cancer *Clin. Chem.* **59** 168–79
[60] Lou H and Dean M 2007 Targeted therapy for cancer stem cells: the patched pathway and ABC transporters *Oncogene* **26** 1357–60
[61] Morrison R, Schleicher S M, Sun Y, Niermann K J, Kim S, Spratt D E, Chung C H and Lu B 2011 Targeting the mechanisms of resistance to chemotherapy and radiotherapy with the cancer stem cell hypothesis *J. Oncol.* **2011**
[62] Vinogradov S and Wei X 2012 Cancer stem cells and drug resistance: the potential of nanomedicine *Nanomedicine* **7** 7–615
[63] Kawasaki B T, Hurt E M, Mistree T and Farrar W L 2008 Targeting cancer stem cells with phytochemicals *Mol. Interv.* **8** 174
[64] Gupta P B, Onder T T, Jiang G, Tao K, Kuperwasser C, Weinberg R A and Lander E S 2009 Identification of selective inhibitors of cancer stem cells by high-throughput screening *Cell* **138** 645–59
[65] Zhao Y, Alakhova D Y and Kabanov A V 2013 Can nanomedicines kill cancer stem cells? *Adv. Drug Deliv. Rev.* **65** 1763–83
[66] Baylin S B and Jones P A 2011 A decade of exploring the cancer epigenome—biological and translational implications *Nat. Rev. Cancer* **117** 26–734
[67] Sana J, Faltejskova P, Svoboda M and Slaby O 2012 Novel classes of non-coding RNAs and cancer *J. Transl. Med.* **10** 1–21
[68] Fukushige S and Horii A 2013 DNA methylation in cancer: a gene silencing mechanism and the clinical potential of its biomarkers *Tohoku J. Exp. Med.* **229** 173–85
[69] Jones P A 2012 Functions of DNA methylation: islands, start sites, gene bodies and beyond *Nat. Rev. Genet.* **13** 484–92
[70] Calin G A and Croce C M 2006 MicroRNA signatures in human cancers *Nat. Rev. Cancer* **6** 857–66
[71] Liu S 2012 Epigenetics advancing personalized nanomedicine in cancer therapy *Adv. Drug Deliv. Rev.* **64** 1532–43
[72] Gajewski T F 2011 Molecular profiling of melanoma and the evolution of patient-specific therapy *Semin. Oncol.* **38** 236–42
[73] Nathanson K L 2010 Using genetics and genomics strategies to personalize therapy for cancer: focus on melanoma *Biochem. Pharmacol.* **80** 755–61
[74] Jithesh P V, Risk J M, Schache A G, Dhanda J, Lane B, Liloglou T and Shaw R J 2013 The epigenetic landscape of oral squamous cell carcinoma *Br. J. Cancer* **108** 370–9
[75] Schoenborn J R, Nelson P and Fang M 2013 Genomic profiling defines subtypes of prostate cancer with the potential for therapeutic stratification *Clin. Cancer Res.* **19** 4058–66
[76] Uppal D S and Powell S M 2013 Genetics/genomics/proteomics of gastric adenocarcinoma *Gastroenterol. Clin.* **42** 241–60
[77] Lange C P and Laird P W 2013 Clinical applications of DNA methylation biomarkers in colorectal cancer *Epigenomics* **5** 105–8
[78] Chmelarova M, Dvorakova E, Spacek J, Laco J, Mzik M and Palicka V 2013 Promoter methylation of GATA4, WIF1, NTRK1 and other selected tumor suppressor genes in ovarian cancer *Folia Biol.* **59** 87–92 PMID: 23746174
[79] Xu J, Wang X, Yan C and Chen W 2019 A polyamidoamine dendrimer-based electrochemical immunosensor for label-free determination of epithelial cell adhesion molecule-expressing cancer cells *Sensors* **19** 1879

[80] Valverde A, Povedano E, Montiel V R, Yáñez-Sedeño P, Garranzo-Asensio M, Barderas R, Campuzano S and Pingarrón J M 2018 Electrochemical immunosensor for IL-13 Receptor α2 determination and discrimination of metastatic colon cancer cells *Biosens. Bioelectron.* **117** 766–72

[81] Muñoz-San Martín C, Pedrero M, Gamella M, Montero-Calle A, Barderas R, Campuzano S and Pingarrón J M 2020 A novel peptide-based electrochemical biosensor for the determination of a metastasis-linked protease in pancreatic cancer cells *Anal. Bioanal. Chem.* **412** 6177–88

[82] Oliveira M, Conceição P, Kant K, Ainla A and Diéguez L 2021 Electrochemical sensing in 3D cell culture models: new tools for developing better cancer diagnostics and treatments *Cancers* **13** 1381

[83] Li M, Xi N, Wang Y C and Liu L Q 2021 Atomic force microscopy for revealing micro/nanoscale mechanics in tumor metastasis: from single cells to microenvironmental cues *Acta Pharmacol. Sin.* **42** 323–39

[84] Nasrollahpour H, Naseri A, Rashidi M R and Khalilzadeh B 2021 Application of green synthesized WO3-poly glutamic acid nano biocomposite for early stage biosensing of breast cancer using the electrochemical approach *Sci. Rep.* **11** 23994

[85] Deng X *et al* 2018 Application of atomic force microscopy in cancer research *J. Nanobiotechnol.* **16** 1–5

[86] Deliorman M, Janahi F K, Sukumar P, Glia A, Alnemari R, Fadl S, Chen W and Qasaimeh M A 2020 AFM-compatible microfluidic platform for affinity-based capture and nanomechanical characterization of circulating tumor cells *Microsyst. Nanoeng.* **6** 20

[87] Park S 2016 Nano-mechanical phenotype as a promising biomarker to evaluate cancer development, progression, and anti-cancer drug efficacy *J. Cancer Prev.* **21** 73–80

[88] Guerrero C R, Garcia P D and Garcia R 2019 subsurface imaging of cell organelles by force microscopy *ACS Nano* **13** 9629–37

[89] Efremov Y M, Suter D M, Timashev P S and Raman A 2022 3D nanomechanical mapping of subcellular and sub-nuclear structures of living cells by multi-harmonic AFM with long-tip microcantilevers *Sci. Rep.* **12** 529

[90] Hessler J A, Budor A, Putchakayala K, Mecke A, Rieger D, Banaszak Holl M M, Orr B G, Bielinska A, Beals J and Baker J 2005 Atomic force microscopy study of early morphological changes during apoptosis *Langmuir ACS J. Surf. Colloids* **21** 9280–6

[91] Park J, Kravchuk , Prishnaprasad A, Roy T and Kang E H 2022 graphene enhances actin filament assembly kinetics and modulates NIH-3T3 fibroblast cell spreading *Int. J. Mol. Sci.* **23** 509

[92] Rother J, Nöding H, Mey I and Janshoff A 2014 Atomic force microscopy-based microrheology reveals significant differences in the viscoelastic response between malign and benign cell lines *Open Biol.* **4** 140046

[93] Kogure A, Yoshioka Y and Ochiya T 2020 Extracellular vesicles in cancer metastasis: potential as therapeutic targets and materials *Int. J. Mol. Sci.* **21** 4463

[94] Sharma S, Das K, Woo J and Gimzewski J K 2014 Nanofilaments on glioblastoma exosomes revealed by peak force microscopy *J. R. Soc. Interface* **11** 2013115

[95] Liu L, Zhang S X, Liao W, Farhood H P, Wong C W, Chen c c, Ségaliny A I, Chacko J V, Nguyen L P and Lu M 2017 Mechanoresponsive stem cells to target cancer metastases through biophysical cues *Sci. Transl. Med.* **9** eaan2966

[96] Moscetti I, Cannistraro S and Bizzarri A R 2019 Probing direct interaction of oncomiR-21-3p with the tumor suppressor p53 by fluorescence, FRET and atomic force spectroscopy *Arch. Biochem. Biophys.* **671** 35–41

[97] Kanno S, Hirano S, Kato H, Fukuta M, Mukai T and Aoki Y 2020 Benzalkonium chloride and cetylpyridinium chloride induce apoptosis in human lung epithelial cells and alter the surface activity of pulmonary surfactant monolayers *Chem.-Biol. Interact.* **317** 108962

[98] Li C, Teixeira A F, Zhu H J and Ten Dijke P 2021 Cancer associated-fibroblastderived exosomes in cancer progression *Mol. Cancer* **20** 154

[99] Maia J, Caja S, Strano Moraes M C, Couto N and Costa-Silva B 2018 Exosome-based cell-cell communication in the tumor microenvironment *Front. Cell Dev. Biol.* **6** 18

[100] Wu Q, Zhou L, Lv D, Zhu X and Tang H 2019 Exosome-mediated communication in the tumor microenvironment contributes to hepatocellular carcinoma development and progression *J. Hematol. Oncol.* **12** 53

[101] Smith D S, Humphrey P A and Catalona W J 1997 The early detection of prostate carcinoma with prostate specific antigen: The Washington University experience *Cancer* **80** 1852–6

[102] Reid B, Nuccitelli R and Zhao M 2007 Non-invasive measurement of bioelectric currents with a vibrating probe *Nat. Protoc.* **2** 661–9

[103] Baker B J, Mutoh H, Dimitrov D, Akemann W, Perron A and Iwamoto Y 2008 Genetically encoded fluorescent sensors of membrane potential *Brain Cell Biol.* **36** 53–67

[104] Mutoh H, Perron A, Akemann W, Iwamoto Y and Knöpfel T 2011 Optogenetic monitoring of membrane potentials *Exp. Physiol.* **96** 13–8

[105] Shen B, Xiang Z, Miller B, Louie G, Wang W and Noel J P 2011 Genetically Encoding unnatural amino acids in neural stem cells and optically reporting voltage-sensitive domain changes in differentiated neurons *Stem Cells* **29** 1231–40

[106] Tsutsui H, Karasawa S, Okamura Y and Miyawaki A 2008 Improving membrane voltage measurements using FRET with new fluorescent proteins *Nat. Methods* **5** 683–5

[107] Tantama M, Hung Y P and Yellen G 2011 Imaging intracellular pH in live cells with a genetically encoded red fluorescent protein sensor *J. Am. Chem. Soc.* **133** 10034–7

[108] Simon D T, Gabrielsson E O, Tybrandt K and Berggren M 2016 Organic bioelectronics: bridging the signaling gap between biology and technology *Chem. Rev.* **116** 13009–41

[109] Tseng A S, Beane W S, Lemire J M, Masi A and Levin M 2010 Induction of vertebrate regeneration by a transient sodium current *J. Neurosci.* **30** 13192–200

[110] Fang Y, Li X and Fang Y 2015 Organic bioelectronics for neural interfaces *J. Mater. Chem.* **3** 6424–30

[111] Löffler S, Melican K, Nilsson K P R and Richter-Dahlfors A 2017 Organic bioelectronics in medicine *J. Intern. Med.* **282** 24–36

[112] Rivnay J, Owens R M and Malliaras G G 2014 The rise of organic bioelectronics *Chem. Mater.* **26** 679–85

[113] Someya T, Bao Z and Malliaras G G 2016 The rise of plastic bioelectronics *Nature* **540** 379–85

[114] Tian B, Xu S, Rogers J A, Cestellos-Blanco S, Yang P and Carvalho-de-Souza J L 2018 Roadmap on semiconductor-cell biointerfaces *Phys. Biol.* **15** 031002

[115] Strakosas X, Bongo M and Owens R M 2015 the organic electrochemical transistor for biological applications *J. Appl. Polym. Sci.*` **132** 41735

[116] Tian B, Cohen-Karni T, Qing Q, Duan X, Xie P and Lieber C M 2010 Three-dimensional, flexible nanoscale field-effect transistors as localized bioprobes *Science* **329** 830–4
[117] Jayaram D T, Luo Q, Thourson S B, Finlay A H and Payne C K 2017 Controlling the resting membrane potential of cells with conducting polymer microwires *Small* **13** 10.1002
[118] Rana M A, Yao N, Mukhopadhyay S, Zhang F, Warren E and Payne C 2016 Modeling the effect of nanoparticles & the bistability of transmembrane potential in non-excitable cells *2016 American Control Conf. (Boston, MA)* (Piscataway, NJ: IEEE) 400–5
[119] Warren E A and Payne C K 2015 Cellular binding of nanoparticles disrupts the membrane potential *RSC Adv.* **5** 13660–6
[120] Liu X, Gilmore K J, Moulton S E and Wallace G G 2009 Electrical stimulation promotes nerve cell differentiation on polypyrrole/poly (2-methoxy-5 aniline sulfonic acid) composites *J. Neural Eng.* **6** 65002
[121] Lee J Y, Lee J W and Schmidt C E 2009 Neuroactive conducting scaffolds: nerve growth factor conjugation on active ester-functionalized polypyrrole *J. R. Soc. Interface* **6** 801–10
[122] Jeong S I, Jun I D, Choi M J, Nho Y C, Lee Y M and Shin H 2008 Development of electroactive and elastic nanofibers that contain polyaniline and poly(llactide-co-epsilon-caprolactone) for the control of cell adhesion *Macromol. Biosci.* **8** 627–37
[123] Guo B and Ma P X 2018 Conducting polymers for tissue engineering *Biomacromolecules* **19** 1764–82
[124] Thourson S B and Payne C K 2017 Modulation of action potentials using PEDOT: PSS conducting polymer microwires *Sci. Rep.* **7** 10402
[125] Balint R, Cassidy N J and Cartmell S H 2014 Conductive polymers: towards a smart biomaterial for tissue engineering *Acta Biomater.* **10** 2341–53
[126] De Felice D and Alaimo A 2020 Mechanosensitive piezo channels in cancer: focus on altered calcium signaling in cancer cells and in tumor progression *Cancers (Basel)* **12** 1780
[127] Han Y, Liu C, Zhang D, Men H, Huo L and Geng Q 2019 Mechanosensitive ion channel piezo1 promotes prostate cancer development through the activation of the Akt/mTOR pathway and acceleration of cell cycle *Int. J. Oncol.* **55** 629–44
[128] Fukuta T, Nishikawa A and Kogure K 2020 Low level electricity increases the secretion of extracellular vesicles from cultured cells *Biochem. Biophys. Rep.* **21** 100713
[129] Lakkaraju A and Rodriguez-Boulan E 2008 Itinerant exosomes: emerging roles in cell and tissue polarity *Trends Cell. Biol.* **18** 199–209
[130] Rabinowits G, GerÁ el-Taylor C, Day J M, Taylor D D and Kloecker G H 2009 Exosomal microRNA: a diagnostic marker for lung cancer *Clin. Lung Cancer* **10** 42–6
[131] Silva J, Garcia V, Rodriguez M, Compte M, Cisneros E and Veguillas P 2012 Analysis of exosome release and its prognostic value in human colorectal cancer *Genes Chromosomes Cancer* **51** 409–18
[132] Zhang Z, Li Q, Du X and Liu M 2020 Application of electrochemical biosensors in tumor cell detection *Thorac. Cancer* **11** 840–50
[133] Ghosh G 2020 Early detection of cancer: focus on antibody coated metal and magnetic nanoparticle-based biosensors *Sens. Int.* **1** 100050
[134] Hassan R Y A and Wollenberger U 2019 Direct determination of bacterial cell viability using carbon nanotubes modified screenprinted electrodes *Electroanalysis* **31** 1112–7
[135] Magar H S, Hassan R Y A and Mulchandani A 2021 Electrochemical Impedance Spectroscopy (EIS): principles, construction, and biosensing applications *Sensors* **21** 6578

[136] Hassan R Y A, Febbraio F and Andreescu S 2021 Microbial electrochemical systems: principles, construction and biosensing applications *Sensors* **21** 1279

[137] Hussein H A, Hassan R Y, Chino M and Febbraio F 2020 Point-of-care diagnostics of COVID-19: from current work to future perspectives *Sensors* **20** 4289

[138] Magar H S, Brahman P K and Hassan R Y 2022 Disposable impedimetric nano-immunochips for the early and rapid diagnosis of vitamin-D deficiency *Biosens. Bioelectron.:* X **10** 100124

[139] Anusha T, Bhavani K S, Kumar J S, Brahman P K and Hassan R Y 2022 Fabrication of electrochemical immunosensor based on GCN-β-CD/Au nanocomposite for the monitoring of vitamin D deficiency *Bioelectrochemistry* **143** 107935

[140] Yu J, Yang A, Wang N, Ling H, Song J, Chen X, Lian Y, Zhang Z, Yan F and Gu M 2021 Highly sensitive detection of caspase-3 activity based on peptide-modified organic electrochemical transistor biosensors *Nanoscale* **13** 2868–74

[141] Deng D, Hao Y, Yang S, Han Q, Liu L, Xiang Y, Tu F and Xia N A 2019 signal-on electrochemical biosensor for evaluation of caspase-3 activity and cell apoptosis by the generation of molecular electrocatalysts on graphene electrode surface for water oxidation *Sensors Actuators* B **286** 415–20

[142] Fraczyk T 2021 Phosphorylation impacts Cu (II) binding by ATCUN motifs *Inorg. Chem.* **60** 8447–50

[143] Shamsipur M, Pashabadi A, Molaabasi F and Hosseinkhani S 2017 Impedimetric monitoring of apoptosis using cytochrome-aptamer bioconjugated silver nanocluster *Biosens. Bioelectron.* **90** 195–202

[144] Zhou S, Wang Y and Zhu J J 2016 Simultaneous detection of tumor cell apoptosis regulators Bcl-2 and Bax through a dual-signal-marked electrochemical immunosensor *ACS Appl. Mater. Interfaces* **8** 7674–82

[145] Li X L, Shan S, Xiong M, Xia X H, Xu J J and Chen H Y 2013 On-chip selective capture of cancer cells and ultrasensitive fluorescence detection of survivin mRNA in a single living cell *Lab Chip* **13** 3868–75

[146] Tan S J, Yobas L, Lee G Y, Ong C N and Lim C T 2009 Microdevice for the isolation and enumeration of cancer cells from blood *Biomed. Microdevices* **11** 883–92

[147] Nagrath S *et al* 2007 Isolation of rare circulating tumour cells in cancer patients by microchip technology *Nature* **450** 1235–9

[148] Kapeleris J, Ebrahimi Warkiani M, Kulasinghe A, Vela I, Kenny L, Ladwa R, O'Byrne K and Punyadeera C 2022 Clinical applications of circulating tumour cells and circulating tumour DNA in non-small cell lung cancer—an update *Front. Oncol.* **12** 859152

[149] Vaux D L 2011 In defense of the somatic mutation theory of cancer *Bioessays* **33** 341–3

[150] Zhang Y *et al* 2013 miR-126 and miR-126* repress recruitment of mesenchymal stem cells and inflammatory monocytes to inhibit breast cancer metastasis *Nat. Cell Biol.* **15** 284–94

[151] Vidal S J, Rodriguez-Bravo V, Galsky M, Cordon-Cardo C and Domingo-Domenech J 2014 Targeting cancer stem cells to suppress acquired chemotherapy resistance *Oncogene* **33** 4451–63

[152] Eyler C E and Rich J N 2008 Survival of the fittest: cancer stem cells in therapeutic resistance and angiogenesis *J. Clin. Oncol.* **26** 2839

Rishabha Malviya, Deepika Yadav, Sonali Sundram, Seifedine Kadry and Gurvinder Singh Virk

Chapter 10

Wireless microrobots: the next frontier in medical advancements

Historically, microbots have been regarded as particularly potent instruments in the field of minimally invasive treatment. Researchers from all around the world have been delving into this topic in recent years to expand the usefulness of microbots in the medical field. Using these tools, surgeons may access and operate on the inner workings of the human circulatory system. These microdevices are designed to remove clots, administer medications, and perhaps target particular cells or areas for diagnosis and treatment as they move through the microvascular system. Despite the large body of literature on this topic, there has not been any experimental investigation of the way in which microbots' shapes affect the hemodynamics of targeted human circulatory locations. Certain human physiological factors have been accounted for in numerical studies; nonetheless, experimental validation is essential and calls for more research. The dynamic performance of microbots is influenced by multiple variables, such as the non-Newtonian properties of blood, its particulate matter characteristics at smaller scales, flow disruptions resulting from the cardiac cycle, and the anatomical features of specific arteries, such as sub-divisions and tortuosity in particular regions. This chapter provides a comprehensive examination of the existing scientific research about the phenomenon of pulsing blood circulation in relation to microrobotics.

10.1 Introduction

Significant progress has been made in the last ten years within the emerging field of microscopic and nanoscale machines and robots (micro- and nanorobots) [1]. The utilization of intelligent materials which are specifically engineered to respond to particular conditions such as pH levels or protein levels, along with advancements in actuation approaches (both onboard and external) and the integration of cognitive physical abilities and computational intelligence, have collectively played a

doi:10.1088/978-0-7503-6019-7ch10

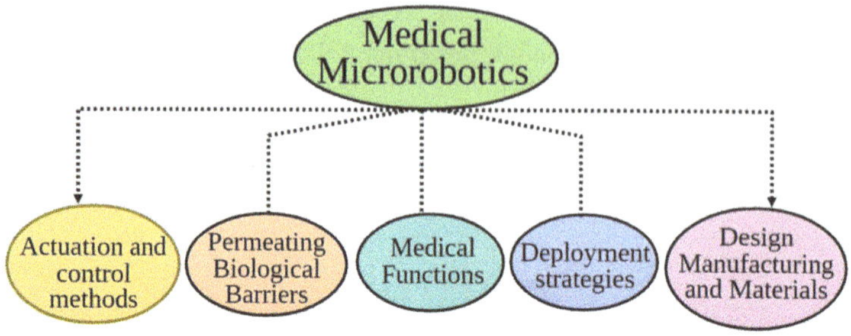

Figure 10.1. The application of medical microrobotics in various fields.

significant role in enhancing the abilities of these robots. Furthermore, the development of intriguing advanced additive manufacturing methods, particularly three-dimensional (3D) printing techniques, has effectively addressed the constraints associated with dimensions [2–4]. Figure 10.1 depicts the utilization of medical microrobotics in several domains. These robotic systems are increasingly being recognized as a burgeoning technology for various medical uses that have the potential to revolutionize fields such as minimally invasive surgery (including microsurgery), object detection, manipulation, assembly, isolation [5, 6], targeted cell/drug deliveries [7–10], and maneuverable navigation in viscous media [11] (including bodily fluids such as plasma and other biological fluids) for visualization and analysis purposes.

The layers of a 3D-printed item are laid down sequentially according to a digital model. The rapid development of microtechnology has witnessed significant advancements, particularly in the development of lab-on-a-chip and organ-on-a-chip technologies, and 3D printing has made important contributions throughout the biomedical spectrum. In comparison with other conventional approaches used for microrobot manufacture, such as lithographic printing methods, accumulation strategies based on electrical engineering [12–14] or chemical vapour deposition [15, 16], assembly procedures, rolled-up technological advances, electroless plating, and an additional strain engineering procedure, 3D printing represents a more affordable procedure that has smaller turnaround times between design modifications [17–20]. Metals, polymers, and bioinks (biocompatible materials with or without embedded cells and composites) are just a few of the many materials that may be 3D printed [21–34]. Hence, 3D printing is becoming the preferred approach for producing microrobots, especially among users who lack exceptional micromanufacturing skills, due to its relatively high accessibility and greater degree of repeatability [35, 36].

In the future, artificial intelligence (AI) is expected to contribute to the process of materials selection by considering the chemical characteristics of the target site. Furthermore, artificial intelligence will enhance the design of microrobots by effectively optimizing design parameters, surpassing the capabilities of human experts. A prime instance of this is the determination of the optimal parameters to minimize diving friction in specific biological fluids [37, 38]. Moreover, AI may be used to predict whether a design will be printed successfully and to fine-tune 3D printer settings for optimal printing. For instance, illumination-induced approaches involve modifying the amount of light, while extrusion-based methods involve manipulating pressure or temperatures. Following the manufacturing process, AI has the potential to assist in the regulation of miniature robots within *in vitro* or *in vivo* environments. This assistance would involve refining the actuation parameters to ensure that the microrobots successfully navigate to their intended destination, even in the presence of unforeseen variations in external factors, such as unexpected alterations in blood flow rate within a blood vessel. However, precision intelligence (PI) may also give microrobots agency by letting them independently sense and respond to their surroundings (e.g. to release a drug when a certain pH level is detected) [39]. Although there have been significant advancements in the manufacture and actuation of microrobots, it is still difficult to transfer these medical devices from the laboratory to clinical use. Microrobots encounter challenges from the time they enter the body until the time at which they reach their intended location, and this is all before the problem of mass-producing devices on such a small scale has ever begun to be tackled. An example of such a challenge is the phenomenon of being subjected to assault and subsequent elimination by the immune system of an organism [40]. In addition, the time and money needed to implement today's test requirements for microrobot safety and performance is a major roadblock to the rapid commercialization of microrobots for use in clinical settings.

This chapter summarizes recent progress in 3D-printed microrobot actuation and construction. It also illustrates how 3D-printed microrobots are utilized in the field of sustainability, namely in the process of water treatment. In addition, it highlights several applications of these microrobots in the field of biomedical sciences, such as drug delivery, surgical procedures, cancer prevention and treatment, image processing, particle surveillance and monitoring, sensing, and tissue regeneration. The potential applications of intelligent materials [41, 42] and AI/PI in the development of smart microrobots are emphasized, along with the challenges that now impede the translation of these advancements from the research laboratory to clinical settings.

10.2 Microrobots and their potential therapeutic applications

10.2.1 The imaging of functional capabilities for disorder diagnosis

Today, active visual imaging, often known as optical imaging, is one of the most essential diagnostic technologies available. This type of imaging covers both endoscopic and laparoscopic operations. Nowadays, visual disease diagnosis is provided by flexible endoscopes and catheters; however, these tools are invasive and are only useful for quick screenings. The utilization of endoscopic instruments in the form of pill-sized capsules has gained significance in the field of minimally invasive and long-term optical image processing, as well as in accessing previously unreachable areas, such as the gastrointestinal tract. Such commercial capsule cameras feature a camera, wireless transmission hardware, and a battery. They take pictures and send them to an external recording device. Capsule millirobots made using such passive imaging devices might allow for long-term, minimally invasive active imaging in otherwise inaccessible locations. For this reason, several research groups have proposed various forms of robotic capsule millirobots for active imaging. To achieve controlled locomotion within the alimentary canal, capsule robots have been constructed and driven by employing micromotors that incorporate leg or fin systems, employing an internal actuation method. Multiple groups of researchers have utilized remote magnetic actuation as a means to impede, propel, or maneuver capsule millirobots throughout the digestive tract via an external actuation methodology [43]. The former strategy reduces the imaging time from hours to minutes, since it does not need bulky external devices for actuation, whereas the latter strategy uses motors that consume more power than imaging alone. Nevertheless, external actuation or power transmission does not have this problem, although it may be more costly and restrict the patient's range of motion by surrounding them with cumbersome apparatus.

During active imaging, knowledge of the millirobot's precise 3D location (and orientation) is crucial to facilitate precise diagnosis and the development of innovative techniques. For instance, the application of 3D visual mapping techniques in the intestinal tract involves the integration of 3D positional data with two-dimensional sensor images. First, it is worth noting that diagnostic imaging methods such as fluorescence utilize low-dose x-rays to capture images of the capsule's region at a rate of 1–2 frames per second [43]. In addition, ultrasonic photography [44–46], positron emission tomography (PET) [43, 47], and magnetic resonance imaging (MRI) [43] are also viable options for accurately determining the precise position of millirobots within the alimentary tract. Researchers accomplished a reduction in the average positioning error to approximately 38 mm by incorporating a wireless transmitter into readily accessible passive capsule endoscopic devices and deploying numerous receiver antennae throughout the patient's entire body [43]. In addition, researchers have employed Hall-effect sensor arrays positioned outside the patient's internal organs to determine the precise position of the instrument [43, 48], which was accomplished by introducing a small magnet into the millirobot. Nevertheless, the presence of additional magnets or electromagnetic coils on capsule robots affects their sensors, hence creating challenges for the implementation of Hall-effect sensing-based methods in capsule robots that employ magnetic actuation. Several research investigations have endeavored to address this problem and have determined that the utilization of Hall-effect sensing of the capsule or elsewhere in the patient's body remains a viable method for achieving 3D localization [49, 50]. The position of an external magnet may also be used to determine the location of a soft capsule robot equipped with a Hall-effect sensor [51].

Another proposal entailed the utilization of capsule millirobots and magnetically operated soft capsule endoscopes equipped with an incorporated complementary metal–oxide–semiconductor (CMOS) camera to proactively examine stomach-type 3D surfaces by remote magnetic manipulation [32]. The capsule's soft body allowed for safe operation (no tissue damage caused by high stress), more degrees of freedom in actuation, and the capacity to change form. To navigate and regulate its location within the stomach, the multi-agent system for collaborative e-learning (MASCE) was rolled using an external magnet after it was swallowed and arrived there in a matter of seconds. Numerous localization algorithms have been proposed to determine the precise 3D position and two-dimensional orientation of robots engaged in imaging [50, 51]. Active imaging with such a millirobot is possible *in vitro* within a stomach phantom used in surgical simulations. The use of active imaging capabilities is currently limited to millimeter scale healthcare robots, as the most compact CMOS sensors and lenses manufactured by Awaiba GmbH are of diminutive dimensions. Smaller, lower-resolution cameras with built-in illumination and lenses may one day allow mobile microrobots to actively examine hitherto inaccessible microscopic places. Within the body of an individual, various anatomical features can be found, including the gastrointestinal tract, spinal column fluid, and the cerebral hemispheres.

10.2.2 Mobile situational awareness for disease diagnosis and health management

To keep track of a patient's or healthy person's health status in real time, today's passive biomedical sensors may be placed either within or outside the body. Sensors of this type could be used to diagnose and provide information about any pathological or abnormal medical condition in real time by measuring or detecting variables such as various physiological parameters that can be monitored to assess the functioning of the human body. These parameters include carbohydrate levels, pH, temperatures, oxygen concentration, viral or bacterial activities, bodily motion (inertia), equilibrium, arterial blood pressure, the rate of respiration, muscular activity, neuronal activity, and pulse rate, among others [52]. A prospective portable healthcare sensor network for proactive health surveillance could be provided inside the human body by incorporating long- or short-range motion as well as management abilities into these sensors by mounting them on healthcare milli/microrobots. In this way, several mobile sensors might be sent on a simultaneous mission to patrol various organs without causing too much disruption. In contrast to the visual monitoring described in 10.2.1, little research has been done on the potential biomedical applications of milli/microrobots. Ergeneman *et al* introduced a magnetically operated untethered magnetic microrobot in their paper [53], which has the potential to perform optical oxygen sensing for ocular measurements.

10.3 Targeted therapy

Targeted treatment has the potential to enhance the concentration of therapeutics, such as drugs, mRNA, genes, radioactive seeds, imaging contrast agents, stem cells, and proteins, in a specific anatomical site inside the body. This localized enrichment can be achieved while minimizing systemic adverse effects. In addition, the therapeutic window of the medication's concentration may be adjusted by manipulating the release kinetics, thus extending the duration of a single dose's effects. Therapeutic biological and chemical substances may be delivered to a specified target region in measured doses using mobile milli/microrobots, reducing the risk of adverse effects while maximizing the benefits of the treatment [54].

Drug delivery to specific areas of the gastrointestinal tract, arteries, etc. using small-scale mobile robots has emerged as the primary targeted therapeutic application. Active capsule endoscopes, which operate at the millimeter scale, have been utilized to administer medications through the gastrointestinal system via passive or active drug release mechanisms [8]. Numerous drug delivery capsules incorporate an external trigger system that initiates an operation facilitating the simultaneous dispensation of a medication at a precisely calculated dosage. The drug release mechanism can be activated by various stimuli such as fluorescent or near-infrared (NIR) radiation, ultrasound, or electromagnetic fields [54]. Joule electrical heating of a shape memory alloy wire can also be utilized to activate a pharmacological mechanism [55]. Micromotor-based actuation [56] and remote-triggered ignition of a propellant-based micro thruster [57] have been used in a capsule robot for the one-shot ejection of pharmaceuticals. Liquid medications might be ejected within the stomach in a controlled manner and administered several times by compressing a magnetically actuated soft capsule millirobot along its long axis [32, 58]. As a semi-implantable drug delivery platform, the same soft capsule robot could transform into a spherical shape within the stomach and remain there for an extended period to release its payload of pharmaceuticals by passive diffusion [15]. After the medication delivery procedure was complete, the capsule could be retrieved by reverting it to its original cylindrical form, allowing it to be eliminated normally by peristalsis.

Initial investigations have been conducted employing micron-scale, autonomous microrobots to deliver pharmaceuticals or other substances into the circulatory system and ocular region [59]. Millimeter-scale robots may be controlled by magnetic field gradients in human arteries with dimensions between 4 and 25 mm and blood flow velocities between 100 and 400 mm s^{-1} [60, 61]. Magnetic resonance navigation was proposed to move a spherical magnet with a diameter of 1.5 mm through the carotid artery of a pig [62]. Later, a technique quite similar to this was used to inject doxorubicin into the hepatic artery of rabbits. This magnetic navigation system has a higher switching rate than that of a spherical permanent magnet system, allowing for closed-loop control [60].

The utilization of rotational magnetized microswimmers equipped with an inflatable helical tail, similar to the flagella found in bacteria, has been proposed as a viable method for achieving efficient swimming locomotion in environments characterized by minimal Reynolds numbers [64–66] to reach capillaries smaller than arterioles (150 m). The microswimmers have the potential to encapsulate drugs for localized administration, either through a passive diffusion process [66] or an active release mechanism. Furthermore, certain investigations have proposed the use of biohybrid microrobots, wherein bacteria are harnessed to transport cargo, such as pharmaceutical particles or molecules, to specific locations [14, 59]. This transportation is achieved via either remote-controlled mechanisms or by leveraging the bacterial ability to sense and respond to the surrounding environment. Here, bacteria operate as onboard actuators by harnessing cellular or extracellular chemical energy and as onboard microsensors by monitoring changes in pH, oxygen levels, and temperature [67]. The utilization of remote magnetic steering control enables the magnetometric dynamic unipolar MC-1 bacterium to transport a considerable number of liposomes, each of which has a diameter of less 200 nm, encapsulating pharmaceuticals. This transportation process does not result in a substantial decrease in the bacterium's swimming velocity. A further investigation of this phenomenon employed a swarm of chemotactic bacteria to carry microparticles of a potential medication that contained embedded superparamagnetic nanoparticles and then used remote magnetic fields to steer the microparticles to their destination, where they released their payload. In uniform 10 mT magnetic fields, the swimming speed of microparticles with a diameter of 6 nm that were pushed by bacteria reached 7.3 m s^{-1}. The rapid and cheap production of biohybrid microrobots would pave the way for their use in microrobot swarms for targeted medicine delivery in the future [68].

10.4 The applications of microrobotics in medicine, particularly in the human cardiovascular system and the bloodstream

Chronic vascular diseases kill more individuals each year than any other medical condition. Vascular occlusions, most often due to thrombus development or atherosclerotic plaques [1, 18], are among the leading causes of mortality from cardiovascular disease. Atherosclerotic plaques narrow arteries, restrict blood flow to essential organs and increase the risk of clots that may cause catastrophic bleeding. The cardiovascular system carries oxygen and nutrients throughout the body. Heart attack, stroke, critical limb ischemia, and deep thrombosis/pulmonary embolism are all possible outcomes of vascular system failure [69]. Several treatment approaches are now employed to treat CVDs. The selection of a specific surgical intervention is contingent upon the state of the cardiovascular ailment and the specific region of the circulatory system that is impacted. An obstruction in the coronary arteries, which feed blood to the heart muscle, is an example of an acute illness. A coronary artery bypass graft (CABG) is a major surgical procedure [70]. To access the cardiac region, a surgical incision must be made in the patient's chest. Pharmaceutical intervention is employed to induce cardiac arrest, followed by the utilization of a heart–lung bypass apparatus to redirect blood circulation away from the obstructed artery. As a result of this procedure, the heart's blood supply can be repaired. A minimally intrusive direct coronary artery bypass graft (MIDCAB) is an alternate approach to traditional open chest surgery. This technique involves the creation of a sequence of small incisions on the individual's left side, specifically between the ribs. This operation is performed to bypass the heart by rerouting blood arteries. The drawbacks of CABG are well-known and include the high risk of surgical death, the high expense, and the extended recovery period [20]. Where feasible, noninvasive methods such as percutaneous coronary intervention (PCI) are favored. Combining coronary angioplasty with the installation of a stent is a dependable technique that is substantially less invasive and costly than CABG [71–73]. During PCI, a balloon or stent coated in a drug-eluting material is used to make a hole in the artery wall and expand it, thereby eliminating the blocked blood vessel. Fragment separation, vascular injury, elastic recoil, restenosis, and infection are some of the most common adverse events [72]. The utilization of ultrasound imaging has yielded a notable enhancement in the efficacy of thrombolytic drugs, resulting in a reduction in treatment duration. This advancement has the potential to enhance stroke therapy. Researchers have successfully devised intravascular catheters that incorporate ultrasound transducers operating at megahertz frequencies, thereby facilitating the dissolution of blood clots. Cavitation, however, is a side effect of ultrasonic exposure that creates dosimetry and control issues. There is a need for further investigation of this technique's potential relevance and full scope of clinical use in thrombolysis. Reference [74] contains a comprehensive inventory and detailed explanation of contemporary therapeutic methodologies employed in the removal of arterial blockages. These procedures offer an appealing alternative to the conventional approaches of catheterization and stenting. The authors describe the underlying physical mechanisms associated with each solution, providing examples of tools, devices, and procedures that are currently recognized as minimally invasive approaches for removing thrombi and atherosclerosis. They systematically classify and organize the therapeutic strategies into distinct categories, namely mechanical, laser-based, chemical, and hybrid removal strategies, based on their respective operational principles.

There have been major developments in the field of minimally invasive surgery during the last decade. The use of miniature robots for vascular network surgery is a prime illustration of this trend. The potential for future, precise medical therapies to be performed by microbots is enormous (figure 10.2). They may be able to perform operations that are challenging or impossible using today's methods. When powered by the body's circulatory system, these tiny robots might one day reach hitherto inaccessible parts of the human body. The future of minimally invasive therapies in the cardiovascular system is bright, and Miloro's categorization [75] is a wonderful place to start learning about them. In the vascular system, mechanical removal is

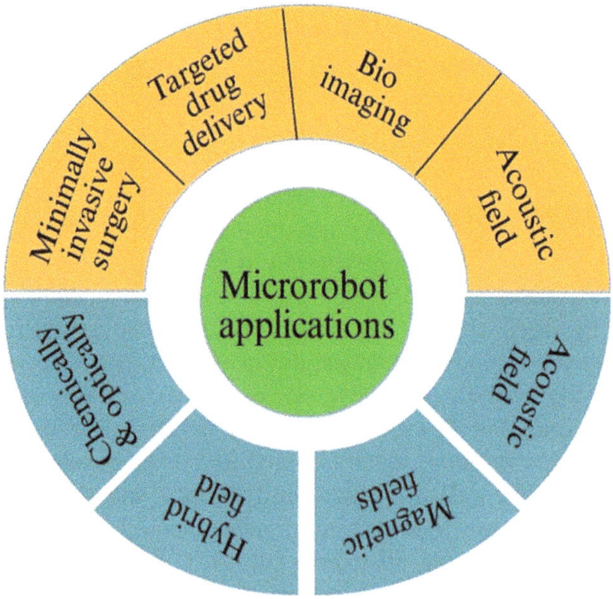

Figure 10.2. The effective construction of microrobotic devices with multiple applications can be achieved by the implementation of self-assembly instructions for their constituent elements.

one treatment method, according to Miloro's categorization [72]. To remove an arterial blockage, this method integrates the application of a mill or microdevice using a range of both mechanical or fluid-mediated procedures (such as crushing, maceration, dragging, scraping, suction, compression, and ultrasound) [72]. A comprehensive investigation was conducted to comprehensively analyze the physiological ramifications associated with the elimination of arterial blockages by diverse thrombectomy/atherectomy techniques, alongside ultrasonic thrombolysis and ultrasound angioplasty. Depending on the devices/tools used and the activities involved, both thrombectomy and atherectomy may cause certain clinical problems despite their minimal invasiveness, ease of use, and low cost. The most commonly observed issues are: endothelial denudation; vascular perforation/dissection; the obstruction of small vessels due to larger thrombi, resulting in distant embolization; limitations in cutter size, leading to an inability to remove thrombi/atheroma; and hemodynamic problems.

Miloro's categorization suggests that laser removal (which includes the use of all treatment types including photochemical, photothermal, and photomechanical operations to eliminate vascular blockages) is another promising technique [72]. The limitations of laser–material interactions in the vascular system and ultrasonic therapy are discussed. In comparison to laser treatments that rely on a photothermal process, those that use ultraviolet (UV) light to trigger photochemical processes are more effective. In conjunction with a lytic agent that directly disrupts molecular bonds, UV light ablates thrombi and prevents platelet aggregation. In contrast, during the thermal phase, the laser energy establishes dynamic contact with the surface of the obstruction and causes gradual erosion. There is a risk of contraction, shrinkage, coagulation, or carbonization if temperatures exceeding 43 °C–45 °C are used [76–78]. Consequently, deliberate efforts are made to prevent heat-related impacts on the circulatory system. These require further investigation, particularly in the context of resolving vascular obstructions.

It is worth noting that microbots may be best suited to carry out certain duties using mechanical, laser, or hybrid removal techniques. They might be modified using dedicated design software, or they could serve as static, convenient, or even autonomous structures. They might be utilized in a rotational motion to scrape fatty material off the inside of a blood artery, or a resonant mechanical structure could be used to produce ultrasonic pressure waves to remove calcified material that is blocking a blood vessel [76–78]. The microbots, in their inert state, might function like a drug-delivered stent, navigating to the site of interest and remaining there to maintain blood flow through a blocked artery. A microrobot that mimics an occlusion and blocks off a blood artery to deliberately deprive an area of nutrients is another intriguing possibility for a permanent construction [77]. It is possible to configure microrobots to provide aneurysm treatments wirelessly or at the touch of a button.

Elimination could also occur through the use of biochemical processes, such as the dissolution or breakdown of a proteolytic agent's target or through the annihilation of the biological framework of an obstruction. Although these clinical therapies (intravenous thrombolysis, intra-arterial thrombolysis) are effective, their only objective is to specifically address blood clots in both arteries and veins, which may result in potential adverse effects such as cerebral hemorrhage, systemic hemorrhage, immunological problems, low blood pressure, and cardiac infarction. [79]. Targeted treatment using microbots is mentioned in the works of several writers [76–78]. With the ability to increase the medication concentration in a given area while decreasing its effects elsewhere, microbots might be used for targeted treatment [77, 78]. Microbots might be used for targeted retinal medication administration to eliminate common barriers in the retinal vascular system caused by clot formation [79].

The use of magnetic field-controlled microbots for targeted medication administration has been shown to be plausible and achievable [79]; however, the authors recommended further investigation of the technique's clinical usefulness. Indeed, sophisticated coating processes are required to load the pharmaceuticals into microbots, and drug delivery kinetics must be better regulated to achieve targeted medication delivery.

Finally, researchers have provided a different approach that emphasized the synergy between the mechanical and chemical processes mentioned above.

10.5 Biomechanical restrictions that impede microrobots

The path a microrobot takes *in vivo* from its place of deployment to its site of action is fraught with danger. To reach its destination, a microrobot must first overcome biological obstacles. The multifaceted nature of the biological barriers and the potential techniques to overcome them are strongly affected by factors such as the site of administration, the tissue that is targeted or involved, and its desired physiological function [80]. The protein corona refers to the spontaneous formation of an adsorbed layer around a microrobot when it is introduced into the human body; it facilitates interactions with diverse proteins [81, 82]. This is a thermodynamic process in which the enthalpy decreases and the entropy rises as a result of the energetically preferred binding of proteins to nanoparticles [83]. Over more than ten years, extensive research into nanoparticles and solid surfaces has demonstrated the significance of several physical design factors in the formation of the protein-based corona. These factors include the chemical composition of the surface, charge, water-retaining capacity, microscopic surface topography, exposed length, and hydrophilic properties [81, 84]. Some of the surface-governed behavior of microrobots may need to be rethought, depending on the properties of this dynamic thin layer. To begin, a microrobot's swimming speed may be modified by changing the polarity of its surface [85]. Second, microrobots may be eliminated from the body through an immunological response if the coronal development causes a physicochemical process involving the improper folding and agglomeration of proteins. Ultimately, the microrobot's interface has the potential to impede its medicinal or physiological functionalities, including the kinetics of its drug release and the identification of surrounding stimuli. Due to their dynamic nature, microrobots may retain their protein corona while they are transferred from one bodily fluid to another [86]. This indicates that the entry point of microrobots may significantly affect the make-up of the protein corona and hence the functional behavior of the robots further down the line. Protein corona formation may also be significantly affected by the shear stress experienced by the microrobots during their active mobility or when they are circulating in the body's bloodstream. Shear stress may cause catch-and-slip linkages in the margination of blood cells and their extravasation from blood arteries [87]. As a direct result of these physical processes, the protein coronas surrounding microrobots *in vitro* and *in vivo* may vary in terms of their protein composition, surface coverage, protein abundance, and coronal dynamics [86, 87]. The system of complementary antibodies, which constitutes a component of the natural immune system, functions as the initial barrier of the human body that responds to external pathogens [88]. Its components make up a key immunological component of the protein corona that surrounds a microrobot in the bloodstream. The presence of opsonin proteins inside the bloodstream of a patient has the potential to trigger the process of opsonization. This procedure involves the activation of the complementary system, which is located on the outermost layer of the microrobot. One of the most significant biological hurdles to microrobots in circulation is the enhanced capacity of leukocytes to detect them as foreign. After initial activation, opsonization may progress to the activation of mast cells and other immune cells, leading to subsequent inflammatory responses. A chain reaction might hinder the microrobots' capacity to go where they need to go and carry out their medicinal duties. Nanoparticles have been greatly aided by designing the surfaces of microrobots to have neutrally charged and long hydrophilic polymers, such as derivatives of poly (ethylene glycol) (PEG) [88]. PEG chains often form a hydrophilic coating surrounding the nanoparticles, which prevents and delays the initial phase of the opsonization process by inhibiting the absorption of opsonin proteins through steric repulsion forces [89, 90]. However, it is worth noting that PEG-conjugated medicines may also trigger an immunological response in certain individuals [90].

The immunological response is not uniformly strong or extensive everywhere throughout the body. The term 'immune privilege' refers to the ability of some anatomical locations to maintain a low-key immunological profile to prevent potentially harmful inflammation. Hence, foreign antigens may be introduced at such locations for extended periods without triggering an inflammatory immune response. The immunological predominance of certain regions, such as the brain and spinal cord (central nervous system (CNS)), the eye, and the feto-maternal system, is widely acknowledged in the scientific community [91–93]. The materials and structural design of microrobots may exhibit a certain amount of flexibility based on factors such as clinical circumstances, tissue characteristics, disease progression, and duration of exposure. Yet, using the patient's own biomaterials to create microrobots might be the best way to avoid the risks associated with an unchecked immune response. Such an individual approach, in which the body recognizes the microrobots as part of itself, has the potential to dramatically dampen the immunological response. As an example, converting natural red blood cells or platelets (with a mean diameter of 7.8 μm and a thickness of 1–2.5 μm) into functioning microrobots might be an effective strategy [94–96]. The blood contains a large number of these cells (4.5–5.5 × 10^9 red blood cells and 1.5–3.0 × 10^8 platelets per milliliter of blood, respectively) [97]. The usage of RBCs as a foundational material may be intriguing and valuable for manufacturing large numbers of microrobots that are now impossible to produce using conventional microfabrication methods. Moreover, under stress, erythrocytes may be bent without undergoing plastic deformation [98].

Since blood travels all across the body, it can even go to far-flung places if it has to. Yet, intravenously administered microrobots face additional obstacles in the bloodstream beyond opsonization and immunological clearance. They are rooted primarily in the physiology of the circulatory system and the fluid characteristics of blood. An important fluidic flow barrier prevents microrobots from functioning reliably in the circulatory system, which is used for propulsion and steering. Arteries are responsible for the transportation of oxygen-rich blood from the heart to various regions of the human body, whereas veins facilitate the return of blood from the body's tissues back to the heart. The arteries have a pulsating blood flow of between 100 and 400 mm s^{-1}. To facilitate the exchange of nutrients and gases, large arteries divide into smaller vessels called arterioles. The blood is recirculated back to the heart through venules, which are junctions between capillaries. While the flow velocity decreases with branching, the slowest flow rate in capillaries is still around 100 μm s^{-1} [99]. The size, hemorheological flow characteristics, and shear stress of these various vessels are all distinct. Since the smallest capillaries may be just a few micrometers in diameter, this sets a lower bound on the size of microrobots that are intended to traverse the whole vascular network. Therefore, it could be inferred that microrobots with a circumference of 5 μm will encounter challenges in navigating through the smallest capillaries. However, larger microrobotic devices possessing soft and relatively pliable structures, similar to those of red blood cells, could potentially traverse these capillaries without inflicting harm. The potential consequences of a high concentration of these robots within the arteries that supply blood to the brain or the pulmonary capillaries include the development of strokes or an embolism of the lungs. Most microrobot speeds are many orders of magnitude slower than the blood's velocity in the blood vessels. Nonetheless, operation in arteries is still possible through the use of supplementary technologies, despite the high flow rates. The application of an inflatable catheter within a porcine carotid artery, observed using a clinical MRI system, has demonstrated that microrobots can maneuver to regulate and reduce the rate of flow [100].

Using the blood's flow as a motorway might be another technique to get around the intravascular flow barrier. An example of this is the utilization of magnetic nanomotors to specifically target blood clots through the influence of fluid dynamics, consequently enhancing the therapeutic efficacy of tissue plasminogen activator (tPA) by inducing rotational motion via a magnetic field. A mouse model was used to show that the thrombolytic process might be sped up by using rotating nanomotors to improve the local mixing and interaction of co-administered tPA with a blood clot [101]. In a similar way, magnetic microrods carrying tPA were employed to target clots in the center of the cerebral artery. The combination of blood circulation and magnetic guidance facilitated the precise navigation of the microscopic rods toward the area of injury, hence assisting in the dissolution of the fibrin clot [102, 103]. While the proof of concept has been established, there are still certain issues that need to be addressed before a full-scale animal or human trial can begin. First, the nanoparticles' potential for harmful aggregation inside the magnetic field is heightened if they build up in an unintended vessel. Smart DNA origami with a DNA aptamer targeting the overexpressed nucleoli protein in tumor-supplying blood arteries was employed in a nanoparticle-free robotic technique. Thrombin was transported to tumor-associated blood arteries by blood flow and a targeting moiety, where it caused intravascular thrombosis and slowed tumor development [103]. Micromotors composed of $CaCO_3$, however, employed a combination of lateral propulsion, buoyed rise, and convection mechanisms to navigate in opposition to the blood flow, regardless of the glassy capillaries' horizontal or vertical alignments. Following this, it was shown that the construct could successfully transport coagulation medicines to manage bleeding in an amputated mouse model [104]. These studies show that therapeutic outcomes for intravascular applications may be accomplished with the right usage of microrobots, despite the obstacles that must be overcome. Moreover, the natural propensity of leukocytes to traverse in the circulation [105] means that biohybrid techniques, such as the utilization of one's cells as cellular cyborgs, might sidestep the intravascular mobility barrier. Cells are passively transported by blood flow, but they actively roll and tumble on endothelial surfaces to extravasate into tissues when they contact chemical cues from the endothelium and sense an elevated level of cytokines [106]. Integrating chemical-sensing-based stimulation of robotic mobility and functionality into synthesized topologies will significantly enhance the potential for subsequent unsupervised intelligent behavior in microrobots. When a microrobot successfully reaches its intended organ within the body and needs to escape the vasculature, the capillaries present a particularly rational and suitable means of egress. Arteries and veins have strong walls that make it difficult for microrobots to get through them into tissues. Uncontrolled internal bleeding may also occur if these vessels are broken.

The rheological characteristics of blood circulating in the vasculature are influenced by various factors, including the arterial dimensions, blood flow rate, and hematocrit value. These factors provide challenges for the effective functioning of microrobots within the bloodstream. The red blood cell volume fraction is the most important factor in determining blood viscosity. Blood is classified as a shearing–thinning fluid that depends on the combined effects of plasma viscosity and temperature. This behavior arises from the ability of red blood cell membranes to undergo deformation and realign themselves parallel to the direction of circulation under high shear rates. Consequently, this alignment leads to a reduction in viscosity. Another obstacle that changes swimming mechanics is the non-Newtonian behavior of blood [107]. To maintain the intended and projected mobility, microrobots must be able to adjust to fluctuating flow parameters and viscosities.

Although there is a possibility of associations with blood cells, the majority of studies on microrobots have mostly focused on their propulsion in Newtonian or low-viscosity fluids, including water, buffered solutions, and serum [108–110].

To gain a comprehensive understanding of the intricate dynamics and behavioral patterns shown by microrobots inside complex and hostile environments, it is imperative to replicate intermittent flow patterns, variations in pressure, and blood composition in both phantoms and microfluidic channels. Magnetic micromotors with helical shapes have been successfully operated within unadulterated human blood, exhibiting a stick-and-slip action as they traverse the blood cells [111].

Endothelial barrier crossing may be necessary for extravascular delivery and other functions to accumulate precisely at the target location. For such cellular barriers, the size impact is more noticeable in the case of microrobots. The aperture size of tight junctions in the brain's uninterrupted vasculature is smaller than 1 nm, posing significant challenges for the transvascular infiltration of microrobots [112]. The blood–brain barrier (BBB) is one of the most strictly controlled biological barriers. Many methods, both invasive and noninvasive, have been used to date to circumvent the BBB and deliver therapeutics to the CNS [113]. The use of focused ultrasound systems (FUSs) to temporarily expand tight connections is one such method that may be compatible with microrobots. Even though the nanometer-sized holes created by FUSs are too small to be penetrated by current microrobots, these pores may be made larger by applying mechanical force to them, much like the way in which leukocytes are extravasated. Nevertheless, albumin, which is toxic to astrocytes, may seep over the BBB and cause neuropathological changes in the brain [114]. Certain pathogens that have BBB-penetrating capabilities, such as certain strains of meningitis-causing bacterium, may have found a transcellular pathway that allows them to penetrate the BBB; this suggests that using the tools already present in nature and following in their footsteps might be beneficial. This requires microrobots that can be actively controlled inside the cytoplasm, which has been proven to be possible. The capacity to move and manipulate helical nanorobots within cells without altering cellular activity has recently been proven [115]. The cerebrospinal canal is another possible route to the brain, although it presents certain challenges due to the body's natural defenses.

10.6 Current challenges facing miniaturized biomedical robots and their potential future applications

Several basic hurdles must be overcome before small mobile robots may be used in high-impact biomedical applications. Millimeter-scale and smaller functional robots call for fundamentally different approaches to design, manufacture, and control than those of larger-scale robots [116]. Other duties, such as receiving input from the surrounding environment and communicating with the operator, will be necessary for medical procedures performed within the human body. From conceptualization through preliminary clinical testing, authors have examined the difficulties of developing smaller, more portable untethered biomedical robots. Considering the recent developments in resolving some of these difficulties, the authors also present a future vision of a solution. A variety of approaches may be taken to address these design issues. The number of milli/microrobots is a major design consideration; alternatives include a single multitasking robot, many robots working in tandem, or a swarm of robots working in concert [117]. While a single microrobot may not be powerful enough to have a substantial theranostic impact on a particular activity, a group of microrobots working together may be able to greatly increase the projected throughput. Each robot in a multirobot setup might be the same (i.e. homogeneous) and perform the same tasks, or it could be distinct (heterogeneous) and do different tasks from the others [118]. The group's motion might be either deterministic or stochastic, depending on whether actuation takes place onboard or remotely [27, 119]. Robots may move about by swimming, crawling, rolling, spinning, or hopping. Micro/nano-sensors and micro/nano-actuators might be combined, together with additional components such as microcontrollers, power sources, wireless communication, etc.

Microrobots with several functions may be successfully designed by instructing their parts to self-assemble (figure 10.2) [120].

Biological organisms consistently employ the ubiquitous process of reprogrammable self-assembly, wherein small parts are organized into larger, more complicated arrangements [121]. Individual parts, or building blocks, provide the instructions for assembling and disassembling structures and performing specialized biological tasks. The utilization of reprogrammable assembly serves as a straightforward and robust method for facilitating the rapid adaptation of organisms to dynamic environmental changes, regardless of the intricate nature of the ultimate assemblage. These highly intelligent biological systems may serve as a rich source of motivation for the development of equally sophisticated artificial designs that can perform many tasks and independently adapt to changing environmental circumstances. Hence, milli/microrobots with optimum functionality may be easily customized and mass-produced through the modular assembly of various micro- and nanocomponents. Although the idea of reprogrammable materials is in its infancy, there is a pressing need for a comprehensive knowledge of, and control over assembly and the associated processes via the use of simple and reliable methods. Coding information into individual building pieces is a significant obstacle to macroscopic self-assembly. Recent efforts [28, 122–126] have developed soft building pieces of varying sizes and forms that can self-assemble. State-of-the-art examples include colloidal patchy particles [127], which may undergo directed and programmable interactions in 3D. Anisotropic and heterogeneous configurations might motivate comparable self-assembly-based robot designs via the spatial-selective surface modification of individual building pieces varying in size from 0.1 to a few micrometers. For this reason, a similar strategy might help to fabricate microrobots made from bigger construction components (10 μm–1 mm). The loss of directionality and the destabilization of structural coherence, however, result from the proliferation of nonspecific interaction sites brought about by a rise in particle size. As a result, there is still more work to be done before the goal of high-fidelity directed bonding between building pieces and a high overall assembly yield is reached. An alternative is to picking and arrange individual building bricks remotely, with the help of a human operator, to assemble them into 2D and 3D constructions [28, 122]. Yet, when construction is done in this fashion, interactions between the constituent parts often stay weak, which does not maintain the overall structural integrity and leads to the ensemble tending to come apart. As a result, an additional step of covalent cross-linking is required to overcome this problem [28]. However, since covalent cross-linking is permanent, it prevents the finished ensemble from ever being reprogrammable again. To construct microrobots according to predetermined manufacturing plans, it will be necessary to achieve bonding stability while keeping the assembly's inherent dynamism intact.

Real-time interactions and feedback between the many parts of a milli/micro-robot are crucial to the overall system's performance. Ideally, an autonomous microrobot's sense of its surroundings would be tightly connected with its movement, cargo release, power supply, and other operational components. As a result, unique sensing techniques that modify robot behavior would conditionally enable operations. To perform noninvasive medical surgery, it is essential to detect the location of a tumor and then 'taxi' microrobots to the place. One of the biggest obstacles to continuous sensing in the real world is the inherent unreliability of biological signals, which may lead to false positives or negatives and, in turn, the unexpected activation of microrobots. Enhanced operational evaluations conducted by milli/microrobots can potentially be accomplished using molecular logic gates, which possess the capability to detect multiple markers conditionally [123, 124]. For each particular task, the best design method and accompanying variables depend on several factors. Following the construction of approximate models of such milli/microrobot systems, rigorous numerical design optimization approaches employing evolutionary algorithms need to be created; this represents a major future challenge.

10.7 Methods for the actuation and control of therapeutic microrobots

The enhancement of microrobots' actuation, navigation, and control capabilities will exert a substantial impact on their transition from laboratory settings to clinical applications. However, there is a requirement to develop integrated actuation and control mechanisms to effectively navigate untethered microrobots through biological settings along predetermined trajectories. These tools should meet at least four criteria [1]. They need to set up a dependable line of communication between the *in vivo* functioning microrobot and the outside world, such as the attending physician. The actuation tools used in the medical field should have enough power and force/torque to propel the device quickly and effectively so that the desired medical procedures may be carried out. Furthermore, these tools must possess biocompatibility. Moreover, a combination of medical imaging and control modalities is essential to enable immediate oversight and feedback-guided robotic maneuvering [4]. It is preferable to use tools that are already available in hospitals, or at least those that are affordable and well-suited for use by clinicians and patients.

Large B fields may safely permeate the human body [125, 126]; they are the most common actuation and control technique offered [23, 127–129]. To control microrobots, scientists have recommended a variety of magnetic field signals. A magnetic spatial gradient can be employed to attract or repel the microrobot, depending on the most rational course of action. To create the magnetic spatial gradient, several

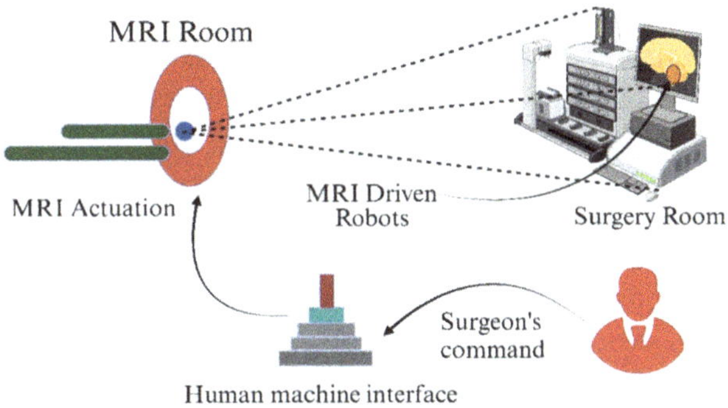

Figure 10.3. The utilization of a clinical MRI system's field applicator in conjunction with an MRI-driven millirobot's magnetic torque to facilitate the insertion of a biopsy needle into the brain.

permanent [129] or electromagnetic coil systems may be used. In particular, incorporating such a strategy into an MRI system, such as interventional MRI [130–135], might significantly turn this popular medical imaging tool into robotic equipment, enhancing its medical capabilities. The magnitude of the field of magnetic attraction (the *B* field) exhibits a slower decay rate (proportional to *L*3) as the distance from the coil rises, in comparison to the magnetic spatial gradients which decay at a faster rate (proportional to *L*4, where *L* represents the distance from the coil). As a result, producing magnetic torque on microrobots and projecting *B* fields into the human body is simplified [136]. Figure 10.3 shows the field application of a clinical MRI system, namely the use of an MRI-driven millirobot's magnetic torque to bore a biopsy needle into the brain [44].

Similarly, the removal of thrombi from blood arteries has been shown to be possible using a similar mechanism [137, 138]. At the micrometer scale, microrobots with a corkscrew form may be driven by a revolving *B* field [139–141], while a microrobot with a tail can be driven by an oscillating *B* field [142]. At the nanoscale, these actuation principles are more effective than gradient pulling [136]. Finally, by adjusting both the *B* field and the *B* field spatial gradient, complicated field signals may be generated. This is very useful for programming complicated movements into magnetic soft milli/microrobots [137–139]. Current microrobotic systems often use isotropic workspaces for their field applicators. The continued progress in high-temperature superconducting materials has the potential to yield notable benefits such as a substantial decrease in coil dimensions and an augmentation in coil quantity within the magnetic arrangement [140]. In this manner, anisotropy might potentially be generated within both the workplace environment and the physiological structure of the human body. Complex movements may be generated by individually controlling numerous microrobots [141, 142] or various parts of the robots. This might pave the way for more complex medical interventions.

The actuation requirements of untethered microrobots within the human body are readily met by sonic waves, since they are external physical force generators [143]. For microrobot-like miniature devices, acoustic actuation may be split into two distinct categories. The first pertains to the confinement of an inflatable on the robot's structure [144–147], while the second concerns the robot's ability to generate reverberation to transmit energy over a certain distance (the latter involves the production of an intricate sound pattern to command several separate entities). In a more precise manner, the construction of holographic acoustic tweezers entails the arrangement of transducers in diverse configurations [148]. A third option for re-creating acoustic waves in any pattern is to employ a transmission holography plate manufactured in 3D [128]. Microrobots that use acoustic waves for control have not been deployed in a clinical setting. A possible explanation for this is that sound waves travel more slowly through solid objects; therefore, it can be challenging to exercise auditory control over microrobots when they are operating inside the human body because of strong reflectors, such as the diaphragm and bones, that might severely interfere with the transmission [149].

Light has been used in conjunction with magnetic and acoustic actuation to actuate and control microrobots in an *in vitro* setting. This approach is preferred due to the ease with which light can be manipulated to form intricate patterns in both temporal and spatial dimensions, hence enabling a substantial level of control and flexibility [150]. NIR light may penetrate the skin to a certain depth, suggesting its future usage beneath the skin or in the eye. Furthermore, it is worth noting that microrobots have the potential to be propelled through the utilization of energy obtained from their surroundings, which can be achieved by unicellular microbes or catalyst-based designs. However, the operation of an autonomous biohybrid or catalytic microrobot necessitates the incorporation of supplementary control mechanisms to facilitate precise steering and accurate localization.

10.8 Conclusions

There is great potential for small, untethered mobile robots to be used in medical and biotechnological settings. They excel in situations where traditional medical instruments, such as those used in operating rooms, would fail because of the limited space or sensitivity of the target area. With their adaptable and modular architectures, these robots may be able to perform a variety of jobs, including theranostic (diagnostic and therapeutic) tasks. Yet, the main obstacles that prevent feasible robotic systems from making the jump from the *in vitro* stage to the preclinical stage are movement, the supply of power, and localization. Clinical practice might undergo a dramatic change with the introduction of perfect self-powered microrobots capable of being actuated autonomously, targeting a particular place to carry out a specified function via real-time reporting to an external operator. Moreover, the anticipated therapeutic result would be much improved by autonomous robots that can organize into swarm-like assemblies for parallel and dispersed tasks. Miniaturized robots need a completely different approach to design and production than that of today's macroscale manufacture, especially at the submillimeter scale. An interdisciplinary team of robotics researchers, chemists, biomedical engineers, and materials scientists is needed for design and manufacture in this size domain due to the dominance of surface–surface interactions over inertial forces. In conclusion, even the most rudimentary examples of untethered mobile milli/microrobots presented so far have opened up new avenues in biomedical applications, paving the way for minimally invasive and cost-effective strategies that have resulted in rapid patient recovery and improved quality of life.

References and further reading

[1] Wang B, Zhang Y and Zhang L 2018 Recent progress on micro- and nano-robots: towards *in vivo* tracking and localization *Quant. Imaging Med. Surg.* **8** 461

[2] Ngo T D, Kashani A, Imbalzano G, Nguyen K T and Hui D 2018 Additive manufacturing (3D printing): a review of materials, methods, applications and challenges *Composites* **B 15** 172–96

[3] Jiménez M, Romero L, Domínguez I A, Espinosa M D and Domínguez M 2019 Additive manufacturing technologies: an overview about 3D printing methods and future prospects *Complexity* **19** 9656938

[4] Ligon S C, Liska R, Stampfl J, Gurr M and Mülhaupt R 2017 Polymers for 3D printing and customized additive manufacturing *Chem. Rev.* **9** 10212–90

[5] Nelson B J, Kaliakatsos I K and Abbott J J 2010 Microrobots for minimally invasive medicine *Annu. Rev. Biomed. Eng.* **12** 55–85

[6] Sitti M, Ceylan H, Hu W, Giltinan J, Turan M, Yim S and Diller E 2015 Biomedical applications of untethered mobile milli/microrobots *Proc. IEEE* **103** 205–24

[7] Ceylan H, Giltinan J, Kozielski K and Sitti M 2017 Mobile microrobots for bioengineering applications *Lab Chip* **17** 1705–24

[8] Medina-Sanchez M, Xu H and Schmidt O G 2018 Micro- and nano-motors: the new generation of drug carriers *Ther. Deliv.* **9** 303–16

[9] Li J X, de Avila B E F, Gao W, Zhang L F and Wang J 2017 Micro/nanorobots for biomedicine: delivery, surgery, sensing, and detoxification *Sci. Robot.* **2** eaam6431

[10] Sitti M 2018 Miniature soft robots—road to the clinic *Nat. Rev. Mater.* **3** 74–5

[11] Sitti M 2017 *Mobile Microrobotics* (Cambridge, MA: MIT Press)

[12] Carlsen R W and Sitti M 2014 Bio-hybrid cell-based actuators for microsystems *Small* **10** 3831–51

Amokrane W, Belharet K, Souissi M, Grayeli A B and Ferreira A 2018 Macro–micro manipulation platform for inner ear drug delivery *Robot. Auton. Syst.* **107** 10–9

[13] Esteban-Fernández de Ávila B, Angell C, Soto F, Lopez-Ramirez M A, Báez D F, Xie S, Wang J and Chen Y 2016 Acoustically propelled nanomotors for intracellular siRNA delivery *ACS Nano* **10** 4997–5005

[14] Lee S, Kim S, Kim S, Kim J-Y, Moon C, Nelson B J and Choi H 2018 A capsule-type microrobot with pick-and-drop motion for targeted drug and cell delivery *Adv. Health. Mater.* **7** 1700985

[15] Yasa I C, Tabak A F, Yasa O, Ceylan H and Sitti M 2019 3D-printed microrobotic transporters with recapitulated stem cell niche for programmable and active cell delivery *Adv. Funct. Mater.* **0** 1808992

[16] Wei X, Beltrán-Gastélum M, Karshalev E, Esteban-Fernández de Ávila B, Zhou J, Ran D, Angsantikul P, Fang R H, Wang J and Zhang L 2019 Biomimetic micromotor enables active delivery of antigens for oral vaccination *Nano Lett.* **19** 1914–21

[17] Fernandes R and Gracias D H 2009 Toward a miniaturized mechanical surgeon *Mater. Today* **12** 14–20

[18] Yu C, Kim J, Choi H, Choi J, Jeong S, Cha K, Park J-O and Park S 2010 Novel electromagnetic actuation system for three-dimensional locomotion and drilling of intravascular microrobot *Sensors Actuators* A **161** 297–304
[19] Jeong S, Choi H, Go G, Lee C, Lim K S, Sim D S, Jeong M H, Ko S Y, Park J-O and Park S 2016 Penetration of artificial arterial thromboembolism in a live animal using an intravascular therapeutic microrobot system *Med. Eng. Phys.* **38** 403–10
[20] Magdanz V, Sanchez S and Schmidt O G 2013 Development of a sperm-flagella driven micro-bio-robot *Adv. Mater.* **25** 6581–88
[21] Stanisz M, Klapiszewski and Jesionowski T 2020 Recent advances in the fabrication and application of biopolymer-based micro- and nanostructures: a comprehensive review *Chem. Eng. J.* **1** 125409
[22] Guo Z, Dong L, Xia J, Mi S and Sun W 2021 3D printing unique nanoclay-incorporated double-network hydrogels for construction of complex tissue engineering scaffolds *Adv. Healthcare Mater.* **10** 2100036
[23] Abedi F, Ghandforoushan P, Adeli F, Yousefnezhad M, Mohammadi A, Moghaddam S V and Davaran S 2023 Development of stimuli-responsive nanogels as drug carriers and their biomedical application in 3D printing *Mater. Today Chem.* **1** 101372
[24] Ćurić L *et al* 2023 Development of a novel NiCu nanoparticle-loaded polysaccharide-based hydrogel for 3D printing of customizable dressings with promising cytotoxicity against melanoma cells *Mater. Today Bio* **1** 100770
[25] Ma K Y, Chirarattananon P, Fuller S B and Wood R J 2013 Controlled flight of a biologically inspired, insect-scale robot *Science* **340** 603–7
[26] Diller E, Zhuang J, Lum G Z, Edwards M R and Sitti M 2014 Continuously distributed magnetization profile for millimeter-scale elastomeric undulatory swimming *Appl. Phys. Lett.* **104** 174101
[27] Diller E and Sitti M 2014 Three-dimensional programmable assembly by untethered magnetic robotic micro-grippers *Adv. Funct. Mater.* **24** 4397–404
[28] Tassioglou S, Diller E, Guven S, Sitti M and Demirci U Untethered micro-robotic coding of three-dimensional material composition *Nat. Commun.* **5** 3124
[29] Zhou Y, Regnier S and Sitti M 2014 Rotating magnetic miniature swimming robots with multiple flexible flagella *IEEE Trans. Robot* **30** 3–13
[30] Ghane N, Beigi M H, Labbaf S, Nasr-Esfahani M H and Kiani A 2020 Design of hydrogel-based scaffolds for the treatment of spinal cord injuries *J. Mater. Chem.* **B***8 10712–38*
[31] Schmidt B V 2022 Multicompartment hydrogels *Macromol. Rapid Commun.* **43** 2100895
[32] Zhu Z, Chen T, Zhu Y, Huang F, Mu K, Si T and Xu R X 2023 Programmable pulsed aerodynamic printing for multi-interface composite manufacturing *Matter* **7** 2034–51
[33] Kapoor D N, Bhatia A, Kaur R, Sharma R, Kaur G and Dhawan S 2015 PLGA: a unique polymer for drug delivery *Therap. Deliv.* **6** 41–58
[34] Behkam B and Sitti M 2007 Bacterial flagella-based propulsion and on/off motion control of microscale objects *Appl. Phys. Lett.* **90** 023902
[35] Yesin K B 2006 Modeling and control of untethered bio micro-robots in a fluidic environment using electromagnetic fields *Int. J. Robot. Res.* **25** 527–36
[36] Peyer K E, Tottori S, Qiu F, Zhang L and Nelson B J 2013 Magnetic helical micromachines *Chemistry* **19** 28–38
[37] Martel S, Tremblay c c, Ngakeng S and Langlois G 2006 Controlled manipulation and actuation of micro-objects with magnetotactic bacteria *Appl. Phys. Lett.* **289** 233904

[38] Frutiger D R, Vollmers K, Kratochvil B E and Nelson B J 2009 Small, fast, under control: wireless resonant magnetic micro-agents *Int. J. Robot Res.* **29** 613–36

[39] Urso M and Pumera M 2022 Micro-and nanorobots meet DNA *Adv. Funct. Mater.* 2200711

[40] Jiang G L 2010 Development of rolling magnetic micro-robots *J. Micromech. Microeng.* **20** 085042

[41] Pelrine R 2012 Diamagnetically levitated robots: an approach to massively parallel robotic systems with unusual motion properties *Proc. 2012 IEEE Int. Conf. Robot. Automation (ICRA) (St. Paul, MN, USA)* 739–44

[42] Snezhko A and Aranson I S 2011 Magnetic manipulation of self-assembled colloidal asters *Nat. Mater.* **10** 698–703

[43] Vikram Singh A and Sitti M Targeted drug delivery and imaging using mobile milli/microrobots: a promising future towards theranostic pharmaceutical design *Curr. Pharm. Design.* **1** 1418–28

[44] Fluckiger M and Nelson B J 2007 Ultrasound emitter localization in heterogeneous media *Proc. 29th Annu. Int. Conf. IEEE Eng. Medicine Biology Society (Lyon, France)* 2867–70

[45] Rubin J M 2006 Sonographic elasticity imaging of acute and chronic deep venous thrombosis in humans *J. Ultrasound Med.* 1179–86

[46] Sitti M, Ceylan H, Hu W, Giltinan J, Turan M, Yim S and Diller E 2015 Biomedical applications of untethered mobile milli/microrobots *Proc. IEEE* **103** 205–24

[47] Sadelli L, Fruchard M and Ferreira A 2017 2D observer-based control of a vascular microrobot *IEEE Trans. Autom. Control* **62** 2194–206

[48] Sliker L, Ciuti G, Rentschler M and Menciassi A 2015 Magnetically driven medical devices: a review *Exp. Rev. Med. Devices* **2** 737–52

[49] Than T D, Alici G, Zhou H and Li W 2012 A review of localization systems for robotic endoscopic capsules *IEEE Trans. Biomed. Eng.* **59** 2387–99

[50] Umay I, Fidan B and Barshan B 2017 Localization and tracking of implantable biomedical sensors *Sensors* **17** 583

[51] Than T D, Alici G, Zhou H and Li W 2012 A review of localization systems for robotic endoscopic capsules *IEEE Trans. Biomed. Eng.* **18** 2387–99

[52] Chen G, Wang H, Chen K, Li Z, Song Z, Liu Y, Chen W and Knoll A 2020 A survey of the four pillars for small object detection: multiscale representation, contextual information, super-resolution, and region proposal *IEEE Trans. Syst., Man, Cybernet.: Syst.* **52** 936–53

[53] Ergeneman O, Dogangil G, Kummer M P, Abbott J J, Naseeruddin M K and Nelson B J 2008 A magnetically controlled wireless optical oxygen sensor for intraocular measurements *IEEE Sens. J.* **8** 29–37

[54] Zhang A, Jung K, Li A, Liu J and Boyer C 2019 Recent advances in stimuli-responsive polymer systems for remotely controlled drug release *Prog. Polym. Sci.* **1** 101164

[55] Li Z, Ye E, Lakshminarayanan R and Loh X J 2016 Recent advances in using hybrid nanocarriers in remotely controlled therapeutic delivery *Small* **12** 4782–806

[56] Said S S, Campbell S and Hoare T 2019 Externally addressable smart drug delivery vehicles: current technologies and future directions *Chem. Mater.* **31** 4971–89

[57] Pao Y H and Rentzias P 1965 Laser-induced production of free radicals in organic compounds *Appl. Phys. Lett.* **6** 93–5

[58] Fang F, Aabith S, Homer-Vanniasinkam S and Tiwari M K 2017 *In 3D Printing in Medicine* ed D M Kalaskar (Cambridge: Woodhead Publishing) 9 167–206

[59] Singh A V, Ansari M H, Laux P and Luch A 2019 Micro-nanorobots: important considerations when developing novel drug delivery platforms *Exp. Opin. Drug Deliv.* **2** 1259–75
[60] Delaporte P and Allowance A P J O 2016 Laser-induced forward transfer: a high-resolution additive manufacturing technology *Opt. Laser Technol.* **78** 33–41
[61] Visser C 2015 Toward 3D printing of pure metals by laser-induced forward transfer *Avometer* **27** 4087–92
[62] Bullock A B and Bolton P R 2006 Laser-induced back ablation of aluminum thin films using picosecond laser pulses *J. Appl. Phys.* **85** 460–5
[63] Luo J, Pohl R, Lehua Q I, Römer G-W, Sun C, Lohse D and Visser C W 2017 Printing functional 3D microdevices by laser-induced forward transfer *Small* **13** 1602553
[64] Ouyang Y, Huang G, Cui J, Zhu H, Yan G and Mei Y 2022 Advances and challenges of hydrogel materials for robotic and sensing applications *Chem. Mater.* **18** 9307–28
[65] Gu D D, Meiners W, Wissenbach K and Poprawe R 2012 Laser additive manufacturing of metallic components: materials, processes and mechanisms *Int. Mater. Rev.* **57** 133–64
[66] Apsite I, Salehi S and Ionov L 2021 Materials for smart soft actuator systems *Chem. Rev.* **27** 1349–415
[67] Goodridge R D 2011 Processing of a polyamide-12/carbon nanofiber composite by laser sintering *Polym. Test.* **30** 94–100
[68] Wang X, Jiang M, Zhou Z, Gou J and Hui D 2017 3D printing of polymer matrix composites: a review and prospective *Composites* B **110** 442–58
[69] Mehta J L, Calcaterra G and Bassareo P P 2020 COVID-19, thromboembolic risk, and Virchow's triad: lesson from the past *Clin. Cardiol.* **43** 1362–7
[70] Kadara R O, Jenkinson N, Li B, Church K H and Banks C E 2008 Manufacturing electrochemical platforms: direct-write dispensing versus screen printing *Electrochem. Commun.* **10** 1517–9
[71] De Cannière D, Jansens J L, Goldschmidt-Clermont P, Barvais L, Decroly P and Stoupel E 2001 Combination of minimally invasive coronary bypass and percutaneous transluminal coronary angioplasty in the treatment of double-vessel coronary disease: two-year follow-up of a new hybrid procedure compared with 'on-pump' double bypass grafting *Am. Heart J.* **1** 563–70
[72] Shirazi S F S 2015 A review on powder-based additive manufacturing for tissue engineering: selective laser sintering and inkjet 3D printing *Sci. Technol. Adv. Mater.* **16** 033502
[73] Bakhai A, Hill R A, Dundar Y, Dickson R C and Walley T 2005 Percutaneous transluminal coronary angioplasty with stents versus coronary artery bypass grafting for people with stable angina or acute coronary syndromes *Cochrane Database Syst. Rev.*
[74] De Gans B J, Duineveld P C and Schubert U S 2004 Inkjet printing of polymers: state of the art and future developments *Adv. Mater.* **16** 203–13
[75] Miloro P, Sinibaldi E, Menciassi A and Dario P 2012 Removing vascular obstructions: A challenge, yet an opportunity for interventional microdevices *Biomed. Microdevices* **14** 511–32
[76] Farina L, Nissenbaum Y, Cavagnaro M and Goldberg S N 2018 Tissue shrinkage in microwave thermal ablation: comparison of three commercial devices *Int. J. Hyperthermia* **19** 382–91
[77] Gregory D A, Zhang Y, Smith P J, Zhao X and Ebbens S J 2016 Reactive inkjet printing of biocompatible enzyme powered silk micro-rockets *Small* **12** 4048–55

[78] Jean B and Bende T 2003 Mid-IR laser applications in medicine *Solid-State Mid-Infrared Laser Sources* (Berlin: Springer) Topics in Applied Physics 89 530–65
[79] Raman R 2016 Bioprinting: high-resolution projection micro stereolithography for patterning of neo vasculature *Adv. Healthc. Mater.* **5** 622
[80] Hwang S, Reyes E I, Moon K S, Rumpf R C and Kim N S 2015 Thermo-mechanical characterization of metal/polymer composite filaments and printing parameter study for fused deposition modeling in the 3D printing process *J. Electron. Mater.* **44** 771–7
[81] Fu D, Wang Z, Tu Y and Peng F 2021 Interactions between biomedical micro-/nano-motors and the immune molecules, immune cells, and the immune system: challenges and opportunities *Adv. Healthcare Mater.* **10** 2001788
[82] Rahimi E, Sanchis-Gual R, Chen X, Imani A, Gonzalez-Garcia Y, Asselin E, Mol A, Fedrizzi L, Pané S and Lekka M 2023 Challenges and strategies for optimizing corrosion and biodegradation stability of biomedical micro-and nanoswimmers: a review *Adv. Funct. Mater.* **12** 2210345
[83] Roels E 2020 Additive manufacturing for self-healing soft robots *Soft Robot* **7** 711–23
[84] Sun H C M, Liao P, Wei T, Zhang L and Sun D 2020 Magnetically powered biodegradable microswimmers *Micromachines* **11** 404
[85] Ng W M, Che H X, Guo C, Liu C, Low S C, Chieh Chan D J, Mohamud R and Lim J 2018 Artificial magnetotaxis of microbot: magnetophoresis versus self-swimming *Langmuir* **8** 7971–80
[86] Lauga E, DiLuzio W R, Whitesides G M and Stone H A 2006 Swimming in circles: motion of bacteria near solid boundaries *Biophys. J.* **90** 400–12
[87] Bunea A I 2021 Light-powered microrobots: challenges and opportunities for hard and soft responsive microswimmers *Adv. Intell. Syst.* **3** 2000256
[88] Chatzipirpiridis G, Avilla E, Ergeneman O, Nelson B J and Pané S 2014 Electroforming of magnetic microtubes for micro-robotic applications *IEEE Trans. Magn.* **50** 1–3
[89] Lee H, Kim D I, Kwon S h and Park S 2021 Magnetically actuated drug delivery helical microrobot with magnetic nanoparticle retrieval ability *ACS Appl. Mater. Interfaces* **13** 19633–47
[90] Medina-Sánchez M, Schwarz L, Meyer A K, Hebenstreit F and Schmidt O G 2016 Cellular cargo delivery: toward assisted fertilization by sperm-carrying micromotors *Nano Lett.* **16** 555–61
[91] Cerritelli F, Frasch M G, Antonelli M C, Viglione C, Vecchi S, Chiera M and Manzotti A 2021 A review on the vagus nerve and autonomic nervous system during fetal development: searching for critical windows *Front. Neurosci.* **20** 721605
[92] Tamriel M, Dabbagh S R and Tassioglou S 2021 Hemp-based microfluidics *Micromachines* **12** 182
[93] Bhagirath A Y, Medapati M R, de Jesus V C, Yadav S, Hinton M, Dakshinamurti S and Atukorallaya D 2021 Role of maternal infections and inflammatory responses on craniofacial development *Front. Oral Health* **6** 735634
[94] Vartholomeos P, Bergeles C, Qin L and Dupont P E 2013 An MRI-powered and controlled actuator technology for tetherless robotic interventions *Int. J. Robot. Res.* **32** 1536–52
[95] Pouponneau P, Bringout G and Martel S 2014 Therapeutic magnetic microcarriers guided by magnetic resonance navigation for enhanced liver chemoembolization: a design review *Ann. Biomed. Eng.* **42** 929–39

[96] Ceylan H, Yasa I C, Kilic U, Hu W and Sitti M 2019 Translational prospects of untethered medical microrobots *Prog. Biomed. Eng.* **6** 012002
[97] Erin O, Giltinan J, Tsai L and Sitti M 2017 Design and actuation of a magnetic millirobot under a constant unidirectional magnetic field *2017 IEEE Int. Conf. on Robotics and Automation (ICRA) (IEEE)* 3404–10
[98] Ostrem J L, Ziman N, Galifianakis N B, Starr P A, Luciano M S, Katz M, Racine C A, Martin A J, Markun L C and Larson P S 2016 Clinical outcomes using Clear Point interventional MRI for deep brain stimulation lead placement in Parkinson's disease *Neurosurgeon* **124** 908–16
Abbott J J, Peyer K E, Lagomarsino M C, Zhang L, Dong L, Kaliakatsos I K and Nelson B J 2009 How should microrobots swim? *Int. J. Robot. Res.* **28** 1434–47
[99] Formaggia L, Quarteroni A and Veneziani A (ed) 2010 *Cardiovascular Mathematics: Modeling and Simulation of the Circulatory System* (Berlin: Springer Science & Business Media) p 27
[100] Lee S, Lee S, Kim S, Yoon C-H, Park H J, Kim J Y and Choi H 2018 Fabrication and characterization of a magnetic drilling actuator for navigation in a three-dimensional phantom vascular network *Sci. Rep.* **8** 3691
[101] Zhang L, Abbott J J, Dong L, Kratochvil B E, Bell D and Nelson B J 2009 Artificial bacterial flagella: fabrication and magnetic control *Appl. Phys. Lett.* **94** 064107
[102] Huang H W, Sakar M S, Petruska A J, Pane S and Nelson B J 2016 Soft micromachines with programmable motility and morphology *Nat. Commun.* **7** 12263
[103] Liu Y, Jiang P, Capkova K, Xue D, Ye L, Sinha S C, Mackman N, Janda K D and Liu C 2011 Tissue factor–activated coagulation cascade in the tumor microenvironment is critical for tumor progression and an effective target for therapy *Cancer Res.* **15** 6492–502
[104] Lum G Z, Ye Z, Dong X, Marvi H, Erin O, Hu W and Sitti M 2016 Shape-programmable magnetic soft matter *Proc. Natl Acad. Sci. USA* **113** E6007–15
[105] Schmidt C K, Medina-Sánchez M, Edmondson R J and Schmidt O G 2020 Engineering microrobots for targeted cancer therapies from a medical perspective *Nat. Commun.* **5** 5618
[106] Vannozzi L, Yasa I C, Ceylan H, Menciassi A, Ricotti L and Sitti M 2018 Self-folded hydrogel tubes for implantable muscular tissue scaffolds *Macromol. Biosci.* **18** 1700377
[107] Rahman M and Rahaman M 2015 A review on high-Tc superconductors and their principal applications *J. Adv. Phys.* **4** 87–100
[108] Ceylan H, Yasa I C, Kilic U, Hu W and Sitti M 2019 Translational prospects of untethered medical microrobots *Prog. Biomed. Eng.* **16** 012002
[109] Gao C, Wang Y, Ye Z, Lin Z, Ma X and He Q 2021 Biomedical micro-/nanomotors: from overcoming biological barriers to *in vivo* imaging *Adv. Mater.* **2** 2000512
[110] Zhou D, Wang C, Hert A, Yan L, Dou B and Ouyang L 2023 3D printing of multicomponent hydrogels for biomedical applications *Multicomponent Hydrogels: Smart Materials for Biomedical Applications* (London: The Royal Society of Chemistry) 22 231–87
[111] Ahmed D, Lu M, Nourhani A, Lammert P E, Stratton Z, Muddana H S, Crespi V H and Huang T J 2015 Selectively manipulable acoustic-powered microswimmers *Sci. Rep.* **5** 9744
[112] Ahmed D, Dillinger C, Hong A and Nelson B J 2017 Artificial acoustic-magnetic soft micro swimmers *Adv. Mater. Technol.* **2** 1700050
[113] Tajes M, Ramos-Fernández E, Weng-Jiang X, Bosch-Morato M, Guivernau B, Eraso-Pichot A, Salvador B, Fernandez-Busquets X, Roquer J and Munoz F J 2014 The blood–

brain barrier: structure, function and therapeutic approaches to cross it *Mol. Membr. Biol.* **1** 152–67
[114] Kaynak M, Ozcelik A, Nourhani A, Lammert P E, Crespi V H and Huang T J 2017 Acoustic actuation of bioinspired micro swimmers *Lab Chip* **17** 395–400
[115] 2017 *Smith's Anaesthesia for Infants and Children* ed P J Davis, J H Marcy and F P Cladis (Amsterdam: Elsevier) 9th edn
[116] Zeng H, Wasylczyk P, Parmeggiani C, Martella D, Burresi M and Wiersma D S 2015 Light-fuelled microscopic walkers *Adv. Mater.* **27** 3883–7
[117] Palagi S *et al* 2016 Structured light enables biomimetic swimming and versatile locomotion of photo-responsive soft microrobots *Nat. Mater.* **15** 647–53
[118] Rahman M A, Cheng J, Wang Z and Ohta A T 2017 Cooperative micromanipulation using the independent actuation of fifty microrobots in parallel *Sci. Rep.* **7** 3278
[119] Sridhar V, Park B-W and Sitti M 2018 Light-driven Janus hollow mesoporousTiO_2–Au micro swimmers *Adv. Funct. Mater.* **28** 1704902
[120] Soto F, Karshalev E, Zhang F, Esteban Fernandez de Avila B, Nourhani A and Wang J 2021 Smart materials for microrobots *Chem. Rev.* **122** 5365–403
[121] Zhao Y, Sakai F, Su L, Liu Y, Wei K, Chen G and Jiang M Progressive macromolecular self-assembly: from biomimetic chemistry to bio-inspired materials *Adv. Mater.* **25** 5215–56
[122] Li W, Palis H, Mérindol R, Majimel J, Ravaine S and Duguet E 2020 Colloidal molecules and patchy particles: complementary concepts, synthesis and self-assembly *Chem. Soc. Rev.* 1955–76
[123] van Dommelen R, Fanzio P and Sasso L 2018 Surface self-assembly of colloidal crystals for micro- and nano-patterning *Adv. Colloid Interface Sci.* 97–114
[124] Gröschel A H and Müller A H 2015 Self-assembly concepts for multicompartment nanostructures *Nanoscale* 11841–76
[125] Li W, Palis H, Mérindol R, Majimel J, Ravaine S and Duguet E 2020 Colloidal molecules and patchy particles: Complementary concepts, synthesis and self-assembly *Chem. Soc. Rev.* **49** 1955–76
[126] van Dommelen R, Fanzio P and Sasso L 2018 Surface self-assembly of colloidal crystals for micro- and nano-patterning *Adv. Colloid Interface Sci.* **251** 97–114
[127] Wang B, Kostarelos K, Nelson B J and Zhang L 2021 Trends in micro-/nanorobotics: materials development, actuation, localization, and system integration for biomedical applications *Adv. Mater.* **33** 2002047
[128] Ceylan H, Yasa I C, Kilic U, Hu W and Sitti M 2019 Translational prospects of untethered medical microrobots *Prog. Biomed. Eng.* **1** 012002
[129] Carlsen R W and Sitti M 2014 Bio-hybrid cell-based actuators for microsystems *Small* **10** (**19**) 3831–51
[130] Ozturk C, Guttman M, McVeigh E R and Lederman R J 2005 Magnetic resonance imaging–guided vascular interventions *Topics in Magnetic Resonance Imaging: TMRI* **16** 369
[131] Krieger A 2009 *Advances in Magnetic Resonance Image Guided Robotic Intervention* Johns Hopkins University
[132] Yang Z, Yang H, Cao Y, Cui Y and Zhang L 2023 Magnetically actuated continuum medical robots: a review *Adv. Intell. Syst.* **5** 2200416
[133] Linte C A, Davenport K P, Cleary K, Peters C, Vosburgh K, Navab N, Jannin P, Peters T M, Holmes D R and Robb R A 2013 On mixed reality environments for minimally invasive

therapy guidance: systems architecture, successes and challenges in their implementation from laboratory to clinic *Comput. Med. Imaging Graph.* **37** 83–97

[134] Zhang J 2021 Evolving from laboratory toys towards life-savers: small-scale magnetic robotic systems with medical imaging modalities *Micromachines* **12** 1310

[135] Kikinis R, Pieper S D and Vosburgh K G 2013 3D slicer: a platform for subject-specific image analysis, visualization, and clinical support *Intraoperative Imaging and Image-Guided Therapy* (New York: Springer) 277–89

[136] Le Doussal P and Sen P N 1992 Decay of nuclear magnetization by diffusion in a parabolic magnetic field: An exactly solvable model *Phys. Rev.* B **46** 3465

[137] Kapoor S, Opneja A and Nayak L 2018 The role of neutrophils in thrombosis *Thromb. Res.* **170** 87–96

[138] Engelmann B and Massberg S 2013 Thrombosis as an intravascular effector of innate immunity *Nat. Rev. Immunol.* **13** 34–45

[139] Peyer K E, Zhang L and Nelson B J 2013 Bio-inspired magnetic swimming microrobots for biomedical applications *Nanoscale* **5** 1259–72

[140] Hou Y, Wang H, Fu R, Wang X, Yu J, Zhang S, Huang Q, Sun Y and Fukuda T 2023 A review on microrobots driven by optical and magnetic fields *Lab Chip* **23** 848–68

[141] Palagi S and Fischer P 2018 Bioinspired microrobots *Nat. Rev. Mater.* **3** 113–24

[142] Li S, Bai H, Shepherd R F and Zhao H 2019 2014 Bio-inspired design and additive manufacturing of soft materials, machines, robots, and haptic interfaces *Angew. Chem. Int. Ed.* **58** 11182–204

[143] Yu J, Yang L and Zhang L 2018 Pattern generation and motion control of a vortex-like paramagnetic nanoparticle swarm *Int. J. Robot. Res.* **37** 912–30

[144] Sui W, Guo S, Zheng L, An R and Tendeng A 2020 Development of the insect-inspired biomimetic underwater microrobot for a father–son robot system *2020 IEEE Int. Conf. on Mechatronics and Automation (ICMA)* 13 862–6

[145] Blattner M M, Sumikawa D A and Greenberg R M 1989 Earcons and icons: Their structure and common design principles *Hum.–Comput. Interact.* **4** 11–44

[146] De Bot K 2020 A bilingual production model: Levelt's' speaking model adapted *The Bilingualism Reader* **24** 384–404

[147] Marzo A, Seah S A, Drinkwater B W, Sahoo D R, Long B and Subramanian S 2015 Holographic acoustic elements for manipulation of levitated objects *Nat. Commun.* **6** 8661

[148] Ceylan H, Yasa I C, Kilic U, Hu W and Sitti M 2019 Translational prospects of untethered medical microrobots *Prog. Biomed. Eng.* **13** 1602553

[149] Athanassiadis A G, Ma Z, Moreno-Gomez N, Melde K, Choi Goyal R and Fischer P 2021 Ultrasound-responsive systems as components for smart materials *Chem. Rev.* **122** 5165–208

[150] Leijten J *et al* 2017 Spatially and temporally controlled hydrogels for tissue engineering *Mater. Sci. Eng.: R: Rep.* **11** 1–35

Rishabha Malviya, Deepika Yadav, Sonali Sundram, Seifedine Kadry and Gurvinder Singh Virk

Chapter 11

Revolutionizing cancer treatment using micro/nanorobotic devices

Nanotechnology and microfabrication techniques are crucial to the creation of innovative tools for the treatment of human illness. The increasing focus on micro-/nanorobots stems from their promising outcomes *in vivo* and preclinical studies, which have led to their potential utilization in personalized and precise remedial assessment, monitoring, medicine delivery, and surgical procedures. The exploration of MNR-based technologies for the precise administration of medication to particular organs and cells is an emerging and highly encouraging field of medical research. Considerable progress has been made in augmenting the functionalities of small-scale MNRs to meet the requirements of biological applications, mostly due to several scientific advancements in development, manufacture, and operational technology. This chapter reviews a range of nanoscale devices, such as nanoswimmers, nanoengines, 3D-motion nanomachines, biologically inspired microbots, nanofish, and nanorockets. It provides a historical account of the creation of these devices and explores their possible applications in medicine for future generations. It discusses the healing possibilities offered by advanced technological devices in many contexts. We discuss the ways in which the quick development of these innovative gadgets for medication delivery applications has affected society. In addition, we also discuss the existing obstacles and primary impediments that must be addressed in the processes of manufacture, scaling up, and clinical translation. The emphasis is on ensuring patient safety and implementing personalized healthcare techniques, which in turn require the creation of secure and inventive materials. Due to the novelty of MNRs, researchers must first ensure that they are ethically sound before contemplating clinical studies of their behavior, function, biocompatibility, toxicity, biodistribution, and effectiveness. The burgeoning possibilities for magnetic nanorobots as prospective medicinal instruments for diverse biological applications are steadily expanding, notwithstanding the nascent stage of this science.

doi:10.1088/978-0-7503-6019-7ch11

11.1 Introduction

Manipulatable at the micrometer scale and the nanometer scale, respectively, microrobots and nanorobots have found applications across disciplines and are of particular interest in the medical area. Because of their compact size, these tools may be employed in healthcare settings instead of invasive techniques such as surgery or common chemical or radiation treatments [1]. They reduce the potential risks of disease, complications, and negative consequences and shorten recuperation times for patients [2–4]. They have several additional uses in the biomedical lab, including genetic and tissue engineering, imaging, and research into the characteristics of biological fluids [5–7]. Nevertheless, their diminutive stature also restricts the range of possible power supply and manipulation mechanisms, and onboard energy storage and conversion present several conceptual challenges. Numerous academic studies have recently been published, offering a comprehensive examination of the diverse methodologies employed in the manipulation and actuation of milli/micro/nanorobots. These approaches encompassed chemically powered motors, acoustic propellers, and ultrasonic energy. In addition, these evaluations have investigated the wide-ranging applications of these technologies, including drug delivery, precision surgery, detection, and the process of detoxification [4, 8–12]. While some of the papers presented here focus specifically on actuator methods [13], others present a concise summary of the diverse array of microscale and nanoscale technologies and millimeter-scale robots available, each with its own set of actuation options. This chapter primarily concentrates on magnetic-field-actuated microscale and nanoscale robots, providing a comprehensive synopsis of their actuation methods and discussing their potential applications in the area of biomedicine. When the amplitude of a magnetic field is less than three teslas (T), the body is transparent to magnetic fields, making its application in biomedical manipulation advantageous [14].

Magnetized nanoparticles (MNPs) have been widely employed in the initial healthcare implementations of magnetized nanotechnology [14, 15]. Their modulation is predominantly contingent upon the response of magnetized substances to magnetic field gradients (figure 11.1). Their numerous applications include the labeling of cells, the magnetic segregation of chemicals for laboratory synthesis and analysis, image processing, electromagnetic medication targeting, the removal of excessive heat, and medical diagnosis [16–19]. Yet, biomedical microrobots are often required to operate in low-Reynolds-number fluidic settings to carry out their duties. Because of their diminutive size, they are subject to significant drag forces and inertial vacuum under such conditions. The utilization of electromagnetic gradients for propulsion under such circumstances may lead to imprecise control and erratic mobility [18]. As a result, it is imperative to improve actuation methods and enhance propulsion efficacy beyond the conventional utilization of electromagnetic differences for manipulation.

In the last few decades, various actuation techniques have been developed, such as magnetic torque, rotating and oscillating magnetic fields, and others. These approaches have been specifically designed to enhance the propulsion of nanorobots and augment their navigational capabilities in both 2D and 3D [21]. The propulsion mechanisms of many of these devices draw inspiration from nature, such as the

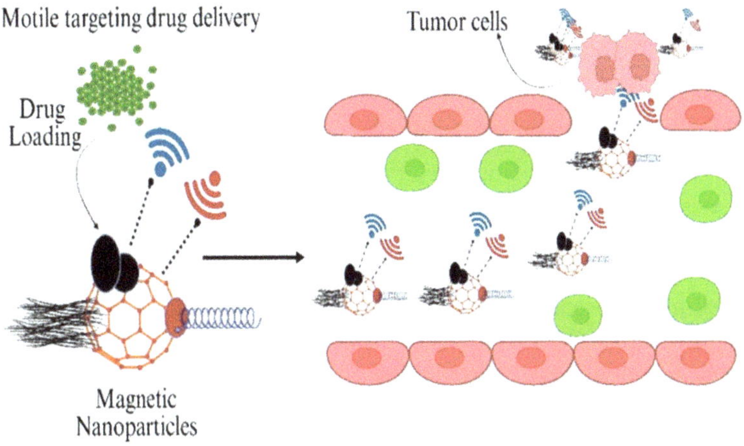

Figure 11.1. Magnetized nanoparticles (MNPs) were extensively utilized in the early instances of magnetized nanotechnology in healthcare. The manipulation of MNPs primarily relies on the reaction of magnetized materials to magnetic field gradients. Reproduced from [20]. CC BY 4.0. © 2022 Zhang, Liu, Guan, and Mou.

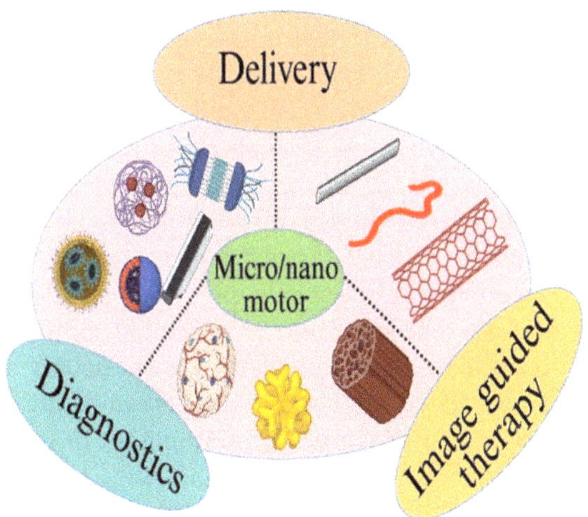

Figure 11.2. An illustration of the contemporary status of medically employed magnetic nanorobots and microrobots, including an analysis of their propulsion systems, manufacturing techniques, existing applications, and technological progress.

hexagonal flagella observed in particular microbes and the tail-like flagella present in spermatozoa as well as in other structures that imitate the underwater movements of salmon within aquatic ecosystems [22–25]. Individuals that can traverse terrain and possess the ability to swim using two arms are among the unique designs that have been suggested in previous studies [11, 26].

The magnetic MNRs used in biomedicine are an innovative technology, and they are still in an early stage of development. The data presented in figure 11.2 describes the contemporary status of medically employed magnetic nanorobots and microrobots, including an analysis of their propulsion systems, manufacturing techniques, existing applications, and technological progress.

11.2 Nano/microrobots for drug delivery

The present state of micro/nanocarriers in the context of the delivery of drugs is limited to passive mass transport and is thus incapable of localized distribution or tissue penetration [27]. Drug delivery vehicles should have certain capabilities, such as propulsion, guided navigation, cargo towing and release, tissue penetration, and specific targeting of disease areas to guarantee the secure and efficient provision of therapeutic payloads to the appropriate locations [28]. These are still problems with existing medication delivery technologies, but MNRs are a promising new class of delivery vehicles that might solve them (figure 11.2). The utilization of motorized MNRs promises to augment the effectiveness of medical procedures and alleviate the widespread negative consequences linked to highly toxic medications. This can be achieved by the rapid and targeted transportation of medicines to diseased areas and the customization of such delivery to individual patients [29].

The medicinal capacities of these microrobots and nanorobots, in addition to their efficiency, have been established in a variety of physiological and laboratory studies [30]. An impermeable membrane was used as a structural framework to fabricate a polymerized nanomotor with multiple layers, which effectively encapsulated a chemotherapeutic agent. The medicated substance was conveyed by the nanomotor to the vicinity surrounding the cancerous cells. A dynamically powered Janus nanomotor was proposed for use as a component of a proactive nanoscale payload transport mechanism to enhance diffusion by a magnitude of 100 compared to the diffusion achieved by passive targeting in the absence of propulsion [31]. Another study introduced a biocompatible pharmaceutical-loaded Janus micromotor made of magnesium. The micromotor exhibited autonomous movement in simulated bodily fluid (SBF) and blood plasma without the need for extra fuel. However, the study also revealed the accidental leakage of the medication payload in response to variations in temperature [32]. A fragment of evidence supported the feasibility of utilizing magnetically micromotor vehicles for targeted drug administration. This was achieved through the use of pharmaceutical-loaded magnetic polymeric particles, which were successfully delivered to HeLa cells [33]. A recent investigation carried out by Walker and his colleagues showed that magnetized micropropellers possessing enzymatic activity exhibited a high degree of effectiveness in penetrating mucin gels [34]. A study conducted by scientists and published in the journal Science demonstrated the potential of ultrasound-induced nanoscale motors to enhance the delivery of medication to cancerous cells. The release of pharmaceuticals was found to be triggered by light stimulation [35]. In the field of magnetoelectric materials in nanororobotic platforms, a recently developed novel design allows the device to perform on-demand magnetoelectrically assisted drug release to cells in addition to being able to be precisely guided towards a targeted location using wireless magnetic fields. This approach has promise for tailored drug delivery applications based on magnetic-field-induced medication delivery [36].

MNRs for drug delivery have a highly robust development pipeline, as evidenced by the large number of new systems now being tested. Within this group, intracellular delivery stands out as a particularly promising field of study; here, nanorobots are used to bypass the cells' membranes and deposit a wide range of medicinal chemicals within them. In one case, ultrasonically driven gold nanowire motors were used to speed up the delivery of siRNA inside living cells by rapidly internalizing and relocating inside cells [37, 38]. These studies demonstrated that the siRNA-loaded nanowires exhibited rapid cellular uptake across different cell lines, significantly enhancing the efficacy and speed of gene suppression in comparison to the performance of immobile nanowires. In addition, the precise transportation of plasmid genetic material to human embryonic kidney cell lines has been achieved through the utilization of magnetic helical microswimmers [39]. Upon contacting the cells, the pDNA-loaded motors discharged their genetic payload.

Most of these investigations were conducted *in vitro*; however, preliminary *in vivo* trials have shown promising outcomes [32–35, 40]. Micro/nanorobotic systems designed for *in vivo* applications have generated significant interest, particularly those whose propulsions are provided by bodily fluids comprising fresh water and gastric acid. Furthermore, in addition to their efficient propulsion capabilities, these motors possess the ability to convey a diverse range of payloads, autonomously and responsively deploy them, and ultimately decompose them into nontoxic compounds. A study was conducted by researchers for the inaugural *in vivo* examination of chemically propelled micromotors. A comprehensive examination was conducted to examine the distribution of motors in the gastrointestinal tract, their ability to retain cargo, and transport it effectively, and their acute toxicity profile in a murine model. The utilization of acid-driven propulsion within the gastric environment resulted in enhanced adherence and prolonged retention of zinc-based micromotors on the gastric mucosa. After dissolving in the stomach acid, the micromotors' bodies released their cargoes on their own. This study demonstrated the ability to accurately position and maintain a micromotor within specific sections of the gastrointestinal (GI) tract of a live mouse [33]. The drive mechanisms described consisted of a cylindrical framework constructed of magnesium and coated with an endoscopic polymeric layer. These motors have the potential to be highly efficient instruments in the field of nanobiotechnology for customized gastrointestinal delivery. The results obtained from *in vivo* experiments demonstrate that these motors are accurately activated within the gastrointestinal tract and are capable of effectively maneuvering through the fluids present in the gastrointestinal tract. Localized tissue absorption and the retention of these motors in certain portions of the gastrointestinal system can be accomplished by selectively activating their propulsion. This can be performed by altering the degree of thickness of the pH-dependent polymeric layer, which does not cause substantial damage. In a recent study, the aforementioned research team demonstrated that micromotors constructed utilizing magnesium can transiently neutralize gastric acid independently. This is achieved by the utilization of efficient chemical propulsion mechanisms, which rapidly deplete protons in localized regions [40]. The findings of experiments conducted using a mouse model confirm that a motor-driven alteration in pH levels can lead to the release of a sensor payload. Micromotors possessing the ability to regulate pH levels have the potential for dual-function activity, simultaneously inhibiting protons and ion-transporting components. These machines do not use fuels that are triggered by external stimuli, including magnetic or auditory fields, and exhibit the potential to be used in various important physiological settings, serving as a valuable alternative to chemically powered motors. Servant *et al* provided a comprehensive description of the *in vivo* imaging and control of a collective of circular microswimmers within deep tissue based on the use of rotating magnetic fields [41]. Fluorescence imaging was used to monitor the microswimmers while they were magnetically guided through the peritoneal cavity of an anesthetized mouse. These findings point to the potential use of magnetic motors of this kind for directing medicine delivery to a specific spot utilizing an external magnetic field. Moreover, it was demonstrated that magneto-aerotactic microorganisms, including the *Magnetococcus marinus* strain MC-1, exhibit potential for the precise transportation of drug-loaded nanoliposomes to hypoxic tumor settings [42]. These bacteria are naturally found swimming in the direction of low oxygen concentrations and local magnetic field lines. Up to 55% of the MC-1 bacteria injected with drug-containing nanoliposomes gained access to hypoxic regions within HCT116 colorectal cancer cells in xenografted tumors in tumor-bearing mice using a magnetic field to direct them to the tumor [43]. The active medicines were shown to penetrate deeper into the xenografted tumors than the controls. These findings point to the possibility that the efficacy of medication-delivering nanocarriers in hypoxic tumor zones might be greatly enhanced by harnessing swarms of magneto-aerotactic microorganisms.

The advancements in micro/nanorobot technology and their potential for *in vivo* delivery have opened up new possibilities for therapeutic uses that surpass the limitations of passive delivery methods. These miniature machines can serve as active transport vehicles, thereby enabling a broader range of therapeutic interventions that were previously unattainable.

11.3 Cancer-targeted drug delivery systems

11.3.1 Enhancing treatment precision using passive drug delivery

In the realm of tumor treatment, the effectiveness of inadvertently targeted drug delivery systems relies heavily on the enhanced permeation and retention (EPR) effect. This consequence is closely associated with the unique pathophysiological features of tumors, the structural characteristics of the nanotechnologies used, and relevant variables associated with blood circulation, such as circulation time and phagocyte degradation [20]. To achieve the desired therapeutic outcome, researchers have developed a diverse array of passive drug delivery systems that are designed according to pharmacological and nanomaterial characteristics that influence the EPR effect. Four primary pathophysiological characteristics are commonly observed throughout the majority of tumors. The observed phenomena are: (i) the occurrence of angiogenesis on a significant scale, (ii) a compromised system of lymphatic circulation and recovery, (iii) elevated manufacture of mediators that increase permeability, and (iv) an atypical vascular structure characterized by poorly aligned endothelial cells. In addition, individuals exhibit compromised function of their angiotensin 2 receptors as well as defects in their smooth muscle barriers. Scientists employ these distinct characteristics of tumors to enhance the effectiveness of personalized medication delivery systems. Furthermore, the physical attributes of the drug, including its dimensions, form, surface charge, and moisture absorption, are all significant factors that contribute to the drug delivery process.

To date, five primary groups of nanocarriers have been identified. The nanoparticles constructed from lipids commonly utilized in scientific research and applications include: (i) lipids in the form of liposomes, (ii) nanostructures composed of polymers such as micelles, which are dendrimers consisting of particulates, (iii) nanomaterials made of carbon, as well as (iv) metal-based and (v) magnetized nanoparticles [44]. The beneficial characteristics of liposomes, which are spherical capsules that undergo self-assembly and can exist as either uniflagellar or multilamellar forms, include the following: (i) the ability to effectively deliver both hydrophilic and hydrophobic therapeutic agents, (ii) the protection of encapsulated pharmaceuticals from unfavorable environmental conditions, and (iii) the potential for functionalization to achieve various benefits such as ligand-mediated particular targeting, structural customization, and an extended duration in the circulation. Micelles made of polymers, which have a size of only 100 nm and a hydrophilic corona, can avoid renal excretion and resist absorption by mononuclear phagocytes under ideal conditions [45]. Dendrimers are polymeric molecules that have well-established host–guest trapping capabilities, definite molecular weights, and a large number of surface functional groups. They are made up of several identically branching monomers that radiate outward from a central point. Carbon nanotubes (CNTs) are a type of carbonaceous miniaturized carrier that can be conceptualized as cylindrical structures formed by rolling up sheets of graphene. CNTs' ability to enter any kind of cell, including those that are notoriously difficult to transfect, is a major plus. To facilitate their conjugation with antibodies, ligands, and medicines of interest, metallic nanoparticles may be produced and modified using a wide range of chemical functional groups. The benefits of these materials have been shown in a variety of biological contexts, including magnetic separation, targeted drug administration, and diagnostic imaging. Nevertheless, their use *in vivo* is constrained by issues of biocompatibility and toxicity. The potential of technology is evident in various domains such as targeted pharmaceutical delivery, the utilization of particles with magnetic properties as contrast materials for diagnostic purposes, as well as their application in the remediation of contaminated water supplies.

Despite the numerous advantages of passively targeted drug delivery systems (PTDDSs) compared to conventional chemotherapeutic drugs, such as prolonged *in vivo* circulation times, decreased absorption by vascular cells and phagocytes, and improved drug efficacy, they still exhibit several limitations and encounter various obstacles that necessitate further investigation for resolution [46].

11.3.2 Enhancing treatment precision using active drug targeting

Actively targeted drug delivery systems (ATDDSs) rely on the coupling of ligands to the pharmaceutical delivery vehicle, which then interacts with particular receptors to achieve specific binding to the intended target cells. ATDDSs have employed a diverse array of ligands, encompassing both smaller molecules (e.g. folic acid; FA) and macromolecules (e.g. peptides) as delineated in the aforementioned list. Consequently, these entities can be regarded as nanocarriers that selectively deliver their cargoes using ligands [47]. The administration of ATDDSs has been shown to enhance the bioavailability of chemotherapeutic agents while concurrently reducing their off-target effects. Sophisticated active drug carriers possess the ability to react to both naturally occurring variables, such as the pH level or hypoxia, as well as external stimuli such as ultrasound imaging, sunlight, warmth, and magnetic fields. This enables the production of a drug delivery system that responds to the surrounding environment or one that administers and transports drugs to specific target locations [48]. Scholars have dedicated significant time and resources to the examination of ATDDSs.

So far, nanomaterial-based targeted drug delivery systems (TDDs) have shown promise as a novel approach to treating cancer. Nanocarriers' potential benefits in reaching tumor tissues and releasing medications steadily and predictably stem from their features. Examples of such features include their nanoscale diameters, which are far smaller than those of conventional particles, resulting in a high surface-to-volume ratio. This ratio is advantageous, as it allows for increased interactions with surrounding molecules. In addition, nanoparticles exhibit favorable drug release patterns, enabling the controlled and targeted delivery of therapeutic agents. Furthermore, nanoparticles can be modified and adapted to suit specific requirements, allowing for precise adjustments to their properties [49–52]. Yet, there are still issues and obstacles with the conventional methods of targeted medication administration. First, the bioenvironment may have an unfavorable effect on nanocarriers by causing them to undergo structural, size, surface property, and charge changes (or even destroying them). Second, accurately evaluating the toxicity of nanocarriers presents challenges due to the multitude of parameters that impact their characterization, including but not limited to their material composition, dimensions, morphology, surface properties (e.g. domain, charge, and permeability), and hydrophobic nature [53]. Third, knowing where they are and where they are distributed in real time is a challenge. Obstacles to their clinical translation include their biostability, their mechanisms of elimination from the human body, and the way the body handles them [54]. Since they rely on passive diffusion and short-range recognition (0.5 nm) to target tumors, the produced PTDDSs and ATDDSs are only effective at hitting their targets to a small degree (a median of 0.7%).

11.3.3 Surgical advancements with micro/nanorobotic assistance

Robotic systems have been developed and used to alleviate the risks and improve the success rate of complicated surgical operations. The discipline of robot-assisted surgery is expanding fast, providing surgeons with new tools and techniques for a wide range of minimally invasive treatments [55, 56]. Little robots have the potential to address a wider range of health issues than their larger counterparts because of their greater mobility and access to anatomical regions that were previously unreachable within human beings.

A lot of hope has been placed on the potential of MNRs to overcome these obstacles and to be used for precise surgical procedures. The application of MNRs in high-precision surgical procedures that are minimally invasive offers notable advantages due to their dimensions, which closely resemble those of the diminutive biological features that they are intended to specifically target [57]. MNRs equipped with microscopic operational components have the ability to access and manipulate intracellular tissues to perform precision surgical procedures. These robotic devices can be driven by a diverse range of energy sources. Microrobots possess a distinct edge over their larger equivalents due to their capability to travel via the most minute blood arteries within the human body and perform cellular-level therapeutic interventions. The development of tetherless microgrippers is a significant milestone on the path to creating fully autonomous robotic instruments for microsurgery [16, 58]. Tissues and cells in inaccessible locations are no obstacle to these portable microgrippers. Traditional microgrippers are limited in size and flexibility because they must be connected to other devices (such as cables or tubes) to receive mechanical or electrical inputs from control systems. Untethered microgrippers often open and close throughout the gripping action, much like their huge tethered counterparts. A set of less invasive microsurgical instruments has been created that includes responsive microgrippers that may be independently triggered by a wide range of environmental conditions [37]. The large-scale manufacture of these microgrippers can be facilitated through the utilization of ordinary layered photolithography, drawing inspiration from the design principles observed in biological appendages. The fingers of these devices are flexibly arranged in many formations encircling the central palm [59]. These soft microgrippers obviate the need for additional tethers by utilizing an inherent self-folding actuator response that is triggered by the surrounding biological environment. The autonomous activation of self-folding microgrippers in certain settings has allowed the microgripper to withdraw from a capillary tube while still holding the collected cells, proving its use for *in vitro* tissue biopsy. Ablation is only one example of how this technology might be used in the medical field [60].

Due to the ability of magnetic fields to permeate dense biological tissues, microrobots that are magnetically activated have shown great promise for *in vivo* minimally invasive surgical procedures. A study has confirmed the efficacy of utilizing an implantable magnetic tubular microrobot to perform surgical procedures in the temporal regions of the human eye [61]. A 23-gauge needle was used to inject the electrochemically synthesized microrobot into the central vitreous fluid of the eye, while an ophthalmoscope and built-in camera were used to observe its progress. An intracranial magnetized microrobot was remotely controlled and moved within the vitreous humor of a live rabbit eye. These magnetic microtubes, or something similar, might be produced and used as implanted devices to target various illnesses in other restricted areas of the human body.

Microrobots powered by ultrasonic actuators have recently emerged as a prominent area of study. Such microrobots are capable of penetrating tissues at an impressive rate. Research has shown that rapid evaporation of a biocompatible fuel (e.g. perfluorocarbon) can activate high-velocity 'bullet-like' propulsion in conjunction with ultrasound [62]. Ultrasound stimulation causes these conically formed tubular microbullets, which carry the fuel source, to travel at rates of over 6 m s^{-1}. Very powerful thrust may be generated at such a high velocity, allowing for the penetration, ablation, and destruction of deeply buried tissue. These extraordinary speeds at which nanobullets may be fired from tubular microscale cannons were achieved by using cannons activated by sound waves to vaporize perfluorocarbon fuel [63]. High-velocity nanobullets might be fired from these micro ballistic instruments, penetrating deeply into diseased tissues. Recent proof-of-concept investigations have shown that unrestrained microscopic nanorobots are capable of performing surgeries at the level of single-cell differentiation. The utilization of minuscule instrumentation in the form of independent and autonomously operated enzymatic InGaAs/GaAs/(Cr)Pt microjets has been documented [64]. Cylindrical structures characterized by dimensions ranging from 280 to 600 nm were propelled within hydrogen peroxide solutions at velocities reaching up to 180 m s^{-1}. The aforementioned tubing possessed the capability to penetrate and integrate with biological material, even at the cellular level, by transforming the rotational energy produced by a chemical reaction into an oscillation simulating that of a corkscrew. However, the aforementioned researchers also reported magnetic microdrills that did not require fuel and could be rolled up; they were operable from a distance using a rotating electromagnetic field. This result implies that the utilization of hydrogen peroxide might not be suitable for applications involving live cells [65]. The performance of self-folding magnetic microtools with cutting edges in drilling and related incision procedures was evaluated in *ex vivo* pig liver tissues. Furthermore, this study demonstrated the efficacy of magnetically accelerated microdaggers in cellular incision and subsequent drug release, which enabled precise and targeted drug administration [66]. The findings of these studies underscore the potential advancements of MNRs in the field of surgical procedures, particularly in achieving precise interventions at the subcellular and molecular levels. The potential of tiny laparoscopic robotic devices can be greatly optimized through a thorough examination of the propulsion procedure, the incorporation of simultaneous pattern recognition and mapping, and the implementation of a reliable control framework. These developments would enable nanorobots to effectively infiltrate and resect tissues as well as detect specific targets.

11.3.4 Robotic biosensing

MNRs have exhibited considerable promise in executing several intricate cellular recognition tasks; therefore, they have the potential to make notable contributions to precise medical diagnostics. The aforementioned promise stems from the unique attributes exhibited by these entities, such as autonomous movement, facile surface modification, and the effective capture and isolation of specific chemicals within intricate biological settings. Synthetic nanomotors equipped with multiple receptors (as shown in figure 11.3) can facilitate the movement of MNRs within a specimen, hence enabling the real-time identification and analysis of macromolecules [12, 14]. Scientists have utilized receptor-functionalized micro/nanomotors to effectively

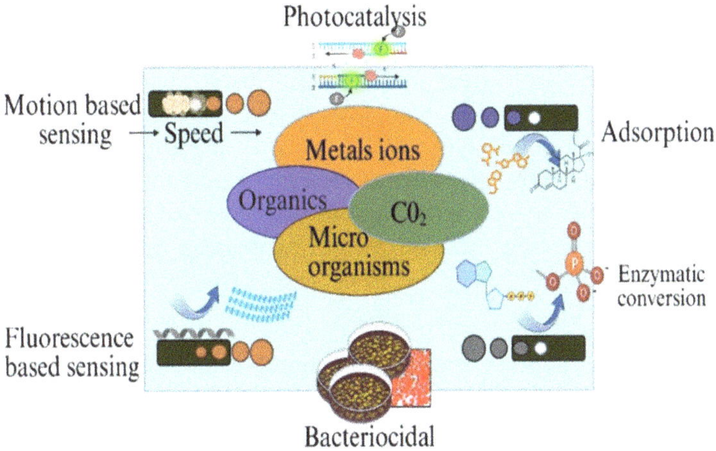

Figure 11.3. The utilization of MNRs for various sensing purposes.

detect and separate biologically relevant targets such as DNA, protein, and cancerous cells in raw body fluids [32, 67–69].

The continual mobility exhibited by customized synthesized motors can significantly enhance the sensitivity and speed of biological testing. The resulting movement facilitates the efficient mixture of solutions in microliter clinical specimens, hence improving the overall performance of test procedures [67]. The precise motion control of such self-propelled nanomotors inside microchannel networks, in addition to their effective cargo towing capacity, might pave the way for novel active-transport-powered medical diagnostic microchips [68]. Several micro- and nanomotors have been designed with receptors to detect and isolate certain analytes. Such research has shown that oligonucleotide-probe functionalized micromotors may efficiently perform DNA hybridization 'on the fly' in complex conditions, enabling the precise and discerning identification of target DNA sequences at concentrations that are as small as nanomolar levels. [69]. A comparable degree of effectiveness was demonstrated by employing tubing microengines customized with aptamers to extract thrombi from biological specimens in a precise and discriminating manner [70]. Cancer cells may be recognized and isolated 'on the fly' through the use of tubular microrockets functionalized with targeting ligands such as antibodies [38]. These micromotors provide enough thrust to propel the trapped target cells through an unmodified biological medium. Lab-on-a-chip diagnostic devices may easily include the micromotor-based target isolation technique, allowing for the integration of autonomous capture, active transport, release, and detection activities inside the devices' many reservoirs and constrained microchannels [68, 71, 72]. Results obtained through the identification of targeted dementia biomarkers demonstrated that the substantial integration brought about by the acceleration of unaltered autonomous propellers significantly increased the specificity of the immunoassay microarray technology [73].

The utilization of tiny robotic devices for intracellular sensing, as well as for the identification and transport of microscopic biological entities in extracellular environments, involves the internalization and mobility of these nanorobots within cells. A novel cellular 'off–on' fluorescence technique was introduced to quantify the naturally occurring levels of target miRNA-21. This strategy involved the application of an ultrasound-propelled nanomotor that was customized with single-stranded DNA (ssDNA) [74]. Dye–ssDNA probes were displaced from the surface. Quenched dye-labeled ssDNA-specific probes recovered their fluorescence quickly when the target miRNA was present. Nanomotor biosensing has the potential to be a useful tool for assessing the single-cell expression of miRNAs in several therapeutic settings.

11.3.5 Enhancing drug delivery with micro/nanorobot mobility

The majority of the current TDDSs rely on the active targeting of drugs using chemical recognition that has a threshold range of 0.5–08 nm, in addition to covert targeting using a phenomenon known as EPR. The efficacy of pharmaceutical administration is a significant concern, as solid tumors only take up approximately 0.7% of nanoparticle doses [75]. The expeditious process of blood vessel formation within tumors, the immune system's mononuclear phagocyte system, and the elimination of malignant tissue through the kidneys all provide significant obstacles in the context of medical treatments. High interstitial fluid pressure, which limits the penetration of medication into tumor tissue; hypoxia, which may restrict certain therapeutic agents; the thick extracellular matrix; and aberrant tumor vasculature all contribute to the challenging tumor environment. Due to these difficulties, successful treatment results are uncommon [76]. One of the hottest topics in tumor treatment is the development of MNR-based 'motile-targeting' drug delivery systems to increase antitumor efficacy while decreasing harm and side effects. Researchers are predicting that microrobot-based mobile microscopic carriers will be able to convey and manage large payloads, such as cells and drug capsules, under complex biological conditions due to their strong propulsive force, precise control of movement, and ability to carry a significant number of drugs [77]. In addition, magnetic nanorobots offer unique advantages in terms of traversing cell-based barriers and facilitating internalization into cells during the administration of drugs. The aforementioned advantages persist even when the magnetic nanorobot dimensions are reduced to the nanoscale range. In addition, magnetic nanorobots experience arbitrary diffusive motions in biological environments, primarily due to the unpredictable Brownian effect that gradually becomes the dominant factor in their motion dynamics [78]. For this reason, the utilization of motile magnetic navigation and resonance has attracted considerable interest as a prospective drug delivery method that has the ability to actively target specific sites.

The insertion of drugs into magnetic nanorods is often achieved via one of three prevalent techniques: post-loading, co-loading, or pre-loading. By considering the specific qualities of a nanocarrier, such as its material, framework, and exterior properties, one can make an informed decision regarding the most effective technique for loading it with medication. The process of loading drugs onto nanocarriers can be achieved using several mechanisms, including adsorption, electrostatic attraction, entanglement, and hydrophobic pressure. This is commonly accomplished via the post-loading technique, which entails the combination of pre-synthesized porous nanocarriers with pharmaceutical solutions [79]. The co-loading strategy involves the combination of medications with polymeric molecules or macromolecules, resulting in the self-assembly of drug conjugates into nanocarriers that are loaded with drugs. During the initial stage of pre-loading, the drug transforms nanoparticles. Subsequently, these small particles are enveloped by a layer of additional materials, resulting in the formation of nanocarriers that are characterized by drug cores and protective shell structures. Pharmaceutical-loaded magnetic nanorods can migrate toward specific locations and achieve targeted drug release in response to either intrinsic stimulation, such as chemotherapy, or external stimuli, including electric fields, magnetic fields, ultrasound imaging, or illumination.

11.3.6 Field-guided micro/nanorobotics

In the context of magnetized miniature robots, the term 'ambient-field-powered' refers to a category of fuel-free magnetized miniature robot that can be activated by an external field, including but not limited to illumination, an ultrasound imaging field, an electric field, or a magnetic field. The advantages of external-field-powered magnetically actuated nanorobots in comparison to chemically powered MNRs include enhanced controllability, an extended operational duration, and reduced adverse unintended effects. These attributes contribute to the heightened potential for the use of magnetically actuated nanorobots in various fields [80].

The principal energy sources of magnetic-field-driven magnetic nanorobots are alternating magnetic fields, including rotating fields. This phenomenon involves the periodic variation of magnetic forces, specifically those that alternate between the 'on' and 'off' states. Magnetic fields can induce two distinct directions of motion in magnetic nanoparticles. Moreover, when subjected to a rotational or fluctuating magnetic field, magnetic nanorods can navigate through fluids that have relatively small Reynolds numbers by undergoing non-reciprocal structural distortion. The rotational movement of a microrobot along its helical axis can be transformed into a translational corkscrew motion, enabling the robot to travel in a direction that is opposed to the rotation of the magnetic field [81]. The side of a magnetic nanoparticle that is in proximity to a wall surface experiences more hydrodynamic drag than the side that is further away. However, the application of magnetic fields can potentially enhance the acceleration of magnetic nanoparticles by generating an asymmetric force field within the surrounding region.

Much interest has been shown in ultrasound, since it is a potent, biocompatible energy source that can be readily accessed in clinical and research settings. A surface standing wave may be produced by an interdigital transducer, whereas an ultrasonic standing wave can be produced using a bulk acoustic wave device. An assessment of an event involving the primary radiation force (PRF) and the resulting secondary radiation force (SRF) can be made if magnetized nanoparticles are exposed to an ultrasound-induced magnetic field. The PRF, which is the predominant force in acoustical waves, is responsible for regulating the motion of magnetic nanorobots. On the other hand, the SRF, although less effective than an axial PRF, regulates the repulsion and attraction between magnetic nanorobots [82]. Three distinct hypothesized methodologies employ ultrasound as a means of propulsion. One proposed phenomenon is the self-acoustophoresis process observed in metallic nanowires. This proposal suggests that randomized unidirectional motion can be induced in nanorods by their inherent asymmetries in a substance or structure when exposed to an ultrasonic field. As evidence for the second process, consider a hollow conical microcannon that was created and filled with silica or fluorescent nanosphere nanobullets. A perfluorocarbon emulsion on the microcannon's inner surface instantly evaporated when subjected to ultrasound. This caused nanobullets to be ejected at high speed, allowing the microcannon to move rapidly. This effect could perhaps be useful for tissue penetration. The final process relates to MNRs that have air bubbles trapped inside them. Acoustic jets may be formed and powered by an applied ultrasonic field. The applications of ultrasonic fields extend beyond the mere propulsion of magnetic nanorobots. They have been utilized to regulate the movement of magnetic nanorobots, such as miniature tubes driven by bubbles and to elicit collective behavior known as swarming [83].

The utilization of luminescence as a sustainable energy resource has been demonstrated by its capacity to initiate molecular nanoreactors, govern physical movement, guide collective behavior, and other related phenomena [84–86]. Three major processes can cause magnetized nanoparticles to spontaneously migrate: light-induced chemical interactions, light-induced body deformation, and light-induced physical processes (such as the photothermal effect, the Marangoni effect, and energy transfer) [87]. Therefore, for light-driven MNRs to achieve movement, they must simultaneously generate a localized nonuniform gradient field or undergo periodic body deformations. The generation of a nonuniform gradient field can be achieved through the utilization of either an irregular light field or a deliberately asymmetrical arrangement. To provide an example, when subjected to ultraviolet (UV) rays, isotropic titanium dioxide (TiO_2) micromotors can be propelled by taking advantage of asymmetric photocatalytic activities and chemical gradients that exist between their illuminated and shaded surfaces [88]. The movement associated with body deformations is a result of the interaction between photoresponsive materials and illumination, which resembles the behaviors observed in naturally occurring microorganisms, such as the metachrony of ciliates, the whole-body deformation of marine phytoplankton, and the rotation of *Escherichia coli*. For instance, the ion concentration of the surrounding medium has been reported in previous studies [89, 90]. The swimming patterns of mimicking morphing microswimmers might vary depending on the arrangement of elements and the luminescent field employed. In the presence of organized monochromatic illumination that exhibited an alternating traveling pattern, it was observed that a microrobot with a straightforward cylindrical shape was capable of generating body deformation that followed the traveling wave pattern. This deformation enabled the microrobot to move in a direction opposite to that of the wave [91].

Magnetic nanorobots can also be propelled by electric fields, utilizing four well-established techniques for achieving this functionality. The first approach involves the application of an alternating current (AC) electric field to generate opposing polarizations in the metallic and dielectric portions of a Janus microparticle. This phenomenon subsequently leads to the propulsion of the microparticle away from the metal side through the utilization of asymmetrical electroosmotic fluxes [92–94]. The second methodology uses the rectification capabilities of diodes to convert an AC electromagnetic field into a direct current (DC) electrical field. This process enables the induction of electrokinetic impulses and the achievement of self-actuation [95]. The third strategy entails the utilization of electromagnetic radiation to induce chemical processes. The last approach employs the Quincke effect. Dielectric micromotors can rotate and move towards a specific destination inside a liquid medium with low conductivity when subjected to a magnetic force produced by an electric current that alternates in direction. The utilization of electric-field-propelled magnetic nanorobots offers enhanced precision and adaptability compared to those of their mechanical counterparts such as electric tweezers. However, the effectiveness of these MNRs is hindered by their limited range of movement and their inability to function optimally in highly ionic biomedia. This restricts their potential applications [96].

11.4 Conclusions and prospects

Throughout the last decade, micro/nanorobotics has developed into an innovative and flexible platform for combining the best features of the fields of nanotechnology and automation studies. As a result, research and development in the field of advanced MNRs have involved the application of a wide array of innovative conceptions and propulsion strategies. MNRs possess several distinct and versatile functions, including rapid motion within intricate biological environments; the ability to generate substantial forces, which allows them to tow large cargos over long distances in a specific direction; straightforward surface functionalization, which allows them to accurately capture and isolate the desired targets; and exceptional biocompatibility, which allows them to operate effectively within living organisms. The healthcare sector has successfully utilized the advantageous characteristics and capacity of MNRs in a wide range of applications. These encompass the extremely sensitive identification of biomolecules, the effective removal of harmful chemicals, the precision delivery of payloads to specific targets, and the accurate execution of procedures at the cellular level. The aforementioned advancements have expanded the applications of micro- and nanorobots beyond their traditional usage in chemical laboratories and test tubes into the domain of operational biological systems. *In vivo*, experiments of this nature play a critical role in the advancement of the clinical application of MNRs.

Micro- and nanorobots' potential in the healthcare sector is still in its infancy. Closing the information gap in nanorobotics has the potential to revolutionize several branches of medicine. More research and development are needed before these small robots can be used to undertake sophisticated surgeries in previously inaccessible areas of the body. To replicate the cognitive abilities exhibited by their biological equivalents, such as microorganisms and molecular machines, future MNRs will require a range of essential characteristics. These include a high degree of mobility, a deformation-resistant framework, adaptability, sustainable operation, precise control, the ability to exhibit group behavior through swarm intelligence, the capacity to perform sophisticated functions, and even the potential for self-evolution and self-replication.

Finding alternative energy sources that are biocompatible and able to power autonomous *in vivo* systems for extended periods is a major problem. While there have been advancements in studying the movement of nanoscale particles in water-based environments utilizing different chemical biofuels and external stimulation, it is necessary to develop novel biofuels and propulsion mechanisms to ensure safe and sustainable functioning within the human body over extended periods. The operational scope of catalytic micromotors is currently limited to laboratory settings due to their sole reliance on hydrogen peroxide as a fuel source. The limited lifespan of micromotors powered by active material propellants (such as magnesium, zinc, aluminum, and calcium carbonate) is primarily attributable to the rapid depletion of their propellant during propulsion. Recent research has shown that enzyme-functionalized nanomotors may be driven by the glucose or urea found in blood. For these enzyme-based motors to be used in the real world, their strength and stability need to be increased. Nanoscale surgery would benefit greatly from the fuel-free and on-demand speed control that magnetic and acoustic nanomotors can offer, making them a promising technology.

Taking nanorobots from their current laboratory setting to living beings will take a lot of work in the future. Viscous biological fluids, such as stomach juices or whole blood, have previously been shown to be no match for the power of MNRs. It is important to take a cautious approach to using such small devices in human tissues and organs, which provide far greater obstacles to mobility. Microswimmers have been driven by a rotating magnetic field as weak as 9 mT and their activation has been effectively achieved within the abdominal cavity of a murine model. Magneto-aerotactic bacteria under a directed magnetic field of just 15 G were able to move into hypoxic areas of tumors. Ultrasound-driven micromotors which have strong 'ballistic' characteristics have been developed, allowing for deep tissue penetration. Nanorobots, due to their diminutive size, may prove to be particularly useful for providing power inside living tissues and organs. Within elastic hyaluronan gels, nanoscale magnetic propellers which possess dimensions comparable to the intervals within the mesh structure of the gel provide a notable benefit in terms of propulsion. Conversely, the movement of larger propellers is impeded. Research findings have shown that nanorobots, due to their nanoscale size and well-optimized design, have great promise for attaining efficient mobility in tissues. Smaller nanorobots have proven successful in penetrating cell membranes and gaining access to the cell inside.

The operational capabilities and cognitive abilities of miniature robotics predominantly hinge upon their material components and surface characteristics, hence rendering the development of nanoscale robotics predominantly challenging within the domains of materials research and interface science. Nanorobots with a biomedical focus are built to operate in settings within living organisms, fluids, and tissues where there is a high probability of unexpected biological occurrences and physiological fluctuations. There is a significant demand for a diverse array of smart materials, including biological components, responsive materials, and soft substances that have the required actuation and can achieve multiple goals without inducing permanent impairments in intricate physiologically relevant biological systems. According to a recent study, changing the rotational trap stiffness may prevent macrophages from ingesting a revolving magnetic microrobot. In contrast, the integration of synthesized nanotechnologies into natural biological materials has the potential to mitigate the adverse effects associated with the phenomenon of immune system evasion and biofouling in intricate bodily fluids and is known to contribute to increased maneuverability and lifespan. For MNRs to be able to operate successfully in environments where circumstances are constantly changing, their construction must use responsive materials. Nanorobots that are hard and rigid pose a risk to the human body and tissues; hence, it is desirable for them to be flexible and malleable. In the future, it is recommended that these entities should be constructed using ephemeral biodegradable substances that undergo dissolution after fulfilling their intended function. To facilitate the mass production of healthcare nanorobots with superior quality and cost-effectiveness, it is imperative to explore novel techniques for fabrication and synthesis, including the utilization of three-dimensional nanoimprinting. Hence, next-generation nanorobots will be made possible with the help of novel intelligent materials and state-of-the-art production methods.

Thousands of biomedical nanorobots will presumably work in tandem to zero in on the source of disease. Tasks that require the coordinated activity of numerous nanorobots, such as the efficient delivery of huge medicinal payloads or large-scale detoxification procedures, could one day be conceivable. Although research into nanorobot navigation and group behavior has progressed, it remains difficult to develop systems that can communicate with one another and work in unison as efficiently as a group of humans. To enhance the precise therapeutic abilities of nanorobots, it is necessary to advance their intelligent swarms in the direction of cooperative motion planning and artificial intelligence on the nanoscale. The successful adoption of swarm behavior in dynamic environments necessitates a comprehensive understanding of 'proactive material' and its corresponding quantitative control theory. The contemporaneous imaging and localization of miniature robots inside the human organism utilizing conventional optical microscopy methods present notable hurdles, as evidenced by the results of experiments. To facilitate the utilization of nanorobot systems in medical applications, it will be imperative to integrate advanced imaging technologies and feedback control systems into nanorobots, enabling unconstrained four-dimensional navigation.

We should expect to see an ongoing expansion of research into the creation and utilization of MNRs in the field of medicine. There is a need for enhanced collaboration between nanorobotic investigators and medical investigators to facilitate comprehensive investigations into the behavior and functionality of MNRs. These investigations should encompass various aspects, such as biological compatibility, retention, toxicity, biodistribution, and therapeutic efficacy.

The entire potential of MNRs in the field of medicine can be effectively realized by conducting such studies. It is highly recommended that researchers in the field of nanotechnology undertake a comprehensive examination of the requirements and preferences of medical professionals. This examination should be conducted to develop targeted medical equipment that addresses particular diagnostic or therapeutic challenges. This recommendation is particularly relevant given the recent notable advancements made in the areas of gastrointestinal drug administration and ophthalmic treatments. The rapid clinical application of MNR research will be facilitated by addressing these special requirements.

References and further reading

[1] Lightstone A W, Benedict S H, Bova F J, Solberg T D and Stern R L 2005 Intracranial stereotactic positioning systems: report of the American Association of Physicists in Medicine Radiation Therapy Committee Task Group no. 68 *Med. Phys.* **32** 2380–98

[2] Polderman K H and Herold I 2009 Therapeutic hypothermia and controlled normothermia in the intensive care unit: practical considerations, side effects, and cooling methods *Critical Care Med.* **37** 1101–20

[3] Vincent C A and Coulter A 2002 Patient safety: what about the patient? *BMJ Qual. Saf.* **11** 76–80

[4] Kassin M T, Owen R M, Perez S D, Leeds I, Cox J C, Schnier K, Sadiraj V and Sweeney J F 2012 Risk factors for 30-day hospital readmission among general surgery patients *J. Am. Coll. Surg.* **215** 322–30

[5] Chung S, Sudo R, Vickerman V, Zervantonakis I K and Kamm R D 2010 Microfluidic platforms for studies of angiogenesis, cell migration, and cell–cell interactions: Sixth International Bio-Fluid Mechanics Symposium and Workshop March 28–30 Pasadena, California *Ann. Biomed. Eng.* **38** 1164–77

[6] Ma Z, Mao Z and Gao C 2007 Surface modification and property analysis of biomedical polymers used for tissue engineering *Colloids Surf.,* B **60** 137–57

[7] Armentano I, Dottori M, Fortunati E, Mattioli S and Kenny J M 2010 Biodegradable polymer matrix nanocomposites for tissue engineering: a review *Polym. Degrad. Stab.* **95** 2126–46

[8] Walther D C and Ahn J 2011 Advances and challenges in the development of power-generation systems at small scales *Prog. Energy Combust. Sci.* **37** 583–610

[9] Koohi-Fayegh S and Rosen M A 2020 A review of energy storage types, applications, and recent developments *J. Energy Storage* **27** 101047

[10] Pratley C, Fenner S and Murphy J A 2020 Nitrogen-centered radicals in functionalization of sp2 systems: generation, reactivity, and applications in synthesis *Chem. Rev.* **122** 8181–260

[11] Koleoso M, Feng X, Xue Y, Li Q, Munshi T and Chen X 2020 Micro/nanoscale magnetic robots for biomedical applications *Mater. Today Bio* **8** 100085

[12] Yang M, Guo X, Mou F and Guan J 2020 Lighting up micro-/nanorobots with fluorescence *Chem. Rev.* **123** 3944–75

[13] Khezri B, Villa K, Novotný F, Sofer Z and Pumera M 2020 Smart dust 3D-printed graphene-based Al/Ga robots for photocatalytic degradation of explosives *Small* **16** 2002111

[14] Grover V P, Tognarelli J M, Crossey M M, Cox I J, Taylor-Robinson S D and McPhail M J 2015 Magnetic resonance imaging: principles and techniques: lessons for clinicians *J. Clin. Exp. Hepatol.* **5** 246–55

[15] Zborowski M, Chalmers J J and Lowrie W G 2017 Magnetic cell manipulation and sorting *Microtechnology for Cell Manipulation and Sorting* (Cham: Springer) 15–55

[16] Barakat N S 2009 Magnetically modulated nanosystem: a unique drug-delivery platform *Nanomedicine* **4** 799–812

[17] Stueber D D, Villanova J, Aponte I, Xiao Z and Colvin V L 2021 Magnetic nanoparticles in biology and medicine: past, present, and future trends *Pharmaceutics* **13** 943

[18] Hola K, Markova Z, Zoppellaro G, Tucek J and Zboril R 2015 Tailored functionalization of iron oxide nanoparticles for MRI, drug delivery, magnetic separation and immobilization of bio substances *Biotechnol. Adv.* **33** 1162–76

[19] Chan M H, Hsieh M R, Liu R S, Wei D H and Hsiao M 2019 Magnetically guided theranostics: optimizing magnetic resonance imaging with sandwich-like kaolinite-based iron/platinum nanoparticles for magnetic fluid hyperthermia and chemotherapy *Chem. Mater.* **32** 697–708

[20] Zhang D, Liu S, Guan J and Mou F 2022 Motile-targeting' drug delivery platforms based on micro/nanorobots for tumor therapy *Front. Bioeng. Biotechnol.* **10** 1002171

[21] Mayorga-Martinez C C, Pané S, Zhang L and Pumera M 2021 Magnetically driven micro and nanorobots *Chem. Rev.* **121** 4999–5041

[22] Bente K, Codutti A, Bachmann F and Faivre D 2018 Biohybrid and bioinspired magnetic microswimmers *Small* **14** 1704374

[23] Williams G 2019 *Unravelling the Double Helix: The Lost Heroes of DNA.* (London: Hachette UK Limited) 18

[24] Khan F A 2020 *Biotechnology Fundamentals* (Boca Raton, FL: CRC Press) 3rd edn 4

[25] Santomauro G, Singh A V, Park B W, Rahimi M, Erkoc M, Goering P, Schütz E, Sitti G and Bill M 2018 Incorporation of terbium into a microalga leads to magnetotactic swimmers *Adv. Biosyst.* **2** 1800039

[26] Tanjeem N, Minnis M B, Hayward R C and Shields IV C W 2022 Shape-changing particles: from materials design and mechanisms to implementation *Adv. Mater.* **34** 2105758

[27] Alavi S, Haeri A, Mahlooji I and Dadashzadeh S 2020 Tuning the physicochemical characteristics of particle-based carriers for intraperitoneal local chemotherapy *Pharm. Res.* **37** 1–24

[28] Esteban-Fernández de Li J, Ávila B, Gao W, Zhang L and Wang J 2017 Micro/nanorobots for biomedicine: delivery, surgery, sensing, and detoxification *Sci. Robot.* **2** eaam6431

[29] Suhail M, Khan A, Rahim M A, Naeem A, Fahad M, Badshah S F, Jabar A and Janakiraman a K 2022 Micro and nanorobot-based drug delivery: an overview *J. Drug Target.* **30** 349–58

[30] Soto F and Chrostowski R 2018 Frontiers of medical micro/nanorobotics: *in vivo* applications and commercialization perspectives toward clinical uses *Front. Bioeng. Biotechnol.* **6** 170

[31] Novotný F, Wang H and Pumera M 2020 Nanorobots: machines squeezed between molecular motors and micromotors *Chem.* **6** 867–84

[32] Gao W and Wang J 2014 Synthetic micro/nanomotors in drug delivery *Nanoscale* **6** 10486–94

[33] Gao W *et al* 2012 Cargo-towing fuel-free magnetic nano swimmers for targeted drug delivery *Small* **8** 460–8

[34] Walker D, Käsdorf B T, Jeong H, Lieleg O and Fischer P 2015 enzymatically active biomimetic micro propellers for the penetration of mucin gels *Sci. Adv.* **1** e1500501

[35] Garcia-Gradilla V, Sattayasamitsathit S, Soto F, Kuralay E, Yardımcı C, Wiitala D, Galrani M and Wang J 2014 Ultrasound-propelled nanoporous gold wire for efficient drug loading and release *Small* **10** 4154–9
[36] Chen X-Z *et al* 2017 Magnetoelectric nanowires for nanorobotic applications: fabrication, magnetoelectric coupling, and magnetically assisted *in vitro* targeted drug delivery *Adv. Mater.* **1605458** 1–7
[37] Wang W, Li S, Mair L, Ahmed S, Huang J, T and Mallouk T E Acoustic propulsion of nanorod motors inside living cells *Angew. Chem.* **126** 3265–8
[38] Esteban-Fernández de Ávila B, Angell C, Soto F, Lopez-Ramirez M A, Baez D F, Xie S, Wang J and Chen Y 2016 Acoustically propelled nanomotors for intracellular siRNA delivery *ACS Nano* **10** 4997–5005
[39] Qiu F, Fujita S, Mhanna R, Zhang L, Simona B R and Nelson B J 2015 Magnetic helical microswimmers functionalized with lipoplexes for targeted gene delivery *Adv. Funct. Mater.* **25** 1666–71
[40] Li J *et al* 2017 Micromotors spontaneously neutralize gastric acid for pH-responsive payload release *Angew. Chem.* **56** 2156–61
[41] Servant A, Qiu F, Mazza M, Kostarelos K and Nelson B J 2015 Controlled *in vivo* swimming of a swarm of bacteria-like micro robotic flagella *Adv. Mater.* **27** 2981–8
[42] Felfoul O *et al* 2016 Magneto-aerotactic bacteria deliver drug-containing nanoliposomes to tumor hypoxic regions *Nat. Nano* **11** 941–7
[43] Jiménez-Jiménez C, Moreno V M and Vallet-Regí M 2022 Bacteria-assisted transport of nanomaterials to improve drug delivery in cancer therapy *Nanomaterials* **12** 288
[44] Kumari P, Ghosh B and Biswas S 2016 Nanocarriers for cancer-targeted drug delivery *J. Drug Target.* **24** 179–91
[45] García K P, Zarschler K, Barbaro L, Barreto J A, O'Malley W, Spiccia L, Stephan H and Graham B 2014 Zwitterionic-coated 'stealth' nanoparticles for biomedical applications: recent advances in countering biomolecular corona formation and uptake by the mononuclear phagocyte system *Small* **10** 2516–29
[46] Tang F, Li L and Chen D 2012 Mesoporous silica nanoparticles: synthesis, biocompatibility and drug delivery *Adv. Mater.* **24** 1504–34
[47] Li J, Zhao J, Tan T, Liu M, Zeng Z, Zeng Y, Zhang L, Fu C, Chen D and Xie T 2020 Nanoparticle drug delivery system for glioma and its efficacy improvement strategies: a comprehensive review *Int. J. Nanomed.* **17** 2563–82
[48] Das S S, Bharadwaj P, Bilal M, Barani M, Rahdar A, Taboada P, Bungau S and Kyzas G Z 2020 Stimuli-responsive polymeric nanocarriers for drug delivery, imaging, and theragnosis *Polymers* **12** 1397
[49] Zhang X Q, Xu X, Bertrand N, Pridgen E, Swami A and Farrokhzad O C 2012 Interactions of nanomaterials and biological systems: implications to personalized nanomedicine *Adv. Drug Deliv. Rev.* **64** 1363–84
[50] Amiri M, Salavati-Niasari M and Akbari A 2019 Magnetic nanocarriers: evolution of spinel ferrites for medical applications *Adv. Colloid Interface Sci.* **265** 29–44
[51] Singh B, Kim K and Park M H 2021 On-demand drug delivery systems using nanofibers *Nanomaterials* **11** 3411
[52] Adepu S and Ramakrishna S 2021 Controlled drug delivery systems: current status and future directions *Molecules* **26** 5905

[53] Elia S A and Saravanakumar M P 2017 A review of the classification, characterization, and synthesis of nanoparticles and their application *IOP Conf. Ser.: Mater. Sci. Eng.* **3** 032019

[54] Nel A E, Mädler L, Velegol D, Xia T, Hoek E M, Somasundaran P, Klaessig F, Castranova V and Thompson M 2009 Understanding physiochemical interactions at the nano–bio interface *Nat. Mater.* **8** 543–57

[55] Wu Z, Lin X, Zou X, Sun J and He Q 2016 Biodegradable protein-based rockets for drug transportation and light-triggered release *ACS Appl. Mater. Interfaces* **7** 250–5

[56] Peters C, Hoop M, Pané S, Nelson B J and Hierold C 2016 Degradable magnetic composites for minimally invasive interventions: device fabrication, targeted drug delivery, and cytotoxicity tests *Adv. Mater.* **28** 533–8

[57] Medina-Sanchez M, Schwarz L, Meyer A K, Hebenstreit F and Schmidt O G 2016 Cellular cargo delivery: toward assisted fertilization by sperm-carrying micromotors *Nano Lett.* **16** 555–61

[58] Katuri J, Ma X, Stanton M M and Sánchez S 2017 Designing micro- and nano swimmers for specific applications *Acc. Chem. Res.* **50** 2–11

[59] Wu Z, Wu Y, He W, Lin X, Sun J and He Q 2013 Self-propelled polymer-based multilayer nano rockets for transportation and drug release *Angew. Chem. Int. Ed.* **52** 7000–3

[60] Ma X, Hahn K and Sanchez S 2015 Catalytic mesoporous Janus nanomotors for active cargo delivery *J. Am. Chem. Soc.* **137** 4976–9

[61] Mou F, Chen C, Zhong Q, Yin Y, Ma H and Guan J 2014 Autonomous motion and temperature-controlled drug delivery of Mg/Pt-poly (N-isopropyl acrylamide) Janus micromotors driven by simulated body fluid and blood plasma *ACS Appl. Mater. Interfaces* **6** 9897–903

[62] Breger J C, Yoon C, Xiao R, Rin Kwag H, Wang M O, Fisher J P, Nguyen T D and Gracias D H 2015 Self-folding thermo-magnetically responsive soft microgrippers *ACS Appl. Mater. Interfaces* **7** 3398–405

[63] Chatzipirpiridis G, Ergeneman O, Pokki J, Ullrich F, Fusco S, Ortega J A, Sivaraman K M, Nelson B J and Pané S Electroforming of implantable tubular magnetic microrobots for wireless ophthalmologic applications *Adv. Healthcare Mater.* **4** 209–14

[64] Li J, Esteban-Fernández de Ávila B, Gao W, Zhang L and Wang J 2017 Micro/nanorobots for biomedicine: delivery, surgery, sensing, and detoxification *Sci. Robot.* **2** eaam6431

[65] Zha F, Wang T, Luo M and Guan J 2018 Tubular micro/nanomotors: propulsion mechanisms, fabrication techniques and applications *Micromachines* **9** 78

[66] Singh S S, Behera S K, Rai S, Tripathy S K, Chakraborty S and Mishra A 2022 A critical review on nanomaterial-based therapeutics for diabetic wound healing *Biotechnol. Genet. Eng. Rev.* **30** 1–35

[67] Wang J 2016 Self-propelled affinity biosensors: moving the receptor around the sample *Biosens. Bioelectron.* **76** 234–42

[68] Wang J 2012 and Cargo-towing synthetic nanomachines: towards active transport in microchip devices *Lab Chip* **12** 1944–50

[69] Kagan D, Campuzano S, Balasubramanian S, Kuralay F, Flechsig G and Wang J 2011 Functionalized micromachines for selective and rapid isolation of nucleic acid targets from complex samples *Nano Lett.* **11** 2083–7

[70] Orozco J, Campuzano S, Kagan D, Zhou M, Gao W and Wang J 2011 Dynamic isolation and unloading of target proteins by aptamer-modified micro transporters *Anal. Chem.* **83** 7962–9

[71] Garcia M, Orozco J, Guix M, Gao W, Sattayasamitsathit S, Escarpa A, Merkoci A and Wang J 2013 Micromotor-based lab-on-chip immunoassays *Nanoscale* **5** 1325–31
[72] Restrepo-Pérez L, Soler L, Martínez-Cisneros C, Sánchez S and Schmidt O G 2014 Biofunctionalized self-propelled micromotors as an alternative on-chip concentrating system *Lab Chip* **14** 2914–7
[73] Morales-Narváez E, Guix M, Medina-Sánchez M, Mayorga-Martinez c c and Merkoçi A 2014 Micromotor enhanced microarray technology for protein detection *Small* **10** 2542–8
[74] Esteban-Fernández de Ávila B, Martin A, Soto F, Lopez-Ramirez M A, Campuzano S, Vasquez-Machado G M, Gao W, Zhang L and Wang J Single cell real-time miRNAs sensing based on nanomotors *ACS Nano* **9** 6756–64
[75] Hu C J, Fang R H, Copp J, Luk B T and Zhang L 2013 A biomimetic nanosponge that absorbs pore-forming toxins *Nat. Nanotechnol.* **8** 336–40
[76] Wu Z, Li J, Esteban-Fernández , de Ávila B, Li T, Gao W, He Q, Zhang L and Wang J 2018 Water-powered cell-mimicking Janus micromotor *Adv. Funct. Mater.* **25** 7497–501
[77] Zhu W *et al* 2015 3D-printed artificial microfiche *Adv. Mater.* **27** 4411–7
[78] Ma X, Jannasch A, Albrecht U-R, Hahn K, Miguel-Lopez A, Schaff E and Sanchez S Enzyme-powered hollow mesoporous Janus nanomotors *Nano Lett.* **15** 7043–50
[79] Trushina D B, Borodina T N, Belyakov S and Antipina M N 2022 Calcium carbonate vaterite particles for drug delivery: advances and challenges *Mater. Today Adv.* **14** 100214
[80] Luo M, Feng Y, Wang T and Guan J 2018 Micro-/nanorobots at work in active drug delivery *Adv. Funct. Mater.* **28** 1706100
[81] Luo M, Li S, Wan J, Yang C, Chen B and Guan J 2020 Enhanced propulsion of urease-powered micromotors by multilayered assembly of ureases on Janus magnetic microparticles *Langmuir* **36** 7005–13
[82] Lutgens L, Deutz N, Gueulette J, Cleutjens J, Berger M and Wouters B 2003 Citrulline: a physiologic marker enabling quantitation and monitoring of epithelial radiation-induced small bowel damage *Int. J. Radiat. Oncol. Biol. Phys.* **57** 1067–74
[83] Liu Z, Ding S, Zhang N, Zhou Y, Cheng N and Wang M 2020 Single-atom enzymes linked immunosorbent assay for sensitive detection of A beta 1–40: a biomarker of Alzheimer's disease *Research* 4724505
[84] Manjare M, Yang B and Zhao Y P 2013 Bubble-propelled microjets: model and experiment *J. Phys. Chem.* C **117** 4657–65
[85] Masland R H 2012 The neuronal organization of the retina *Neuron* **76** 266–80
[86] Medina-Sanchez M, Xu H and Schmidt O G 2018 Micro- and nano-motors: the new generation of drug carriers *Ther. Deliv.* **9** 303–16
[87] Menter D, Tucker S, Kopetz S, Sood A, Crissman J and Honn K 2014 Platelets and cancer: a casual or causal relationship: revisited *Cancer Metastasis Rev.* **33** 231–69
[88] Miki K and Clapham D 2013 Rheotaxis guides mammalian sperm *Curr. Biol.* **23** 443–52
[89] Mobasheri A, Kalamegam G, Musumeci G and Batt M E 2014 Chondrocyte and mesenchymal stem cell-based therapies for cartilage repair in osteoarthritis and related orthopaedic conditions *Maturitas* **78** 188–98
[90] Mody V V, Siwale R, Singh A and Mody H R 2010 Introduction to metallic nanoparticles *J. Pharm. Bio Allied Sci.* **2** 282–9
[91] Moreno-Garrido I 2008 Microalgae immobilization: current techniques and uses *Bioresour. Technol.* **99** 3949–64

[92] Mou F, Chen C, Ma H, Yin Y, Wu Q and Guan J 2013 Self-propelled micromotors driven by the magnesium–water reaction and their hemolytic properties *Agnew. Chem. Int. Ed.* **52** 7208–12

[93] Mou F, Chen C, Zhong Q, Yin Y, Ma H and Guan J 2014 Autonomous motion and temperature-controlled drug delivery of Mg/Pt-poly (N-isopropyl acrylamide) Janus micromotors driven by simulated body fluid and blood plasma *ACS Appl. Mater. Interfaces* **6** 9897–903

[94] Mou F, Xie Q, Liu J, Che S, Bahmane L and You 2021 ZnO-based micromotors fueled by CO_2: the first example of self-reorientation-induced biomimetic chemotaxis *Natl. Sci. Rev.* **8** 066

[95] Mou F, Zhang J, Wu Z, Du S, Zhang Z and Xu L 2019 Phototactic flocking of photochemical micromotors *iScience* **19** 415–24

[96] Mourran A m, Zhang H, Vinokur R and Moeller M 2017 Soft microrobots employing nonequilibrium actuation via plasmonic heating *Adv. Mater.* **29** 1604825

[97] Campuzano S, Orozco J, Kagan D, Guix M, Gao W, Sattayasamitsathit S, Claussen J C, Merkoc A and Wang J 2012 Bacterial isolation by lectin-modified micro engines *Nano Lett.* **12** 396–401

[98] Nguyen K V and Minteer S D 2015 DNA-functionalized Pt nanoparticles as catalysts for chemically powered micromotors: toward signal-on motion-based DNA biosensor *Chem. Commun.* **51** 4782–4

[99] Yu X, Li Y, Wu J and Ju H 2014 Motor-based autonomous microsensor for motion and counting immunoassay of cancer biomarker *Anal. Chem.* **86** 4501–7

Chapter 12

Cyborgs and cyberorgans: biosecurity in biorobotics for healthcare—a case study

Cyborgs are often seen as the next stage in human development, due to significant improvements in robotics and artificial intelligence. The field of biosecurity, which encompasses the convergence of cybersecurity, cyber–physical security, and biosecurity, studies a growing threat environment that can significantly impact the economic, social, and political welfare of a country. Moreover, it carries substantial implications for national security. Emerging healthcare applications include cyborgs, which combine AI robots with physicians to conduct remote surgeries from hospitals in patients' homes. Examples of cyborg applications include robot-assisted knee replacement surgeries and real-time performance monitoring systems for thigh medical care. This case study investigates the convergence of biorobotics and biosecurity in the healthcare sector, specifically exploring two emergent concepts: 'cyberorgans' and the larger domain of 'cyborgs.' The incorporation of biorobotics into healthcare systems during a period characterized by rapid technological progress offers considerable potential for significant developments, along with novel obstacles. This chapter investigates the effects of deploying robotic technology, including surgical robots, teleoperated medical equipment, and autonomous healthcare assistants, on healthcare delivery, patient outcomes, and the broader healthcare environment. Moreover, it explores the notion of 'cyberorgans,' a field that combines cybernetics with organ engineering, which has the potential to significantly transform organ transplantation and regenerative medicine. Within the parameters of this dynamic environment, this chapter presents the key aspect of biosecurity, focusing on the susceptibilities linked to networked healthcare systems and the possible hazards to patient data, device integrity, and even patient well-being. It provides a thorough analysis of case studies and practical situations, offering perspectives on the appropriate strategies and technologies for ensuring the security of healthcare settings in the era of biorobotics and modern medical technology. It examines the potential associated with these advances and emphasizes the need to implement effective biosecurity for healthcare.

doi:10.1088/978-0-7503-6019-7ch12

12.1 Introduction

Cyborgs are the next concept to be introduced in biorobotics. In 1960, Manfred Clynes and Nathan S. Kline introduced the term 'cyborg' to describe the idea of self-regulating extraterrestrial humans. However, they probably did not anticipate the rapid progression toward a more advanced form of human–machine symbiosis. This development involves the use of medical biomaterial prostheses to replace lost organs and restore impaired sensory functions. Biomaterial implants made by humans first appeared in the historical record during the Neolithic era. The prostheses used in ancient times mostly consisted of organic substances such as silk, wood, nacre, ivory, and diverse animal tissues. These materials were employed to alleviate the conditions of individuals afflicted with decaying teeth, limb amputation, and ailments affecting the skeletal structure. Technology has led to the use of gold, silver, titanium, and other metallic alloys as implants [1]. However, with the rapid growth in available possibilities, scientists now confront the challenge of which materials to utilize. Multifunctional biomaterials with electrical, magnetic, and biological properties are being used to create smarter and more effective implants. Cyborg systems facilitate the enhancement of handicapped human bodies through technological means, hence enhancing technical efficiency. In addition, they permit the monitoring of healthcare data across various healthcare facilities [2]. Cyborg agents perform a variety of surgical operations on patients using healthcare sensors, such as those located in the thigh, knee, and foot [3–5]. There are two significant and distinct categories of cyborgs in medicine. The first is the type of cyborg designed to repair damaged bodily systems [6]. The second concept refers to an advanced cyborg design that corresponds to the concept of achieving optimum performance. This involves the optimization of output by referring to the knowledge or adjustments acquired, while simultaneously decreasing input, which pertains to the energy consumed throughout the process. The augmented cyborg aims to surpass basic functions or acquire new ones [7]. The phrase 'cyborg soldier' is often used in the military to describe a service member who has a human–machine interface that allows them to use their weapon and other survival devices. The concept of cyborgization in sports has gained national attention in recent years. In the future, genetic alteration may emerge as a significant method for enhancing the physical capabilities of individuals. The field of biomimetics involves the integration of novel structures and processes derived from living organisms into the design and construction of mechanical entities. The field of biomimetics, often known as bionics, has facilitated the development of mechanical systems that exhibit properties similar to those seen in live organisms [8]. Moreover, the wide array of living forms exhibiting varied morphologies serves as a valuable repository of designs that may be integrated into the development of biorobotics.

According to Bandyopadhyay *et al* [9], the machines that are produced exhibit a higher level of performance. On the other hand, when building a mechanical model, strict adherence to biological systems may very seldom generate any useful results [10]. Biorobotics gave us the word 'cyborg,' which means a creature with both natural and manufactured parts [11]. Such creatures raise fundamental concerns about the differences in free will and understanding between humans and their mechanical counterparts. The concept of cyborgs, which refers to a hybrid that combines human and machine traits, is already deeply ingrained in our social reality and our day-to-day lives. By examining the concept of cyborg ontology, researchers have proposed that the implementation of person-centered practice may be realized within the contextualized, embodied, and relational realms of technology. Cyborgs are a combination of humans and machines [12].

However, cyborgs are already an established part of our society and are no longer the preserve of science fiction. Lapum [12] suggests that technologies affect the biological way of being and do not only exist as a combination of humans and machines. Considering cyborg ontology in healthcare raises concerns about the potential risks and benefits of combining humans and machines [12]. Such concerns affect both healthcare providers who use technology to improve patient care and those who become too dependent on technology and lose their humanity. Biorobotics is an academic discipline that focuses on the analysis and examination of biological systems using a biomechatronic perspective. This area of research aims to achieve two primary objectives. One perspective is the advancement of approaches and technology to create and implement bioinspired systems and devices, including humanoid and animaloid robots. In contrast, the secondary objective of biorobotics involves the conceptualization and creation of apparatuses intended for biomedical purposes, including diagnostic procedures, surgical interventions, rehabilitation processes, supportive aids, bionic technologies, and neuro-robotic advancements. In the following discussion, we address the ethical implications that arise from the second purpose of biorobotics. Biosecurity may be broadly characterized as the implementation of measures to ensure the safety and security of living organisms. The article illustrates that the people working in this field, the causes or people they serve, the tools they use, and the outcomes they achieve are all quite different. Certain biosecurity activities may seem ordinary; however, they possess significant implications (such as the use of disinfectants at farm entrances to prevent the transmission of foot and mouth viruses). Cyborgs often possess enhanced sensory capabilities, enabling them to include features that facilitate the quantitative tracking of motions and the efficient administration of customized therapies [13]. The efficient integration of organic and mechanical components in a cyborg presents both potential and problems. Achieving consistency in this integration requires a comprehensive understanding of the unique human participating in the system [14]. In contrast, serious games, which are widely used in virtual reality healthcare content [15, 16], have the potential to enhance environmental experiences by including a range of behavioral reactions [16]. These might also include modifying training situations based on the user's intentions or requirements [17]. Effective virtual cyborg modeling goes beyond replicating the exterior structure of the real-world equivalent. When interacting with the environment, it is important to consider internal body conditions such as muscle tiredness and cognitive load [18]. Cyborgs, which are intimately connected to the human body, may be defined as robotic entities that possess artificial intelligence capabilities. These entities are further integrated with healthcare servers, enabling the monitoring of healthcare-related aspects.

12.2 Biorobotics in healthcare

The term 'biorobotics' refers to systems that either interact with biological components, are inspired by biological systems, or are partially built from biological materials (biohybrid robots). The most prevalent applications of biorobotics are in medication administration, the simulation of biological processes, and the handling of hazardous materials. Biorobotic devices need to be flexible enough to work well with living things and be able to imitate them. Numerous robotic systems used for the replication of biological activities, such as submerged adhesion and muscle mimetics, make use of polymer substrates that bear similarity to those utilized in bioelectronic applications [19, 20]. This section covers popular polymer substrates, their material properties, and restrictions. Various materials are often used in the construction of soft robots. Polyurethane foams are often used as versatile structural materials, offering a wide range of applications. On the other hand, silicone elastomers exhibit properties suitable for the development of flexible actuators. Hydrogels have considerable potential due to their suitability for applications in aqueous environments and interactions with biological entities (figure 12.1). Polymers are often used in contemporary robotic systems due to their elasticity, robustness, and conformability. The viscoelasticity of a polymer chain depends on its micro- and macrostructures, particularly in materials with both viscous and elastic dynamic responses [3]. Biologically relevant Young's moduli are necessary for the smooth interaction and seamless integration of soft electrical devices [21].

The substrate should have a Young's modulus between 1 kPa and 100 MPa. To improve tissue integration and minimize injury, it is important to match mechanical stiffnesses, Young's moduli, and other key material properties such as ultimate elongations, toughnesses, and resilience moduli [22]. Polyurethanes, polydimethylsiloxane, and hydrogels are common polymer substrates. Robot-assisted neurorehabilitation has been used for a long time to improve neuromotor recovery by training paralyzed arms intensively, repeatedly, and in the context of a job while reducing the work of healthcare professionals [23, 24]. It has been shown that using robotic devices to assist people who have motor deficiencies is an effective strategy for accelerating functional rehabilitation [25].

In recent years, there has been an enormous growth of interest in the field of biorobots. Numerous studies have been conducted, resulting in the advancement of devices capable of performing gripping tasks [26], walking [27], pumping [28, 29], and

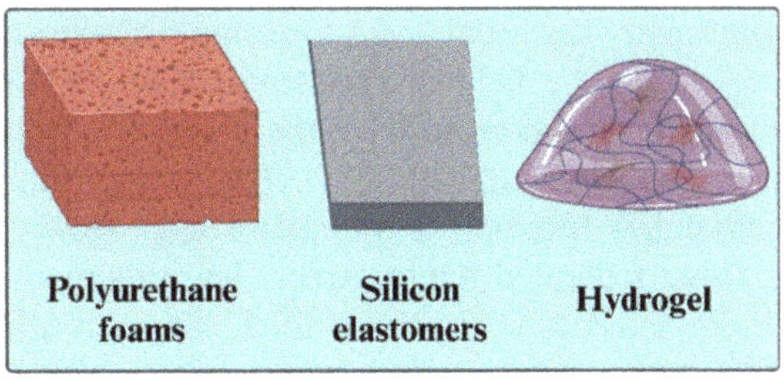

Figure 12.1. Base materials that are often used in the manufacture of soft robots.

swimming [30, 31]. Furthermore, no harmful byproducts are emitted during their manufacture or operation, making these devices ecologically friendly. In addition, they are capable of self-repair, have a small electromechanical footprint, and can meet their energy requirements. [32]. In addition to biorobots that are completely powered by molecular actuators, cell-based biological actuators are utilized in bigger devices to create the necessary force for device performance. Many actuators consist of confluent layers of contractile cells on a thin, flexible substrate [33, 34]. According to Alford *et al* [33], the majority of cells employed for biorobot actuation are those found in the skeletal and cardiac muscles of mammals. Biorobots of various sizes and functionalities have been constructed, with actuation provided by molecular motors. The sizes of these biorobots range from the microscale to the macroscale, i.e. 10^{-9} to 10^{2} m. Prokaryotes, which include bacteria [35, 36], are highly versatile and have been used to perform a wide variety of tasks, from working together as a unit, to driving submillimeter gears [37], or delivering packages along a chemical gradient [38]. Large-scale biorobots based on muscle-powered actuators have been produced for challenging tasks.

12.3 Cyborgs and cyberorgans in healthcare

The word 'cyborg' denotes an organism that has been merged with a synthetic component or technology, is dependent on feedback mechanisms, and has enhanced capabilities. Cyborgs, which are intricately connected to the human body, are robotic entities that include artificial intelligence capabilities. In addition, these entities are equipped with healthcare servers that serve the purpose of monitoring and managing healthcare-related aspects. The growing field of cyborgs and cyberorgans in healthcare is an interesting sector where the domain of human biology intersects with modern technology. Cyborgs, also known as cybernetic beings, integrate components of both humans and machines to increase physiological capacities. These enhancements include a wide range of technologies, such as brain implants that improve cognitive skills and bionic limbs that restore movement. Simultaneously, the integration of cyberorgans, including bioengineered or artificial organs, offers innovative approaches to address the challenges of organ failure, limited availability of transplant organs, and the provision of individualized healthcare. The phenomenon of convergence holds significant promise to enhance patient well-being and quality of life. However, this issue gives rise to significant inquiries about ethical considerations, privacy concerns, and the fundamental essence of human identity. To explore the deep implications of these developments, it is imperative to manage the subtle equilibrium between harnessing their revolutionary potential and addressing the ethical and social concerns they prominently present in the field of modern medicine. The introduction of a cyborg-based system has been shown to have the potential to reduce the limitations faced by individuals in their daily activities [39]. This study examined the implementation of a consumer-centric Internet of Medical Things (IoMT) infrastructure for cyborg applications, using federated reinforcement learning methodologies.

The objective is to implement cyborg-based IoMT apps on mobile cloud networks to facilitate various treatments and healthcare services. Cyborgs provide a range of services that use robotic technology to facilitate medical care through mobile cloud networks for both patients and physicians. IoMT is an innovative model in which various healthcare apps are being developed to assist users in their healthcare practices. Consumer-centric cyborgs incorporate various forms of computing, such as integrated computing, software computing, and infrastructure computing, in which applications consist of multiple layers and components. Embedded systems, such as the Arduino UNO and the Raspberry Pi, are often utilized in the field of healthcare. These boards are used to facilitate the operation of diverse healthcare sensors which are responsible for collecting data from the human body. Subsequently, this data is sent to a server to be used in prediction [40]. Some studies [41] have proposed a healthcare system that is both resource-efficient and sustainable. Efforts were made to reduce resource usage during simulation and forecasting based on cyborg data in a specialized data-processing environment. Numerous methods have been proposed to address prediction problems in distributed cyborg-enabled cloud networks, including the SARSA method (state, action, reward, state, action), Q-learning, policy, and value functions [41–43].

All of the previous studies only focused on optimizing the predetermined characteristics, such as processing latency and service delay, of cyborg applications. However, there are certain aspects, such as processing and resource costs, that need to be optimized for cyborg applications. The term 'cyborganic system' is supported by advancements in cybernetics, cyborganics, and bioelectronics. These systems provide a potential pathway to a future characterized by programmable tissue and biomaterial-like machinery that may function as a protective barrier against age-related illnesses. In 2012, Harvard University made significant contributions that had a crucial role in facilitating the successful integration of electronic components with living tissues. This groundbreaking concept, referred to as 'cyborg tissues,' garnered widespread attention from the media and generated a surge of enthusiasm surrounding the potential advancements in regenerative medicine [44–47]. The field of cyborganic technology and its range of applications have seen significant advancements, with several innovative proofs-of-concept being produced in laboratories at both the microscale and the macroscale. The integration of cyborganic systems and genetically modified circuits into cells is significantly transforming the environment of this scientific area. The emergence of cyborg science has generated much interest and enthusiasm because of its possible medical consequences. The concept of individuals with cyborg-like qualities has captivated the minds of many readers. Nevertheless, certain challenges still hinder progress in this field. The survey conducted in this chapter, while not exhaustive, seeks to demonstrate the wide range of applications enabled by laboratory monitoring, and wearable and implantable cyborganic healthcare equipment.

12.4 Case study

Various case studies of cyborgs, cyberorgans, and biosecurity in the context of biorobotics for healthcare are included in table 12.1.

12.5 Patent list

Various patents related to cyborgs, cyberorgans, and biosecurity in the context of biorobotics for healthcare are included in table 12.2.

Table 12.1. Case studies related to cyborgs, cyberorgans, and biosecurity in the context of biorobotics for healthcare.

S. No.	Author	Case study
1.	Hecht	They successfully created a novel access technology aimed at allowing individuals with disabilities to freely perform tasks for which they previously relied on human assistance. This technology has the potential to significantly reduce the expenses associated with delivering this assistance, hence enhancing accessibility for those requiring such services. However, if the provision of this service was previously performed by a person, the implementation of innovative technology might result in a reduction in employment opportunities. This technology may lack a social component which consumers may have appreciated prior to its introduction but is now inaccessible. Researchers developing this technology must consider both its positive and negative effects on accessibility, employment, and social interaction, as per the guidelines. Researchers may suggest policies or solutions to alleviate adverse consequences, such as remote social support technology integration [48].
2.	Donna Haraway	The cyborg was created as a symbol for activist examination of communal, cultural, and natural collective phenomena. According to a prominent scholar in the field, cyborgs may be seen as representations of power dynamics and individual identities. That is, they are graphs, connected lists, mesh structures, assemblies, layouts, or 'pattern linkages.' The concept of the cyborg embodies a state of consciousness that relies on the destabilization of barriers between biological matter and technology to form its fundamental nature. The cyborg represents a complex kind of subjectivity that intersects several identities and may be analyzed using various concepts and frameworks that have influenced its development [49, 50]
3.	Manfred Clynes and Nathan Kline	The emerging field of biorobotics introduces the concept of cyborgs, which are organisms comprising both natural and artificial components. Cyborgs are depicted as a fusion of organic and artificial components, prompting inquiries into the distinctions between humans and machinery, particularly inquiries about morality, free will, and empathy. Frequently portrayed with superior physical or cognitive abilities compared to their human counterparts, cyborgs are often referred to as individual cyborgs when they possess bionic or robotic enhancements. Otto Bock HealthCare's C-limb system is an innovative example of modern prosthetic applications; it is designed to replace a human limb that has been amputated due to an accident or sickness [51, 52].

(Continued)

Table 12.1. (*Continued*)

S. No.	Author	Case study
4.	Shao	They published a study describing a technical interface that enables wireless management of modified cells' functioning using an Android-operated smartphone. The integration of cyborganic systems and genetically designed systems into cells is significantly altering the physical environment of the field. Specifically, a smartphone equipped with an optogenetic interface sensitive to far-red light (FRL) was used to control insulin synthesis performed by cells housed in an electronic scaffold implanted into diabetic mice. This is a promising precursor to a cyborganic feedback loop that may detect inadequacies and offer biological stimuli to correct critical physical conditions [53].
5.	Jillian Weise	Significant analysis of the cyborg's metaphorical figurativeness. Disabled individuals, including those with pacemakers, dialysis, wheelchairs, and biologics, have been referred to as cyborgs. 'Cyborgs' refers to individuals whose existence and cognitive processes are dependent on and mutually shaped by the presence of a connection between a biological entity and technological components. Weise emphasizes the existence of the manifest cyborg and its significance. Technological impacts on the tangible and observational reality are not intangible or intellectual, but rather necropolitical. The impact of technology and its implementation has an important role in defining the survival or mortality of individuals, operating within the framework of social prejudices, discrimination, oppression, and ideal concepts [54, 55]
6.	Alison Kafer	A researcher in the field of Critical Disability Studies aims to establish a harmonious relationship between the concept of the cyborg and the lived experiences of those with disabilities. The study of medicine and technology is influenced by ideologies about normality and deviance. Scientific interventions assume a normative endpoint for the cyborg body, saving it by approximating the 'whole' and 'perfect' human. Success is determined by deviance from the 'natural' and presenting a superhuman future. Cyborgs that are alive, breathing, and critical do not demand to be identical to contemporaneous individuals in every way; rather, they desire the ability to self-direct and take responsibility for the building of their interfaced bodies [56].
7.	Jasbir Puar	The cyborg combines both multidimensional individuality and a framework that may be navigated in all directions to explore the concepts and constructions that have influenced it.

		In the same way that 3D computer graphics use meshes, the cyborg can be considered as a model that relies on various factors for its produced output. These factors include the perspective, the edges connecting the nodes and the vertices, and the multifaceted coordinates individually related to the node. These coordinates enable the system to process important visual aspects such as the color, shading, reflection, and positioning of each node. In addition, the system takes account of the infinite interstitial space that exists between the nodes [50].
8.	Alicia A	This study discussed alternate perspectives on the influence of assistive technology (AT) on the disability community. These perspectives are grounded in the lived experience of the first author, who identifies as a white handicapped autistic person. Individuals who have been officially labeled with neurodevelopmental disorders, impairments, and chronic diseases often experience systemic violence via normative interventions that prevent society from accepting the vast range of physical embodiments that exist. The interventional objective of aligning the conduct with normative expectations is often framed as a type of access in itself [57].
9.	Botha and Frost	Individuals acquire habits of suppression and concealment as a means of avoiding the negative consequences of stigma, discrimination, and violence. In consideration of the observed collaboration between social stigma and normalization, researchers must contemplate the potential implications of interventions aimed at enhancing 'social skills,' 'behavior shaping,' and achieving a state of being 'indistinguishable from their neurotypical peers' [58].
10.	Cassidy	The observed differences in suicidal thoughts and behaviors (STBs) between those with autism and those without autism may be attributed to the phenomenon of 'camouflaging,' which refers to the act of trying to blend in, disguising one's true self, or making efforts to comply with societal norms and expectations [59].
11.	Singleton	A system of wearable connected devices that aim to support doctors in the surveillance and supervision of residents' behavior and whereabouts. Each resident in the area has the potential to be equipped with a total of five wearable devices, namely one for each ankle and wrist in addition to a central node. The purpose of this assembly of devices is to ascertain the precise position of the patient, evaluate their physiological condition, and systematically categorize and document a range of physical activities. The technique may be useful for counter-surveillance and detecting and reporting the mistreatment of people in institutions. Disabled individuals in institutions face an increased risk of emotional, physical, and sexual abuse. Using technology to hold institution staff accountable for abuses can save lives and help eliminate disability segregation in placements [60].

(Continued)

Table 12.1. (*Continued*)

S. No.	Author	Case study
12.	Warwick (2003, 2004)	Biological creatures are created and developed by artificial techniques. The development of life from nonliving materials, on the other hand, would be a complete biorobotics. This area is often known as synthetic biology or biological nanotechnology. The numerous types of replicants that may be seen in several famous films also pertain to biorobotics. In role-playing games, the name bioroid has occasionally been used for a partly or fully organic robot. A biological brain was made by growing neurons that were originally grown separately in a lab. This biological brain was then put into a robot body [61, 62].
13.	Colombo (2005)	Biorobotics is a revolutionary innovation utilized in different industries, including medicine. The development of a robot-assisted treatment for upper limb rehabilitation in chronic post-stroke patients is a significant advancement in medical research. This method uses admittance-controlled biorobots to promote upper limb mobility in chronic post-stroke patients by addressing motor outcomes. Furthermore, these instruments enable clinical quantitative measurement of therapeutic progress. To enhance patients' motor outcomes, rehabilitation procedures may be designed and adapted appropriately. Reducing disability may improve motor outcomes for these people. The use of biorobots in neurorehabilitation is another human achievement. It allows for the future development of customized rehabilitation methods [63].
14.	A. Abbott	The flexibility inherent in the design of robotic devices enables the creation of many experimental scenarios that may be systematically used to investigate 'cases' that would be impractical or unfeasible to directly investigate in an organism. This strategy may also facilitate the discovery of emergent behaviors that would be difficult to discern through the observation of the organism's behavior alone [64].
15.	Lyotard	The improved cyborg aims to exceed conventional performance and maybe acquire additional functionalities that were not initially inherent. In the military, the phrase 'cyborg soldier' refers to a soldier with integrated weapon and survival systems, forming a human–machine interaction. The concept of cyborgization in sports has gained national attention in recent years. In the field of prosthetics, the topic of cyborgs encompasses other aspects such as the use of steroids, blood doping, and bodily alteration, which warrant inclusion in the discussion. In the future, genetic modification may emerge as a significant method for enhancing the athletic capabilities of those involved in sports. Various forms of art also contribute to the public understanding of cybernetic organisms [7].

Table 12.2. Patent lists related to cyborgs, cyberorgans, and biosecurity in the context of biorobotics for healthcare.

S. No.	Patent number	Description
1.	US9510853B2	To further appreciate the features and benefits of this disclosure, refer to the following thorough description, which includes illustrated embodiments following the principles of the invention, and the accompanying drawings. The many specifics included in describing the invention are not meant to restrict its use but rather to serve as illustrations of its various characteristics. Various modifications, changes, and variations can be made to the method and apparatus of the invention without affecting its spirit and scope [65].
2.	US20210121251A1	New and improved surgical methods have resulted from the use of surgical biorobots. However, previous robotic surgical procedures and equipment may have been suboptimal. Individual diversity in tissue ablation rates and recovery may have been poorly addressed by the previous methods. In addition, the surgical setup and treatment duration might affect results and may not have been adequately addressed by the earlier techniques and equipment [66].
3.	US10092205B2	Advancements in robotic actuators, sensors, innovative materials, control algorithms, and the miniaturization of computers have facilitated the development of wearable lower-body exoskeletal robotic prostheses. These prostheses aim to enhance endurance, strength, and mobility. The Humans Assistive Limb (HAL) exoskeleton developed by Cyberdyne Inc. and the ReWalk system created by Bionics Research Inc. are both designed to assist those affected by stroke, spinal cord injuries, and advanced age to regain the ability to walk. The HAL cyborg robot suit, developed by Cyberdyne, incorporates a voluntary control system that utilizes biosignals detected by sensors on the patient's skin. These signals are then processed by an autonomous robotic system, which in turn creates torque that assists limb motions. The ReWalk system is designed specifically for individuals with lower-limb mobility impairments, provided they possess functional hands, arms, and shoulders, as well as the ability to stand and use crutches. This innovative technology enables wheelchair users to assume a standing position, ambulate, and ascend stairs. The Robotic Exoskeleton (Rex) developed by RexBionics enables persons with mobility limitations to perform various ambulatory tasks, including standing, sitting, walking, turning, and ascending stairs, without the need for assistive devices such as crutches or walkers [67].
4.	US20170245878A1	This invention relates to the area of energy therapy of tissue, and more precisely, to the therapy of an organ such as the prostate using fluid stream energy.

(Continued)

Table 12.2. (*Continued*)

S. No.	Patent number	Description
		In other cases, inadequate removal might be the consequence of the use of older treatment procedures and equipment on patients. For example, traditional prostate surgery sometimes requires a longer recovery period and yields less than ideal results, at least in some cases. Previous tissue imaging techniques and equipment may not be optimal for imaging treated tissue [68].
5.	EP2813194B1	This invention involves the science of limb control, specifically focusing on an artificial limb designed for either human or robotic use. The invention applies to a control unit designed for the electrical control of an electrically controllable limb device. In addition, it encompasses a system that includes said control unit. Furthermore, it involves a method for controlling an electrically controllable limb device and it encompasses a computer program. The innovation described herein has broad applicability in both the realm of human-controlled artificial limbs and robotic limbs. However, the subsequent discussion primarily focuses on the use of this invention in the field of human artificial limbs, specifically arm or hand prostheses. The limb refers to any organ of the body, such as an upper extremity (arm) or a lower extremity (leg) [69].
6.	US20090144095A1	This patent is concerned with approaches and processes that can be used to institute protocols and frameworks for managing biosafety and biosecurity risks. To assess the adherence of people and organizations to these protocols and frameworks, it is necessary to build methods and systems for auditing facilities and testing entities. The organization specializes in the implementation of comprehensive measures and protocols for managing biosafety and biosecurity risks. This includes providing training, consulting services, conducting audits, and certifying companies, facilities, systems, and individuals to ensure compliance. In additionally, the organization conducts thorough analyses of biosafety and biosecurity risks with the aim of minimizing the likelihood of accidental, natural, or deliberate release of potentially dangerous materials and information, as well as for use in making investment decisions and pricing an offering, which are all relevant to this application [70].
7.	US20170319430A1	This invention is related to wearable sensor systems and also involves wireless communication between the users of such systems as well as wearable actuators and control systems. It involves wearable devices containing sensors, actuators, and control systems tailored for application in medical settings and the area of female sexual response and well-being in one specific version.

		The subject of women's health, sexuality, and sexual responsiveness has received a growing amount of attention in recent years. The area of wearable sensors is seeing significant growth, as evidenced by the availability of commercial devices designed for the surveillance of essential physiological indicators, including body temperature, cardiac rhythm, and respiration [71].
8.	US20160078366A1	This invention deals with computerized devices that utilize natural voice capabilities. Specifically, it focuses on a technological system and strategy that enhances the understanding of speech in interactive audio response systems. In addition, it addresses a computer technique and approach that interprets utterances in a speech recognition application, taking into account predefined constraints. A fixed, preset, annotated automatic speech recognition (ASR) corpus file serves as the foundation for the computer system. This document contains a comprehensive compilation of all projected acceptable verbal expressions. This technological innovation is not designed to function as a computer system equipped with artificial intelligence, like that found in a cyborg or an android. The computer system of AI enables cyborgs, androids, machines, mentally ill or neurologically impaired patients, and individuals with mental disabilities to actively participate in society and experience a healthy mental state [72].
9.	US20220037039A1	The invention is designed for use in a healthcare context; it may collaborate with robotic control to aid in patient diagnosis, education, and treatment. Typically, the system has a processor, memory storage, user interface, and controller with three modes of operation: autonomous decision-making, patient interactive, and doctor interactive. The controller analyzes patient, healthcare provider, diagnostic test, and medical database data using artificial intelligence in its operational mode. The controller utilizes the studied data to choose a diagnostic test or clinical advice for a healthcare practitioner or medical robot, and if the data indicates a diagnostic test, the controller may ask a medical robot to conduct it. The system refines the examined data to produce a patient diagnosis and treatment plan. Outpatient emergency department visits may be processed from presentation to discharge by this system [73].
10.	US20200360100A1	The disclosed techniques and equipment enhance tissue therapy, such as tissue resection. Image-guided therapy systems may have a treatment probe and an imaging probe. The imaging probe could detect the target spot as the therapy probe removes tissue. The therapeutic and imaging probes may be attached to robotic arms controlled by computer devices. The imaging probe may be linked to a second robotic arm for computer-controlled movement during target site scanning before and/or during tissue excision by the therapy probe. In a passive mode, one or more computing devices

(Continued)

Table 12.2. (*Continued*)

S. No.	Patent number	Description
		can execute instructions to manually adjust the robotic arms to position the treatment and imaging probes for imaging and treatment in the same or different tissue sites. One or more computer devices may execute instructions to maintain the probe position when the robotic arms are removed from manual adjustment. The robotic arms may retain manually established positions with one or more translational or rotational directions. Some implementations preserve the rotational angle and translational location for each of the three axes, improving imaging and probe treatment precision [74].
11.	US20230077141A1	Medical professionals and robotically assisted surgeons employ several medical tools. The surgeon may use a master controller to remotely control medical tools during robotically assisted surgery. The controller may be far from the patient, such as on the other side of the operating room, in a separate room, or in an entirely other building. In the operating room, it is possible to position a controller in close proximity to the patient. Using a servo motor, the clinician's hand input devices may move a manipulator supporting the medical instrument. The clinician's hand input devices may move a manipulator supporting the medical instrument using a servo motor. The physician may use a robotic system to control a robotic system. The physician may use ultrasonic blades, surgical staplers, needle drivers, electrosurgical cautery probes, and more. Each of these structures helps the physician cut, coagulate, hold, or drive a needle, grip a blood artery, and dissect or cauterize tissue [75].
12.	US9981389B2	This invention is related to the components and functionalities of robotics platforms. It explores the manipulators employed in robotics platforms, as well as the computer and network hardware utilized, the software designs employed in robotics platforms, along with the vision systems and diverse software processes that can be executed on these platforms. These software processes encompass perception, planning, behavior, and control processes, among others. The claimed innovations in this application are more narrowly focused on manipulators for use in robotics platforms with a standard joint architecture. In common use, a robot refers to an electromechanical device controlled by software. Humanoids and industrial robots are only two examples of the wide variety of robots available. Mobile robots are not confined to a single area; rather, they are free to explore their surroundings at will. The development of mobile robots for the traversal of inhospitable terrain is gaining momentum [76].

13.	US20200281667A1	This invention relates to a robotic device for minimally invasive medical interventions performed on a patient's deformable tissues, for example, for the purpose of performing treatment or diagnosing a patient's deformable organs or anatomical structures. Minimally invasive or percutaneous medical interventions (diagnosis, therapy, and/or surgery) are becoming more important, especially in oncology for local cancer treatments that act directly on organ cells such as the liver, kidneys, lungs, pancreas, breasts, prostate, etc. Outside oncology, many medical procedures and applications use a minimally invasive or percutaneous access route, such as needle insertion, biopsies (the collection of tissues for pathological analysis), the placement of drains (for the aspiration of fluids), the injection of therapeutic products (for pain relief), and so on [77].
14.	US20230191614A1	This invention pertains to robotic devices that allow for the spatial guidance of an articulated arm to treat a patient's body. For this reason, the invention focuses on a device that can control a robotic arm's motions in real time based on an analysis of incoming visual data. This invention relates to a robotic device designed to enable the automated guidance of a robotic arm. This device consists of a framework that supports a robotic arm which is articulated along multiple axes of freedom. The robotic arm includes a distal operator device that enables human–machine interaction. In addition, the robot device incorporates an image acquisition system, which comprises at least two optical devices that are an integral part of the framework and positioned at distinct locations on the frame. Each optical device is specifically configured to capture 3D images. The image acquisition system is designed to capture multiple 3D images of a patient's body from optical devices. Furthermore, the robot device includes a computational unit that generates a real-time human body model of the patient based on the acquired 3D images. This computational unit also generates a guiding trajectory that is referenced to the surface of the human body model. Consequently, the movements of the robotic arm are controlled by and synchronized with this guiding trajectory [78].
15.	US20220079613A1	This invention offers enhanced techniques and equipment for conducting tissue resection, specifically in the context of prostate tissue resection. This is achieved by placing an energy source within the urethra. In many cases, a fluid stream is sent toward the tissue to make several clouds that shed. The fluid stream may be scanned to send shedding clouds to distinct overlapping areas. Each of the many falling clouds can take away a small

(*Continued*)

Table 12.2. (*Continued*)

S. No.	Patent number	Description
		piece of tissue. Equipment used to ablate tissue often has a source of pressurized fluid and a nozzle that releases a fluid stream that forms shedding clouds [79].
16.	US20170245878A1	This invention improves prostate tissue excision by placing an energy source in the urethra. Energy is delivered radially outward from the energy source toward tissue that might be a urethral wall inside the prostate. The energy source is displaced to remove a certain amount of tissue around the lumen, and the motion of the energy source is partly regulated by an automated controller. A clinician may examine an image of the prostate tissue to be treated using several user interfaces. The physician may see the proposed therapy on a screen, which may itself comprise many pictures. The treatment probe may consist of an anchor, and the displayed picture may include a reference image marker matching the anchor. The doctor may scale the anticipated tissue removal profile to the prostate's target tissue and change the therapeutic profile. Multiple pictures of the target tissue may be superimposed onto the treatment profile at the same time. In many cases, sagittal and axial views of the tissue are shown, and the treatment profile of the predefined volume is shown on the sagittal and axial views at a scale that is mostly the same as those of the pictures. This makes it possible to plan the treatment [80].
17.	US102119919B2	This innovation offers a prosthetic hand that exhibits the ability to perform several sorts of grasping actions. The prosthetic finger units are designed with under actuation, using a differential mechanism layout to provide control both inside and between the finger units. This patent furthermore presents a technique for additive manufacturing molding to produce the same products. The innovation pertains to a device specifically designed for prosthetic hand functionality. The device consists of a hand frame that incorporates a differential mechanism linked to an index finger unit that can be activated, as well as at least one secondary finger unit and a thumb unit that can be activated. The thumb unit is equipped with multiple lockable positions, each corresponding to a distinct grasping configuration of the prosthetic hand [81].

12.6 Conclusions

Because robotics and artificial intelligence have advanced significantly, cyborgs are frequently viewed as the next stage in human evolution. Cyborg systems, which were formerly merely a notion found in science fiction, are now real and may be utilized to help individuals with neurological abnormalities and improve their quality of life. The emergence of cyborg science is generating considerable interest and enthusiasm because of its possible medical consequences. The concept of individuals with cyborg-like characteristics is appealing to some readers. Nevertheless, certain challenges continue to hinder progress in this field. The survey conducted in this study, while not exhaustive, seeks to demonstrate the wide range of applications enabled by laboratory monitoring and wearable and implantable cyborganic healthcare equipment. The integration of advanced cyborganic diagnostics and precision medicine has the potential to emerge as a crucial foundation of the future healthcare industry. In conclusion, this case study has demonstrated the significant capabilities of cyborg technologies and cyberorgans in the realm of biorobotics for healthcare. However, it also emphasized the crucial need to establish comprehensive biosecurity protocols to avoid any hazards linked to these breakthroughs. As the convergence of human biology and technology progresses, it will become imperative to adopt a proactive stance toward biosecurity. It is important to ensure the secure and responsible integration of biorobotics within the healthcare sector, which will ultimately result in improved patient outcomes and enhanced medical capabilities.

References

[1] Mehrali M *et al* 2018 Blending electronics with the human body: a pathway toward a cybernetic future *Adv. Sci.* **5** 1700931

[2] Fox A 2021 The (possible) future of cyborg healthcare: depictions of disability in Cyberpunk 2077 *Sci. Cult.* **30** 591–7

[3] Luo J *et al* 2022 Rehabilitation of total knee arthroplasty by integrating conjoint isometric myodynamia and real-time rotation sensing system *Adv. Sci.* **9** 2105219

[4] Yanambaka V P, Mohanty S P, Kougianos E and Puthal D 2019 PMsec: physical unclonable function-based robust and lightweight authentication in the internet of medical things *IEEE Trans. Consum. Electron.* **65** 388–97

[5] Joshi A M, Jain P, Mohanty S P and Agrawal N 2020 iGLU 2.0: a new wearable for accurate non-invasive continuous serum glucose measurement in IoMT framework *IEEE Trans. Consum. Electron.* **66** 327–35

[6] Gray C H, Figueroa-Sarriera H and Mentor S 2020 *Modified: Living as a Cyborg* (Milton Park: Routledge)

[7] Lyotard J F 1984 *The Postmodern Condition: A Report on Knowledge* **Vol 10** (Minneapolis, MN: University of Minnesota Press)

[8] Vogel S 1998 *Cats' Paws and Catapults* (London: Penguin Books)

[9] Bandyopadhyay P R 2002 Maneuvering hydrodynamics of fish and small underwater vehicles *Integr. Comp. Biol.* **42** 102–17

[10] Vogel S 2020 *Life in Moving Fluids: The Physical Biology of Flow-Revised and Expanded* 2nd edn (Princeton, NJ: Princeton University Press)

[11] Gough A and Gough N 2023 Education research beyond cyborg subjectivities *Oxford Research Encyclopedia of Education* (Oxford: Oxford University Press)
[12] Lapum J, Fredericks S, Beanlands H and McCay E 2012 A cyborg ontology in health care: traversing into the liminal space between technology and person-centred practice *Nurs. Philos.* **13** 276–88
[13] Nijland R H, Van Wegen E E, Harmeling-van der Wel B C and Kwakkel G 2013 Early Prediction of Functional Outcome After Stroke (EPOS) Investigators. Accuracy of physical therapists' early predictions of upper-limb function in hospital stroke units: the EPOS Study *Phys. Ther.* **93** 460–9
[14] Zanatta F, Giardini A, Pierobon A, D'Addario M and Steca P 2022 A systematic review on the usability of robotic and virtual reality devices in neuromotor rehabilitation: patients' and healthcare professionals' perspective *BMC Health Serv. Res.* **22** 523
[15] Webster-Wood V A, Guix M, Xu N W, Behkam B, Sato H, Sarkar D, Sanchez S, Shimizu M and Parker K K 2022 Biohybrid robots: recent progress, challenges, and perspectives *Bioinsp. Biomim.* **18** 015001
[16] Djaouti D, Alvarez J and Jessel J P 2011 Classifying serious games: the G/P/S model *Handbook of Research on Improving Learning and Motivation Through Educational Games: Multidisciplinary Approaches* (Hershey, PA: IGI Global) 118–36
[17] McClarty K L, Orr A, Frey P M, Dolan R P, Vassileva V and McVay A 2012 A literature review of gaming in education *Gaming Educ.* **1** 1–35
[18] Croatti A, Gabellini M, Montagna S and Ricci A 2020 On the integration of agents and digital twins in healthcare *J. Med. Syst.* **44** 1–8
[19] Wang Y *et al* 2017 biorobotic adhesive disc for underwater hitchhiking inspired by the remora suckerfish *Sci. Robot.* **2** 8072
[20] Kellaris N, Gopaluni Venkata V, Smith G M, Mitchell S K and Keplinger C 2018 Peano-HASEL actuators: muscle-mimetic, electrohydraulic transducers that linearly contract on activation *Sci. Robot.* **3** 3276
[21] Guimarães C F, Gasperini L, Marques A P and Reis R L 2020 The stiffness of living tissues and its implications for tissue engineering *Nat. Rev. Mater.* **5** 351–70
[22] Wallin T J, Pikul J and Shepherd R F 2018 3D printing of soft robotic systems *Nat. Rev. Mater.* **3** 84–100
[23] Marchal-Crespo L and Reinkensmeyer D J 2009 Review of control strategies for robotic movement training after neurologic injury *J. Neuroeng. Rehab.* **6** 20
[24] Watanabe H *et al* 2021 Efficacy and safety study of wearable cyborg HAL (Hybrid Assistive Limb) in hemiplegic patients with acute stroke (EARLY GAIT STUDY): protocols for a randomized controlled trial *Front. Neurosci.* **15** 666562
[25] Bertani R, Melegari C, De Cola M C, Bramanti A, Bramanti P and Calabrò R S 2017 Effects of robot-assisted upper limb rehabilitation in stroke patients: a systematic review with meta-analysis *Neurol. Sci.* **38** 1561
[26] Tanaka Y, Morishima K, Shimizu T, Kikuchi A, Yamato M, Okano T and Kitamori T 2006 Demonstration of a PDMS-based bio-microactuator using cultured cardiomyocytes to drive polymer micropillars *Lab Chip* **6** 230–5
[27] Chan V, Park K, Collens M B, Kong H, Saif T A and Bashir R 2012 Development of miniaturized walking biological machines *Sci. Rep.* **2** 857
[28] Park J, Kim I C, Baek J, Cha M, Kim J, Park S, Lee J and Kim B 2007 Micro pumping with cardiomyocyte–polymer hybrid *Lab Chip* **7** 1367–70

[29] Tanaka Y, Sato K, Shimizu T, Yamato M, Okano T and Kitamori T 2007 A micro-spherical heart pump powered by cultured cardiomyocytes *Lab Chip* **7** 207–12
[30] Herr H and Dennis R G 2004 A swimming robot actuated by living muscle tissue *J. Neuroeng. Rehab.* **1** 6
[31] Holley M T, Nagarajan N, Danielson C, Zorlutuna P and Park K 2016 Development and characterization of muscle-based actuators for self-stabilizing swimming biorobots *Lab Chip* **16** 3473–84
[32] Hess H 2011 Engineering applications of biomolecular motors *Annu. Rev. Biomed. Eng.* **13** 429–50
[33] Alford P W, Feinberg A W, Sheehy S P and Parker K K 2010 Biohybrid thin films for measuring contractility in engineered cardiovascular muscle *Biomaterials* **31** 3613–21
[34] Xi J, Schmidt J J and Montemagno C D 2005 Self-assembled microdevices driven by muscle *Nat. Mater.* **4** 180–4
[35] González L M, Ruder W C, Leduc P R and Messner W C 2014 Controlling magnetotactic bacteria through an integrated nanofabricated metallic island and optical microscope approach *Sci. Rep.* **4** 4104
[36] Peyer K E, Zhang L and Nelson B J 2013 Bio-inspired magnetic swimming microrobots for biomedical applications *Nanoscale* **5** 1259–72
[37] Sokolov A, Apodaca M M, Grzybowski B A and Aranson I S 2010 Swimming bacteria power microscopic gears *Proc. Natl Acad. Sci.* **107** 969–74
[38] Kim D, Liu A, Diller E and Sitti M 2012 Chemotactic steering of bacteria propelled microbeads *Biomed. Microdevices* **14** 1009–17
[39] Oliva M A and Borondo J P 2020 Cyborg as a surgeon: a theoretical framework for cyborg acceptance in healthcare service *Societal Challenges in the Smart Society* (Logroño: Universidad de La Rioja) 57–70
[40] Bharati S, Podder P, Mondal M R and Paul P K 2021 Applications and challenges of cloud integrated IoMT *Cognitive Internet of Medical Things for Smart Healthcare: Services and Applications* (Cham: Springer) 67–85
[41] Tang S and Wiens J 2021 Model selection for offline reinforcement learning: practical considerations for healthcare settings *Proc. Mach. Learn. Res.* **149** 2–35 PMID: 35702420
[42] Baucum M, Khojandi A and Vasudevan R 2020 Improving deep reinforcement learning with transitional variational autoencoders: a healthcare application *IEEE J. Biomed. Health Inform.* **25** 2273–80
[43] Guerrero I, Miró-Amarante G and Martín A 2022 Decision support system in health care building design based on case-based reasoning and reinforcement learning *Expert Syst. Appl.* **187** 116037
[44] Feiner R, Engel L, Fleischer S, Malki M, Gal I, Shapira A, Shacham-Diamand Y and Dvir T 2016 Engineered hybrid cardiac patches with multifunctional electronics for online monitoring and regulation of tissue function *Nat. Mater.* **15** 679–85
[45] Mannoor M S, Jiang Z, James T, Kong Y L, Malatesta K A, Soboyejo W O, Verma N, Gracias D H and McAlpine M C 2013 3D printed bionic ears *Nano Lett.* **136** 2634–9
[46] Feiner R and Dvir T 2017 Tissue–electronics interfaces: from implantable devices to engineered tissues *Nat. Rev. Mater.* **3** 3–16 17076
[47] Dai X, Zhou W, Gao T, Liu J and Lieber C M 2016 Three-dimensional mapping and regulation of action potential propagation in nanoelectronics-innervated tissues *Nat. Nanotechnol.* **11** 776–82

[48] Hecht B *et al* 2021 It's time to do something: mitigating the negative impacts of computing through a change to the peer review process *arXiv preprint arXiv* 09544
[49] Haraway D J 2004 *The Haraway Reader* (London: Psychology Press)
[50] Puar J K 2012 "I would rather be a cyborg than a goddess": Becoming-Intersectional in Assemblage Theory *Philosophia* **2** 49–66
[51] Clynes M E and Kline N S 1960 Cyborgs and space *Astronautics* **14** 26–7
[52] Kristal S, Baumgarth C and Henseler J 2020 Performative corporate brand identity in industrial markets: the case of German prosthetics manufacturer Ottobock *J. Bus. Res.* **114** 240–53
[53] Shao J *et al* 2017 Smartphone-controlled optogenetically engineered cells enable semi-automatic glucose homeostasis in diabetic mice *Sci. Transl. Med.* **9** 387
[54] Williams R M and Gilbert J E 2019 Cyborg perspectives on computing research reform *Extended Abstracts of the 2019 CHI Conf. on Human Factors in Computing Systems* (New York, NY: ACM) 1–11
[55] Mbembé J A and Meintjes L 2003 Necropolitics *Public Culture* **15** 11–40
[56] Kafer A 2013 *Feminist, Queer, Crip* (Bloomington, IN: Indiana University Press)
[57] Broderick A A 2009 Autism,'recovery (to normalcy),' and the politics of hope *Intell. Develop. Disabil.* **47** 263–81
[58] Botha M and Frost D M 2020 Extending the minority stress model to understand mental health problems experienced by the autistic population *Soc. Mental Health* **10** 20–34
[59] Camm-Crosbie L, Bradley L, Shaw R, Baron-Cohen S and Cassidy S 2019 People like me don't get support': autistic adults' experiences of support and treatment for mental health difficulties, self-injury and suicidality *Autism* **23** 1431–41
[60] Singleton G, Warren S and Piersel W 2014 Clinical overview of the need for technologies for around-the-clock monitoring of the health status of severely disabled autistic children *2014 36th Annual Int. Conf. of the IEEE Engineering in Medicine and Biology Society* (Piscataway, NJ: IEEE) 789–91
[61] Warwick K 2004 *March of the Machines: The Breakthrough in Artificial Intelligence* (Champaign, IL: University of Illinois Press)
[62] Warwick K, Gasson M, Hutt B, Goodhew I, Kyberd P, Andrews B, Teddy P and Shad A 2003 The application of implant technology for cybernetic systems *Arch. Neurol.* **60** 1369–73
[63] Colombo R, Pisano F, Micera S, Mazzone A, Delconte C, Carrozza M C, Dario P and Minuco G 2005 Robotic techniques for upper limb evaluation and rehabilitation of stroke patients *IEEE Trans. Neural Syst. Rehab. Eng.* **13** 311–24
[64] Abbott A 2007 Biological robotics: working out the bugs *Nature* **445** 250–4
[65] Luis B, Surjan G, Sasnett M W and Foote J 2016 *Tissue resection and treatment with shedding pulses* 14/816747 United States
[66] Aljuri N, Mantri S and Staid K P 2019 *Artificial intelligence for robotic surgery* US17/250230 United States
[67] Contreras-Vidal J L, Prasad S, Kilicarslan A and Bhagat N 2018 *Methods for closed-loop neural-machine interface systems for the control of wearable exoskeletons and prosthetic devices* 61/842673 United States
[68] Alijuri N, Mantri S, Baez L, Surjan G, Sasnett M W and Foote J 2017 *Automated image-guided tissue resection and treatment* 15/93158 United States
[69] Farina D, Popovic D, Graimann B, Markovic M and Dosen S 2014 *Control of limb device* 131716714 European Patent Office

[70] Shahi G S and Nadershahi A H 2008 *Method and system for assessing and managing biosafety and biosecurity risks* US12/038,643 United States

[71] Shadduck J H 2017 *Wearable sensing and actuator systems, and methods of use* 15/661363 United States

[72] Kaplan B 2016 *Computer system of an artificial intelligence of a cyborg or an android, wherein a received signal-reaction of the computer system of the artificial intelligence of the cyborg or the android, a corresponding association of the computer system of the artificial intelligence of the cyborg or the android, a corresponding thought of the computer system of the artificial intelligence of the cyborg or the android are physically built, and a working method of the computer system of the artificial intelligence of the artificial intelligence of the cyborg or the android* 14/756957 United States

[73] Wein L M 2022 *Robotics medical system having human collaborative modes* 17/311201 United States

[74] Mantri S, Alijuri N, STAID K P and Hemphill J 2020 *Robotic arms and methods for tissue resection and imaging* 16/940100 United States

[75] Scheib C J, Vargas M and Denlinger C 2023 *Robotically controlled uterine manipulator* 17/468754 United States

[76] Kennedy B A, Frost M A, Leichty J M, Hagman M J, Borders J W, Piacentine J S, Bergh C F, Sirota A R and Carpenter K C 2018 *Robotics platforms incorporating manipulators having common joint designs* 14/637278 United States

[77] Blondel L, Badano F and Nahum B 2020 *Robotic device for a minimally invasive medical intervention on soft tissues* 16/762876 United States

[78] Serrat T and Khachlouf A 2023 *Robot device for guiding a robotic arm* 18/010391 United States

[79] Alijuri N, Mantri S, Baez L, Surjan G, Sasnett M W and Foote J 2022 *Stiff sheath for image-guided tissue resection* 17/456108 United States

[80] Alijuri N, Mantri S, Baez L, Surjan G, Sasnett M W and Foote J 2020 *Automated image-guided tissue resection and treatment* 15/593158 United States

[81] Belter J T, Dollar A M, Leddy M, Dale K and Gemmell Jr 2019 *Multi-grasp prosthetic hand* 15/240819 United States